WHAT PSYCHOTHERAPISTS
SHOULD KNOW ABOUT DISABILITY

WHAT PSYCHOTHERAPISTS SHOULD KNOW ABOUT DISABILITY

Rhoda Olkin

THE GUILFORD PRESS
New York   London

© 1999 The Guilford Press
A Division of Guilford Publications, Inc.
72 Spring Street, New York, NY 10012
http://www.guilford.com

Printed in the United States of America

This book is printed on acid-free paper.

Last digit is print number: 9   8   7   6   5   4   3   2

Library of Congress Cataloging-in-Publication Data

Olkin, Rhoda.
  What psychotherapists should know about disability / Rhoda Olkin.
    p. cm.
  Includes bibliographical references and index.
  ISBN 1-57230-227-5 (hbk.) 1-57230-643-2 (pbk.)
    1. Handicapped—Mental health Case studies.   2. Psychotherapy Case
studies.   I. Title.
RC451.4.H35045   1999
362.4—dc21   99-33774
                                                                                       CIP

To Michael, Noah, and Sophia,

who help me find curb cuts
both real and metaphorical

About the Author

Rhoda Olkin, PhD, is a professor in the clinical psychology program at the California School of Professional Psychology in Alameda, California. She is also on the staff of Through the Looking Glass in Berkeley, California, an agency serving families with disabilities, and the National Resource Center for Parents with Disabilities. She has experience in disability from the perspective of an administrator (she founded handicapped services at the University of California, Santa Barbara, in the mid-1970s, and is currently the Faculty Advisor to Students with Disabilities at the California School of Professional Psychology), researcher, clinician, teacher, and spouse (of a man with multiple sclerosis), as well as personal experience (she had polio in 1954). Her short stories have been published in literary magazines, and her most recent story on a disability theme appears in *Bigger Than the Sky: Disabled Women on Parenting* (Trafalgar Square Publishing). Her two children can spot ramps and handicapped parking with the best of them.

Preface

I am bicultural. I live in two worlds—the nondisabled majority and my minority group's world of the disability community. One is the world of stairs, ab-rollers, fishing, careers, mountain climbing, the other of crips, gimps, retards, and spazzes. Guess where I feel more at home?

In the disabled community we refer to people without disabilities as ABs (able-bodied) or TABs (temporarily able-bodied). Notice the vantage point—*non*disabled, *not* like us. We don't call them "normals" because to us they are not the norm. In our world abnormal *is* normal.

Take Nick, for instance. Nick's the kind of guy people automatically avoid. Mothers jerk their children back as they pass him in the street ("Don't point, dear. Shhhh.") Nick uses an electric wheelchair. His limbs go in the wrong direction, as if not attached properly, and his hands are at odd angles. His face seems to grimace for no reason, and his tongue is all too much in evidence. When he speaks the contortions and gyrations extend from head top to toes, and the words are mangled, swallowed, expectorated, some of them intelligible, others obscured by the process of expulsion.

I know a lot of guys like Nick.

This book is only superficially about Nick. Because Nick is fine. He's a lawyer, he has friends, he has "quality of life." Nick's main problem is ABs: The counselor who told Nick's mother that she had to "grieve the loss of the normal child" she didn't have before she could learn to love Nick. The doctor who worked on Nick's limbs oblivious to the fact that they were attached to a whole body, much less a whole person. The mother who assured Nick that he could grow up to be anything he wanted to be, even when Nick wanted to be a football player. The colleges that refused to let him enroll and the law schools that wouldn't even send him an application. The father who didn't want him to marry his daughter. The therapist who told him he had a chip on his shoulder.

People, really well meaning, perfectly nice people, use words to describe Nick such as "resilient," "brave," "adaptable," "plucky," "courageous." Courage requires options.

Where is it written that we get options?

I had polio at the age of 1 and had two major polio-related surgeries in childhood. Throughout my youth I wore a leg brace, sometimes to the top of my thigh, other years to below my knee. I now wear a plastic orthotic to stabilize my right ankle. I've used crutches for distances since age 16 and began using an electric scooter for work, shopping, and walks about 12 years ago. I walk with a pronounced limp and have regular back and foot or ankle pain. I spent the first 30 or so years of my life trying to distance myself from people such as Nick. I wasn't like him; except for the leg brace and surgeries and limp and pain and fatigue and reactions of others, except for those little things, I was normal. Surely I was nearer to the nondisabled world than to Nick's. I could "pass." Until suddenly I couldn't. Until suddenly I had to "come out" as a person with a disability. This happened over time, like so many changes do, but there was a defining moment.

I had been giving workshops on working with clients with disabilities. As had been my wont since puberty I wore pants or long dresses to hide the differences between my two legs (one robust, the other scrawny and emaciated) and the orthotic on my right foot and ankle. And for some reason it suddenly hit me: I am a role model; what am I modeling? I bought a knee-length dress and wore it for the first time in front of an audience of more than 100 people. I was on a raised stage, so they all had a good view.

I had started my long trek home (it's a slow trek when you limp).

Many years ago I attended the first professional meeting in which most of the participants had disabilities. It was a personally and professionally illuminating experience, and several notable issues were raised for me.

This was the first time in my life I had ever been in a professional setting with a preponderance of people with disabilities. In my usual professional settings I am often the only person with a disability. What I see mirrored back to me is the image of nondisabled colleagues. However, at this conference the mirror image was of professionals with disabilities, persons like myself, but reflected back to me in a way I'm not used to. My first response was, Hey, I'm not like "them," they're "disabled"; I can "pass" in a nondisabled world.

But by day 4 I was wearing my red T-shirt with black lettering on the front that reads "Crip Is Hip." What happened?

First, being disabled myself is no immunity to my holding negative attitudes toward disability. In fact, living with a disability heightened my awareness of the pervasiveness of negative attitudes toward disability. It would be hard for me not to have internalized at least some portion of these attitudes. Second, what happened to me is what happens to most people when they come into prolonged contact with a person with a disability—the disability starts to recede, becomes less of a "defining characteristic," and the person as a whole being, for whom disability is just one facet, emerges. Third, the conference itself affirmed the importance of focusing on the capabilities rather than on the disabilities of the participants. Even though this focus has become a cliche, and even an EEOC (Equal Employment Opportunity Commission) hiring slogan, it must not be overlooked as a critical reframing of disability. Fourth, a variety of viewpoints about disability and images of oneself as a person with a disability emerged over the course of the conference, allowing me to feel supported in my own views as well as to feel comfortable with some of my differences.

I was struck throughout the meetings by the dual level of activity taking place at any one time. On the one hand, audiences were extremely polite and quiet, allowing those with particular impairments better access to the speakers. For example, there were American Sign Language interpreters (always accorded seats in the front), a woman who mouthed words for a lip-reading participant with a hearing impairment, a sight-impaired man who kept notes on a Braille typewriter—all these people needed to be able to hear the speakers clearly, without interference from audience whispers. So on one level there was a sense of quiet among the audiences. At another level there was a hum of constant activity—the tap of the Braille machine, the hum of a respirator, the whine of an electric wheelchair, the continual rearranging of furniture to accommodate mobility aids of all shapes and sizes. I had to learn as an audience member to tune these things out; at the same time they were interesting to me. I found myself wondering, Is my scooter as loud as his scooter? Is the wheelbase wider than her wheelchair? Where did she get that handy cup holder?

At the conference I was scheduled to present a paper on hierarchies of acceptability—the fact that all physical disabilities are not created equal and that some are more stigmatized, and less accepted at intimate levels of contact, than are others. I worried inordinately about the impact my presentation might have on the participants. I was anxious about saying out loud to an audience comprising people with various disabilities that in many studies those with paraplegia were viewed as less acceptable than were those with amputations, that persons with multiple sclerosis were viewed much more negatively than were persons who were deaf or blind. We like to pretend that, at least among our peers with disabilities, we are all "equally" disabled in terms of psychosocial factors. This clearly is not the case. This observation, although probably known to most persons with disabilities, is rarely said out loud. However, the findings were not controversial; the audience barely murmured in response to the implications of the data. Perhaps there was something validating in confirming what many of us have already experienced. Yet within a few years I would come to repudiate the assumptions and orientation, questions, methods, and value of my own research.

As the conference went on I became increasingly embarrassed at not being able to sign. As a person who researches issues related to disability, I began to feel that this was a shortcoming on my part rather than on the part of the deaf person, somewhat analogous to studying the culture of Brazil without knowing Portuguese. After all, learning their language (American Sign Language) was an option for me, but learning to speak English is not a viable option for most deaf people. After seeing the same (deaf) woman for 3 days, running into her in the bathroom, I couldn't so much as say, Hi, how are you? or Where do you come from? What the Deaf community has been saying for years truly struck home: If the whole world signed, deafness would not be much of a disability.

Although a tone of openness and acceptance pervaded the conference, not all opinions were welcomed. For example, at a meeting to discuss curricula on disability one woman asked whether having such a curriculum simply drew more attention to ourselves, and after all, wasn't everyone, in one way or another, disabled? A visceral tension swept the room, and the responses of her interlocutors were best summed up by another woman who said that if we were all disabled in one way or another, she'd trade her childhood with an AB's any day. The general feeling expressed by most participants was that the experience of having a disability is unique and is not analogous to, say, having an alcoholic parent, being molested as a child, being Catholic in a Protestant town, and so on.

A second issue that raised much hot debate was whether disability simulations (e.g., having nondisabled students use wheelchairs for a day) were (1) effective in conveying the disability experience, (2) ethical, and (3) warranted. On one side were those who adamantly opposed such exercises (myself included), who argue that disability simulations reduce the experience of disability to a physical condition when it is more an interpersonal and psychosocial experience. On the other side were those who assert that disability simulations are one of the few ways to help the nondisabled "get it" at some level beyond the merely intellectual. It is an argument that no amount of data will resolve; much like religion, one chooses faith by alternate means.

The last issue the conference evoked for me is about the differentiation between assertion and aggression—the fine-line boundaries demarcating righteous anger, appropriate assertiveness, pushiness, and narcissism. These were best exemplified in the tendency of some participants to park their wheelchairs or scooters wherever they chose, with a seeming disregard to the needs of those around them. The result was that if a person in a wheelchair at the front of the room wanted to leave, a long line of wheelchairs and scooters had to back up into the hall. This may seem paradoxical at a conference directly about disability, in which so many participants were persons with disabilities themselves. But in another way it makes perfect sense. Imagine for a moment that everywhere you went you had to search for parking that was close to where you needed to go, allowed enough room for you to use your wheelchair lift, and was near a curb cut. Then, after you gained entrance to the store, you found that the store, even though supposedly "accessible," had aisles filled with merchandise that made passage in a wheelchair impossible. Imagine how ordinary crowds hog sidewalks, UPS trucks block curb cuts, persons without handicapped placards park in handicapped spots, restaurants assure you over the phone that they are accessible only to turn out to have inaccessible bathrooms, so that you can eat but you cannot pee. It doesn't take long before you get used to shoving, pushing, and thrusting yourself forward in life as best you can, not taking other people's word for things, and developing both an anger and a sense of entitlement (why isn't the bathroom on *this* floor accessible?). This anger serves a useful purpose, helping to stave off depression and helplessness and fueling an active militancy to effect changes. But it is not a terribly attractive behavior. On more than one occasion (usually when I'm berating someone for parking illegally in a handicapped zone) I've been told, "It's people like you who give the handicapped a bad name" (we once had a good name?). So should we knock it off? Probably not. But we should address this issue more openly, acknowledge its impact on others and on ourselves, and make an informed choice about what is best for us both as individuals and as a collective group growing impatient with bargaining for what seems like our rights.

Having a disability is the second hardest thing I've ever done in my life (parenting is the first). My disability, like that of most people with disabilities, involves the usual triad of pain, fatigue, and muscle weakness, and let's face it, these are difficult symptoms to live and function with. The profound effects that having a disability have on interpersonal relationships and social interchange are wearing. The physical demands are constant. The time and money needed for accommodations compete with other needs, and the unpredictability of future disability-related needs is worrisome. The lack of accessibility and the inability to take for granted that I can go anywhere are frustrating. These factors mean that a part of me almost always is attending to my disability (though usually out of conscious awareness). If it's true that we can hold in immediate memory only seven bits (plus or minus two), and one bit is taken up by my disability needs, then less is available for remembering other things. It's rather like having a program on a computer that takes up a large part of the RAM; less is available to run other programs or for storing data.

Despite this I never, now or in the past, entertained the question of who I'd be without my disability, how my life would have been different, or how great it would be to be able-bodied. To me that's what "living with a disability" means—refraining from or ceasing to ask those questions. I believe that the goal of treatment of persons with disabilities—when the treatment focus is on the disability itself—is to help people live *with* their disability. Given a menu of events, I would not *choose* disability, but who gets to choose? You get what you get. I still have a partner, two children, a career I love, the chance to write this book—multitudes of small moments of joy. And, as they say, at least I have my health.

Oh, that's right; I don't.

Contents

15 For Teachers and Supervisors   322

Introduction and Overview

A man in his late 20s calls you to set up an initial appointment. It was his wife who suggested he come in, and he didn't think he needed to, but lately he's been concerned because he feels his job performance is impaired. When he arrives at your office he is using a manual wheelchair. He . . .

1. . . . Is unable to get into your building because it is not wheelchair accessible.
2. . . . Complains of depression over the past 6 months and thoughts of suicide. He never mentions his disability or his wheelchair use as part of his depression or reasons for his suicidal ideation.
3. . . . Says that sexual relations with his wife have tapered down to almost nothing.
4. . . . Is preoccupied with whether his decreased job performance is noticeable to his boss, whether he'll be fired, and what would happen to his health insurance if he loses his job.
5. . . . Tells you, in response to your questions, that he takes pain medications daily and drinks five or so beers about 4 days a week.

In this book I hope you will learn (1) whether your building and office have to be in compliance with the accessibility requirements of the Americans with Disabilities Act, and if so, who's responsible for ensuring changes; (2) several ways to address disability issues in treatment and how to understand disability in the context of a specific person; (3) possible effects of disabilities on sexual abilities and pleasure; (4) what bosses tend to fear about hiring persons with disabilities; and (5) facts about substance abuse among persons with disabilities, impediments to treatment, and much more. In fact, I hope you will come to see disability in a whole new way.

You probably didn't wake up this morning and think, "I'd like to learn just a little more about people with disabilities. In fact, I'd like to learn a book's worth." Yet here you are reading this. What you've stumbled upon is exactly a book's worth—what you need to know about disability and persons with disabilities, and only what you need to know, because this book is written for mental health professionals like you.

Why should you read this? First, because some of the clients you work with right now have disabilities (though maybe you don't think of them this way). Second, an increasing proportion of the population is aging, and although aging is not invariably associated with disability, the latter does increase with the former. Third, this book gives you a way to think about and understand disability that will serve you in many circumstances and across many disabilities. Fourth, many of you are in positions of influence in the field, through teaching, research, supervision, consultation, program design and evaluation, and being a provider of clinical services for managed care. (Take heart: This book will barely mention managed care.)

HOW TO USE THIS BOOK

Of course, all authors want you to start at the beginning of their book and read straight through to the end. I do too. The book is meant to be one-stop-shopping for learning about working with clients with disabilities. As such, it is set up to be read completely and in order. But recognizing reality and busy schedules, a word or two to those readers who wish to skim or read only part of the book. By looking at the Contents you will probably choose to read one of the chapters on therapy (Chapters 7–12); I urge you to read Chapters 2 and 3 instead. These will help you understand disability in ways that will enable your own clinical judgment to serve you best. Reading Chapters 7–12 in isolation will provide too mechanical an approach; the hard edges of the techniques, skills, and knowledge in these later chapters must be softened with the reframing of disability that occurs in the early chapters. A second tip to skimmers: Principles for therapists, summaries of key points, longer clinical examples with commentary, or conclusions are listed at the end of most chapters, as a way of synthesizing key material.

You will note from chapter titles that this book is not organized around disorders. Most books on disabling conditions have chapter names such as "Diabetes" and "Cerebral Palsy." The philosophy behind that type of organization is that there are unique features of disorders, and therefore an understanding of the person with the disorder comes from understanding the disorder itself. I disagree with that conclusion. Yes, there are definitely idiosyncracies of each disabling condition, but there is tremendous overlap in the experiences of persons with disabilities that cuts across many types of disorders. There is a "disability experience," and this book discusses that experience. The result is that once you have a grasp of the commonalities of the disability experience, you have the foundation from which to begin, and you can add to it information about the specifics of any one type of disability, the functioning and the severity level for the particular client.

For most of the book (Chapters 1–13) I address clinicians. However, there is a chapter (14) for researchers and another for teachers and supervisors (15). I provide an overview of decades of research in the field with a critique of current research and ending with suggestions for future directions.

WHAT THIS BOOK IS NOT

First, several categories of disability are not included in this book, and comments are not meant to be generalized to these disabilities. An overly simplified method of categorizing disabilities could be as follows: sensory, physical, cognitive, learning, developmental, systemic, psychoemotional (more on categorization in Chapter 2). Three of these are not covered:

1. I do not cover psychiatric or psychoemotional disabilities. I leave you to your own copy of the fourth edition of the *Diagnostic and Statistical Manual of Mental Disorders* (DSM-IV; American Psychiatric Association, 1994) and your years of training and experience in exactly this type of disability. I mention it here only because it is considered a disability in the relevant laws.

2. Several specific disabilities in the DSM-IV are also not covered, namely, several of the developmental disabilities. Although I do include cerebral palsy, which is considered a developmental disability, I have not covered autism, Rhett's disorder, Asperger's disorder, or pervasive developmental disorder not otherwise specified. Special training and clinical experience are necessary for working with persons with these disorders.

3. Generally the Deaf are not covered in this book, although deafness will be included in some of the discussions. The rationale for excluding this type of disorder is based on several considerations. Persons in Deaf culture argue that deafness is not a disability and should

not be included in such discussions. There is a strong Deaf community that overlaps with, but is not synonymous with, the disability community. The Deaf have their own language (American Sign Language; ASL); if the hearing world knew ASL, deafness would barely register as a disability. Also, although having knowledge about disabilities does allow that knowledge to be widely applied across many disabilities it does not transfer in the same way to understanding of deafness or the Deaf community. Finally, it is an assumption here that Deaf clients are best served by Deaf therapists within the Deaf community.

Second, one specific population–the elderly with age-related or late onset disabilities—is not included as a special population. Much of the discussion that follows is applicable to this group. However, there are additional diagnostic and intervention skills relevant to working with geriatric populations, and I pretend no special expertise in this area.

Third, it is assumed that the disabilities discussed herein are not imminently terminal, that is, that lifespan is at or near normal expectancy. Thus there is no discussion of working with terminally ill people. Nonetheless, any compromise to health raises issues of personal vulnerability and mortality, and no discussion of disability would be complete without some discussion of death and dying. These crop up here as well. Nonetheless, this book is not a guide to working with those who are dying or their families.

Fourth, this is not a book of etiquette for interacting with people with disabilities. It is not a "how to" because by reading this book you will be able to decide for yourself how to. When I give workshops on clients with disabilities the most frequent question members of the audience ask me is, "What should I do when . . . " (fill in the blank; examples might be "when a person in a wheelchair comes to my office," "when someone on a scooter comes to a closed door," "when I think the client's disability is part of the presenting problem"). These are unanswerable questions. Or, rather, the answer is simple but not helpful: It depends. You will have to use your clinical judgment. But this book will give you things to think about in making the decision. One way that is sometimes helpful to people in deciding how they would like to handle daily manners with persons with disabilities is to ask themselves what they would do if they were being polite to an elderly person. For example, if you saw an elderly person coming to a door would you open it for him or her? If you were talking with an elderly grandmother seated on a chair would you kneel down to be at her eye level? Would you offer to carry a heavy package for an elderly gentleman? Many people would answer affirmatively to those questions, but you probably would answer "no" to the following questions: Would you scurry around a room expecting everyone to rearrange themselves when an elderly person entered? Would you pat an elderly person on the head? Would you ask the companion of an elderly man, "What would he like for lunch?" The elderly person rule, although not infallible or applicable to all situations, can serve as a broad guide.

Fifth, this is not an inspirational book. As one author with multiple sclerosis (MS) put it, it is not a "feel good" but a "feel real" book (Mairs, 1997). I am not seeking to uplift the spirits of those with disabilities or to help therapists feel better about disability. Being a person with a disability is one of the hardest things to be; every day carries new trials. One person who barely knew me suggested I call the book "Nothing ever gets me down." Nonsense; plenty gets me down, including the pain, fatigue, and weakness associated with having a disability. I am not superwoman, brave, courageous, or plucky. This book does not promote that vision of persons with disabilities; it is not a pity book.

Sixth, this book is not neutral. I am firmly entrenched in the minority model of disability (see Chapter 2) and a stalwart family systems therapist. My theoretical leanings are toward the cognitive-behavioral therapies. All these beliefs are reflected in this work. However, the topics discussed in this book transcend theory. In other words, I raise issues and awareness of the disability experience, give examples of how something might be discussed in treatment, and discuss broad therapeutic guidelines, but the decisions on exactly how these are handled in the therapy remain yours. This is not meant to be a treatment manual. You are a competent therapist and will use your own judgment on how these principles should be applied.

Seventh, this book is not designed to put you at ease. On the other hand, it's not designed to make you feel anxious or incompetent either. It does raise many issues that can heighten emotional responses. Any discussion of outgroups (gays and lesbians, persons with disabilities, ethnic minorities) often becomes quickly passionate. A typical scenario in intergroup discussions is the majority group members asking, "Why must we always deal with your anger?" and minority group members responding, "How can you know us without understanding our rage? Anyway, why is it up to us to put you at ease?" In writing this book I struggled with this rhetorical conversation. You will throughout this book undoubtedly face increased affect—mine, yours, and clients'. This is probably ultimately for the best, because it allows more realistic appraisal and rehearsal for working with clients with disabilities. Confronting disability often invites emotional responses.

Finally, this book is not meant to be either autobiographical or biographical. Although you will read some things about me and my disability, and about my clients, students, supervisees, colleagues, and even friends with disabilities, material has been disguised and altered in an effort not to identify anyone. Even if you think you recognize yourself, I did not write about you, although I may have written about someone who has some features in common with you.

LANGUAGE AND TERMINOLOGY

I use the term "person [client, parent, student] with a disability" throughout. As we shall see when examining the language associated with disability (Chapter 2) this is the current preferred term. It both reflects the fact that the disability is only one aspect of the person, and does not define the whole, and does not imply that the personhood itself is disabled.

Table I.1 lists abbreviations. The chapters define some terms more fully. In a footnote, the table also includes a brief discussion of two of the terms: "activities of daily living" and "instrumental activities of daily living."

TABLE I.1. Abbreviations Used Frequently in This Book

Abbreviation	Stands for:
ABs	Able-bodied people. Also called TABs (temporarily able-bodied)
ADA	Americans with Disabilities Act (1990)
ADL[a]	Activities of daily living (see also IADL)
AIDS	Acquired immune deficiency syndrome
ALS	Amyotrophic lateral sclerosis (also known as Lou Gehrig's disease)
CP	Cerebral palsy
HIV	Human immunodeficiency virus, the virus that causes AIDS
IADL[a]	Instrumental activities of daily living (see also ADL)
IDEA	Individuals with Disabilities Education Act
ILC	Independent living centers
ILM	Independent living movement
LD	Learning disability(ies)
MD	Muscular dystrophy
MS	Multiple sclerosis
MR	Mental retardation
PCA	Personal care attendant
PCP	Primary care physician
SCI	Spinal cord injury
TBI	Traumatic brain injury
TDD or TTY[b]	Telecommunications device for the deaf or teletype

[a]There are at least 12 versions of ADL measures, probably more. Items included are those considered essential for self-care and maintenance: drinking, feeding, transfers (bed to chair/floor to chair), washing, grooming, walking or mobility, dressing and undressing, toileting, climbing stairs, bathing, making a hot drink or snack. Continence is a more controversial item that is sometimes included.

Some scales are extended to include more items. These additional items are sometimes referred to as IADL. These tend to be more outdoor activities, as well as leisure activities. IADL tend to include going outdoors, crossing roads, getting in and out of car, using public transport, carrying hot drinks, washing up, laundry, light housework, gardening, managing money and paying bills, shopping, going out socially, driving, working at employment or volunteer job, doing hobbies, reading, using a telephone, writing letters.

It should be noted that the distinction between ADL and IADL is unclear and variable across states and instruments. The lists are important in that they are used as the basis for eligibility requirements for various services and funds and as measures of improvement or for hospital discharge. Therefore, they are important not only for what they contain but for what they omit, the latter most notably being sexuality, pregnancy, and parenting.

[b]TDDs are also called TTYs, which stands for teletype, the old fashioned kind of device. TDD was adopted to denote the more modern technology. However, some people in the Deaf community dislike the term "telecommunications device for the *Deaf*" (TDD) because the device is as much for the hearing to communicate with those who are Deaf as it is for the Deaf.

ONE

Who Are People with Disabilities?

This chapter addresses the basic question of what is a disability—a seemingly simple question with a complex answer. The chapter considers the distinction between disability and illness and various ways of categorizing disabilities. It explores important features of disability identity and disability community. The next section briefly gives statistics and information about persons with disabilities. Finally, I discuss some clinical implications of these basic data.

DEFINITIONS

Who are people with disabilities? To try to answer this we might pose three questions:

1. What conditions—physical, cognitive, psychoemotional, sensory—would be included in a definition of disability?
2. How do the relevant laws define disability?
3. Under what conditions do people consider themselves a person with a disability?

The first question is actually difficult to answer, one of the problems being the blurry distinction between disability and illness. To illustrate this, think of two continua, one denoting health and the other disability. The two continua are not parallel but get closer as severity increases on each one; that is, the two concepts of health and disability are related, but they are neither completely coincidental nor orthogonal. On the low end of the disability continuum might be nearsightedness or some degree of color blindness. People with such relatively minor loss of function rarely would be considered "disabled" by either their own or other people's definitions. Moving to the middle of the continuum might be mild cerebral-palsy (CP) or minimal aftereffects of polio. At the right end of the continuum we could place serious disabilities with significant degrees of impairment in several major life functions; an example might be amyotrophic lateral sclerosis (ALS). The other continuum focuses on one's health. Its left end is quite separate from the disability continuum. Placed there are minor, routine, and temporary ailments such as colds. Slightly higher on the scale are flu and ear infections—diseases that can, under the wrong conditions, lead to more serious consequences. In the middle might be Kartagener syndrome (heart on right side, crowding other organs), or lower-level spinal cord injury. Examples from the right end would be Duchenne muscular dystrophy (MD), and some conditions leading to dwarfism (there are more than 150 such conditions, but a few of them are fatal).

It is possible to have a disability—for example, CP—and also to be in excellent health. However, more serious disabilities often compromise an individual's health. For example, as mobility and movement decrease, certain health problems increase, such as decubitus ulcers, urinary track infections, and pneumonia. These secondary conditions—that is, the illnesses—are usually the cause of any death, not the disability per se. Conversely, on the more serious end of the health continuum the illness often begins to impair abilities in major life functions; compromised health begets disability. So the overlap between disability and illness becomes increasingly important as the conditions on either or both increase in severity. It is probably not possible to come up with a definition of disability that includes only disability and not illness, and vice versa.

Alternatively, disability can be defined as a condition that limits functioning. This is primarily how disability laws address the problem of definition. The first comprehensive legal definition was in the Rehabilitation Act (1973; see Chapter 6). This definition was taken almost verbatim and used in the more recent Americans with Disabilities Act (ADA) (1990), and is provided in Table 1.1.

One of the important points about the definition is that it is based primarily on *function* rather than on underlying condition or diagnosis. For example, someone might use a wheelchair because of MD, CP, or polio; although these conditions are very different, the functional limitations may be similar. In general, the specific diagnosis often is less important clinically than is an understanding of the ways in which the condition affects functioning. (However, keep in mind that some diagnoses in and of themselves carry high degrees of stigma, such as acquired immune deficiency syndrome [AIDS] or mental retardation.) Functioning is assessed in terms of ability to perform specific tasks. These tasks are referred to as activities of daily living (ADL) or instrumental activities of daily living (IADL).

Since the Rehabilitation Act, and increasingly since the ADA, the courts have been fine-tuning the definition of disability. Conditions such as obesity and height have been tested in the courts and have not always resulted in consistent outcomes. For example, behavioral problems in young children were recently included in a Supreme Court decision that paved the way for new funding sources for working with such children. Conversely, eligibility criteria for school help has been narrowed, excluding kids with more minor disorders (those very kids who could most benefit from limited help). A clear, concise, and consistent definition of disability remains elusive.

A third approach to the question of definition is to ask, "When do people consider themselves persons with disabilities?" Do persons with disabilities so consider themselves, and do persons without disabilities view the target person as one who has a disability? Using some combination of these definitions, we could hypothesize three groups of persons with disabilities (see Figure 1.1).

TABLE 1.1. Definition of Disability in the ADA (Section 1630.2)

The term "disability" means, with respect to an individual—(A) A *physical or mental impairment* that substantially limits one or more of the *major life activities* of such individual; (B) A record of such an impairment; or (C) Being regarded as having such an impairment. *Physical or mental impairment* means: (1) Any physiological disorder, or condition, cosmetic disfigurement, or anatomical loss affecting one or more of the following body systems: Neurological, musculoskeletal, special sense organs, respiratory (including speech organs), cardiovascular, reproductive, digestive, genitourinary, hemic and lymphatic, skin, and endocrine; or (2) Any mental or psychological disorder, such as mental retardation, organic brain syndrome, emotional or mental illness, and specific learning disabilities. *Major life activities* means functions such as caring for oneself, performing manual tasks, walking, seeing, hearing, speaking, breathing, learning, and working. *Substantially limits . . .* means: (i) Unable to perform a major life activity that the average person in the general population can perform; or (ii) Significantly restricted as to the condition, manner, or duration under which an individual can perform a particular major life activity as compared to the condition, manner, or duration under which the average person in the general population can perform that same major life activity.

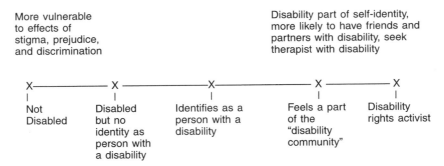

FIGURE 1.1. Disability identities.

Three Disability Identity Groups

The Functional Limitations Group

The first group would be those with significant impairments in one or more major life functions, who might even respond to the term "handicapped" (e.g., have handicapped parking placards) but who do not consider themselves persons with disabilities or members of a disability community. For example, a recent survey (Toms Barker & Maralani, 1997) inquired about disability conditions and the ways in which these affect household and parenting tasks. Some number of the respondents filled out more than 60 questions on disability and disability-related issues, giving diagnoses, functional limitations, and so on, and then wrote in a comment along the lines of the following: "I do not think of myself as a person with a disability." People responded to specifics about their functioning, but their identities did not include the disability. This echoes the findings from a 1985 Harris poll (no. 854009) in which persons with disabilities were asked a series of questions about their self-views. Although almost half the respondents did not think of themselves as disabled or handicapped, and did not think that other people would think so either, almost three-quarters felt a sense of common identity with other persons with disabilities. Thus it seems that a majority of persons with disabilities would fall into this first group. Most people with disabilities are surrounded by people without disabilities, and thus see mirrored back to them nondisabled bodies and movements. If their disabilities are not too severe they are accorded the right to "pass," to be among the nondisabled as if they were not disabled at all; they are treated as if they were "normal." It is not surprising if they identify more with the nondisabled than with the disabled population.

The Disability Identity Group

A second group consists of people for whom the disability is incorporated into the overall self-concept. Like any attribute, it may carry a positive, negative, or ambivalent valence. Persons in this group identify as members of the nondisabled world and try to function and live as "normally" as possible. For guidance they tend to seek assistance from able-bodied peers or professionals, and compare themselves to able-bodied norms. The vulnerability comes from trying to meet able-bodied standards despite the disability.

The Civil Rights Group

Some subgroup of the second group comprise this third group. These are people in the disability community, who participate in the disability rights movement, who view disability as a social construct, and who maintain that those with disabilities are a minority group that has been and is being denied its civil rights. They consider themselves bicultural. This group is most likely to have friends with disabilities and to want to see a therapist who has either a disability or significant disability experience (e.g., an immediate family member).

THE DISABILITY COMMUNITY

Persons with disabilities form a community with some features in common with other out-groups, and many features specific to that community. The disability community has its own history, language, perspectives, priorities, humor, norms, and a sense of pride in its identity. It espouses a particular model of disability (the minority model; see Chapter 2) that stresses collective disability experience rather than separation by diagnosis or medical condition. As an out-group, one labeled deviant and stigmatized, the disability community focuses attention on the interaction between society and its deviants and views disability as a social construction. This perspective on disability shifts attention from rehabilitation to social activism, with an emphasis on disability rights and independent living.

Children with disabilities are often raised to deny their disabilities, to look and behave as able-bodied as possible. Isolation from other children with disabilities and absence of role models and mentors with disabilities place such children in a position of deviance on the fringes of the nondisabled world. They are loved *in spite of*, not *with*, their disabilities. Families may unwittingly bolster the child's outsider position by denying the realities of the disability experience. Commonly families tell children that the disability is a problem only if the child *lets* it be a problem—disability is only a matter of overcoming it in your head.

Imagine that you were standing on the edge of a circle looking in. Wouldn't you want to find a circle in which you could be in the middle? Then, through some happenstance, you start talking to other persons with disabilities, and things you never talked about with anyone before become commonplace topics. You have experiences in common. You feel understood in a way you never have before. You would describe it as "coming home." There you perch, on the edge of one circle, in the middle of another. Now you are bicultural. But your family is not; you have become a part of a community your family might not join, that may be alien to them, that may threaten their views on disability. So now you have two families, your family of origin and the disability community. Where are you going to spend Thanksgiving?

CATEGORIZATION, SEVERITY, AND FUNCTIONING

Disabilities can be categorized by diagnosis (e.g., MS, asthma, or insulin-dependent diabetes), by system affected (e.g., nervous, musculoskeletal, cardiovascular, pulmonary, visual, and auditory systems), by onset (i.e., age at onset and speed of onset), or by function loss (e.g., quadriplegia and paraplegia). But in fact all these factors must be considered in understanding a specific person's disability. Let's see what happens when we take only one dimension of disability out of context. It may seem deceptively easy to answer the question, "How severe is the disability?" but it's actually quite difficult. Consider the following examples:

> Sally, now in her late 40s, had breast cancer 8 years ago, and underwent radiation and chemotherapy. The cancer reoccurred and was also found in more than 15 lymph nodes. Since then, the goal of treatment was to extend her life, but cure was improbable. She had periods of intensive treatments (e.g., hospitalization and isolation after T-cell transfer), but in between these phases she worked three-quarter time as an executive assistant. Her work performance was excellent, and she rarely missed days unexpectedly due to illness. She arranged in advance with her boss when she would be absent for an extended period and made arrangements for her absences by hiring temporary assistants and training them.

Most of us would probably consider Sally's illness severe in the following ways: (1) it is life threatening, and she is more likely to die from the cancer than from other causes; (2) treatment methods are invasive, risky, systemic, and often occur in a hospital; (3) periods of exacerbation or intensive treatment cause complete inability to perform job tasks; (4) Sally feels unwell about 50% of the time. But let's look at a second example:

> Dara, like Sally, is in her late 40s and works as an executive assistant. She is in generally excellent health but gets frequent migraines (about 20 times per year). These last for several days and are debilitating. If she is at work when one comes on she leaves immediately, and if she's not at work she calls in sick. She may be absent for up to 3 days with one episode of migraine. She is unable to predict frequency or onset of migraines and hence misses work at the last minute; others at the office fill in for her, but her boss finds her unplanned absences disruptive.

Using the same criteria as before, how severe is Dara's disability? (1) It is not life threatening and should not affect life expectancy at all; (2) treatment is noninvasive, symptom focused, outpatient, and occurs over short durations; (3) symptoms cause complete inability to perform job tasks; and (4) other than when she has a migraine, Dara feels well and considers herself healthy.

Whose disability is more severe? In the long run the cancer has more serious consequences than the migraines and more profound effects on life. Yet, in the short run, the migraines cause more impairment in job performance, and the boss is more likely to want to fire Dara. Dara finds the migraines disruptive, and she is discouraged about potential for curbing their frequency or severity. She feels her doctors don't take her seriously, yet her quality of life is quite affected by the migraines.

As we see from these examples, understanding only one facet of disability in isolation (e.g., frequency, degree of incapacitation, or pain) fails to give a complete picture. Several authors have proposed ways to think about disabilities that incorporate many factors, including onset, severity, prognosis, and impact on functioning. Rolland (1994) has one of the more complete and well-articulated psychosocial typologies. I have extended his system (see Table 1.2) to include disability phase, the individual's and family's stages of development, and the overall health context of the person with the disability (the last four rows of the table).

DISABILITY STATISTICS

There are several problems in trying to address how many persons with disabilities there are, the nature of the disabilities, and the limitations

TABLE 1.2. Psychosocial Dimensions of Disability

Onset:	Acute		Gradual
Course[a]:	Progressive	Constant	Relapsing
Outcome:	No impact on life expectancy	Shortened lifespan or possible sudden death	Fatal
Degree of incapacitation:	None	Mild Moderate	Severe
Degree of uncertainty[b]:	Completely unpredictable		Completely predictable
Individual's overall health:	Excellent	Compromised	Poor
Disability phase:	Diagnosis	Remission Chronic	Exacerbation
Individual developmental phase:	Dependence	Emancipating	Interdependence
Family's life stage:	Centripetal		Centrifugal

[a]A progressive course of disability does not mean that the course is downward—some disabilities may improve over time.

[b]Note that degree of uncertainty is on a continuum. Although the other variables are also on a continuum, they are "described here in a categorical manner by selection of key anchor points along the continuum" (Rolland, 1994, p. 23).

they impose. The difficulties are related to variability in definitions of what constitutes a disability, the age groups included in the sample, sampling methods, and how data on multiple conditions are collected and analyzed. Further, disability interacts with a number of variables (notably age, gender, ethnicity, income, education, family structure, and social and occupational environment) such that impairments that lead to functional limitations in one set of circumstances or environmental conditions might not in another set of circumstances. Bearing in mind these limitations, what follows is a collation of many sources of disability statistics (Asbury, Walker, Maholmes, Rackley, & White, 1992; LaPlante, 1993, 1996; LaPlante, Miller, & Miller, 1992; Leung, 1991; McNeil, 1993; National Institute of Handicapped Research, 1985; Sisco, 1991; Thompson-Hoffman & Storck, 1991).

Persons with disabilities constitute the largest minority group in the United States (and ASL is the third most common language, after English and Spanish). Most recent reports of the number of Americans with disabilities estimate a figure of 43 million, or 14.3% of the population. Among persons with disabilities, 6% are under 15 years old, 60% are 15 to 64, and 34% are over 64. If we consider only more severe disabilities, the numbers skew to the higher ages (2.2%, 55%, and 43%). Of all Americans, 9% are limited in ability to perform a *major* life function as defined for their ages (*play* in infancy and toddlers, *school* for children, *work* for adults, and *self-care* for all adults).

Of the prime working-age group (16–64), 10% are limited in the amount or kind of work they can do. Even having a more mild disability has a noticeable negative effect on participation in the work force (only 65% of such persons are working, compared with 80% for those without disabilities) and having a severe work limitation has a profound effect on employment (only 12% are in the work force). The unemployment rate of persons with disabilities is conservatively estimated to be about 66%. In the 1980s, earning growth for full-time employment grew only 29% for men with disabilities, compared with 45% for men without disabilities. Men at the lower end of the income scale are more likely to have disabilities, and those with disabilities have lower earnings. Further, disability is associated with less education, which in turn affects earning power.

Women are more disadvantaged by disability than are men. "Women with disabilities have a 33% participation rate in the market in comparison to 60% rate for men with disabilities" (Danek, 1992, p. 9). Women with disabilities earn less than men with disabilities, and less than men or women without disabilities. It seems that gender and disability compound each other, having a synergistic negative effect on employment and income (DeLoach, 1989, 1992). Not surprisingly, disability is associated with lower income but results in a higher rate of poverty for women than for men.

Types of Conditions Causing Disability

The five most common disabling conditions are heart disease, back problems, arthritis, diabetes, and orthopedic impairments of upper or lower extremities. Approximately 1.5 million adults use a wheelchair. This represents 1% of the total adult population, or the same incidence as schizophrenia. About 9% of adults with disabilities use a cane, crutches, or a walker for more than 6 months. Of all adults, 5% have difficulty seeing words and letters in ordinary newsprint, 6% have difficulty hearing normal conversation, and 1% have trouble making their own speech understood by others. A little over 3% have mental health disorders (excluding mental retardation, learning disabilities, and dementia). Most people have more than one condition, with an average of 1.6 conditions per person. Injuries account for 13% of all disabling conditions.[1]

---

[1]An unknown number of disabilities are due to abuse; no data are kept on this. However, one study (Conley-Jung, 1996) found that 2% of visual impairments were caused by or significantly exacerbated by physical abuse as a child.

Disability status is associated with certain patterns of health insurance. Persons with disabilities are less likely to be covered by private health insurance than the nondisabled. Those with severe disabilities are more likely to be covered by government (vs. private) insurance than are people with no or mild disabilities, and persons with mild disabilities are the most likely to be uninsured (36%). This latter group might be analogous to those referred to as the working poor—too much income to qualify for aid and too little income to be sufficient for needs, particularly given increased costs of living with a disability.

Disability is by no means a random event but occurs disproportionately among certain population groups and in turn is affected by demographic variables of the person. Thus to understand disability we have to examine it in relation to the characteristics of the person and environment in which it occurs.

Disability, Gender and Age

The likelihood of disability, of work disability, and that the disability will be severe all increase with age. Persons under age 24 account for 43% of the general population, but less than 15% of the population of persons with disabilities. At the other end, persons 65 years or older comprise 8% of the total population, but almost 33% of the number of persons with disabilities.

Nonetheless, we should remember that most persons with disabilities are under 65. Over half of all persons with disabilities are in the 25 to 64-year-old age range (20% are between ages 25 and 44). "Thus, while disability is highly prevalent among older persons, to overemphasize disability as a phenomenon associated with aging would be to ignore the unique characteristics and needs of younger disabled persons" (Thompson-Hoffman & Storck, 1991, p. 18).

Although women are more likely to have a disability than men (even accounting for women's longer life expectancy), this is not true among the younger ages (up to age 21), where boys outnumber girls in the ranks of those with disabilities. Approximately 4.2% of children under 21 have a chronic activity limitation (4.8% of males, 3.5% of females). Over 4.5 million children (ages 0–21) are enrolled in education programs for the handicapped. The largest group (68%) comprises those with a learning disability or speech impairment; the second largest group is children with mental retardation (17%). Children with disabilities are more likely to be from families with income under $10,000, compared to their peers without disabilities (28% vs. 20%).

The nature of childhood disabilities has changed over time. Virtual eradication of polio in the U.S. since the mid-1950s is but one of the more notable differences. Yet there has been little significant change in the incidence of most birth defects since the early 1970s (except for anencephaly and spina bifida, which have declined by about 40%). The reported percentage of children with activity limitations doubled from 1966 to 1981, but this may be due as much to improvements in reporting as to actual increased incidence.

The most frequent childhood psychiatric diagnosis in the United States is attention-deficit/hyperactivity disorder (ADHD), which is considered a disability under law. The number of children taking medication for ADHD more than doubled from 1990 to 1995. Astonishingly, about 2.8% of children ages 5 to 18 are taking methylphenidate (Ritalin). Typically these children are diagnosed at age 7 or 8, and remain on the drug for 5 to 7 years (a period longer than in the past). Most children with an ADHD diagnosis received it from a pediatrician who, by self-report, spent about 1 hour diagnosing the disorder. Children with untreated ADHD are more likely to drop out of school (about one-third do so), abuse substances, or commit suicide.[2]

Children with disabilities are more likely than those without disabilities to have more and longer overnight stays in the hospital, more doctor visits per year, more days of school missed, and more emotional and behavioral problems. The more severe the disability, the greater the likelihood of each of these factors. Further, families with a child with a disability experience more disruption than do other families (e.g., moving, financial strain, separation or divorce).

Disability, Gender, and Ethnicity

Comparisons of prevalence rates are confounded by differences across ethnicities in life expectancies, birth rates, and immigration patterns. Data in general support the following conclusions:

> There is a higher concentration of disability among blacks, and, in most cases, a lower concentration among Hispanics. Where breakdowns are available on Native Americans, they consistently form the subgroup with the largest percentage of disabled persons. Disability prevalence rates for Asians and Pacific Islanders are markedly below national estimates. In interpreting these data, it should be noted that the prevalence of limitation of activity by race and Hispanic ethnicity is influenced by differences in the age structure of these groups. (Thompson-Hoffman & Storck, 1991, p. 25)

---

[2]A resource for persons with ADHD is CHADD, 8181 Professional Place, Suite 201, Landover, MD 20785; telephone (301) 306-7090.

Disability rates have escalated more in the minority population. Factors that may contribute to this higher rate include "poor prenatal and perinatal care, nutrition and diet, an inaccessible health care system, greater risk for physical injury in terms of living conditions and types of employment situations, and . . . a lack of proper health care knowledge and education" (Asbury et al., 1992, p. 2). Of particular importance is that the effects of disabilities are harsher for women and for ethnic minorities. Such persons with dual- or triple-minority status are less likely to return to the work force and more likely to have lower incomes and to be more severely disabled. Married women who incur a disability are more likely than their male counterparts to become separated or divorced. African American and Hispanic families are more likely to contain a parent with a disability (18.7% and 16.3%) than are Caucasian families (about 10%).

Caucasian children have a higher percentage of less severe disabilities compared to African American children (2.2% versus 1.3%), but the reverse is true for medium (1.8% and 2.4%) and high levels of disability severity (.2% and .3%). Focusing only on teenagers (12–16) with a disability, a higher proportion are African American, are from low-income families, and have less educated parents.

Ethnicity interacts with gender and disability status: Caucasian men are more likely than Caucasian women to have a work disability, but for African Americans with a work disability more are female (54%) than male (46%). Gender and ethnicity further interact with specific types of disabilities:

1. African Americans are about 12% of the U.S. population but 15.5% of persons with a disorder of the nervous system (e.g., mental retardation, CP, epilepsy, Parkinson's, MS).
2. More females than males have a *chronic health condition* (58% are female); this is even more pronounced for African Americans (64% are female).
3. Across all racial/ethnic groups the percentage of those with a *physical disorder* is close to evenly divided between males and females.
4. Under age 65, African Americans and Hispanics are over-represented among persons with *chronic health conditions,* but over age 64 Caucasians are overrepresented in this group. This may reflect factors enabling persons of different ethnicities to reach older ages; life expectancy is less for African Americans and Hispanics compared to Caucasians, and it may be that only the healthier survive past age 65.
5. Because marriage patterns differ across ethnic groups, more Afri-

can Americans than Caucasians with *physical disabilities* are widowed and fewer are married.

Disability, Education, Income, Occupation, and Geography

The effects of lower education levels among persons with disabilities is devastating, and this is one of the key factors in higher poverty, lower income, and greater unemployment. Disabilities create less of a barrier to employment for those jobs associated with higher levels of education. Dropping out before completing high school is particularly disastrous for employment and income for those with disabilities. However, "work disability is an ambiguous concept. The work disability question implies that the only factor affecting the ability to work is the condition of the person" (McNeil, 1993, p. 12). But clearly ethnicity and education interact. In general, Caucasians have more education than do African Americans and Hispanics. Thus, of the 7.2% of persons with physical disabilities who are college graduates, 90% are white and only 4% are African American. Given the relationship between education and employment for persons with disabilities, this results in high unemployment rates for African Americans with a physical disability, and Hispanics with disabilities have the highest proportion of unemployment.

"A disability belt" (U.S. Department of Education, 1993, p. 1) runs through Appalachia and the Mississippi Valley. Proportionately more persons with a work disability live in the South. (This may reflect the types of work available in different locales.) Differences in rates of work disability among states are appreciable—states at the high end have rates up to three and a half times those at the low end; these extremes are not due to differences in age groups among the states. Rates of work disability for each state in 1980 were highly correlated with 1990 data ($r = .9$), indicating a great degree of stability in the relative position of states. Typically states that rank high on work disability have low educational attainment and economic resources. Such states "will experience more difficulty implementing the goals of the ADA and other policy goals aimed toward reducing disability and undesirable societal reactions to disability" (U.S. Department of Education, 1993, p. 19). Two states consistently rank high on disability (West Virginia and Alabama) and two consistently rank low (Connecticut and Alaska). Furthermore, the two high-disability states have low rates of completion of high school (66% each), and the two low-disability states have high rates of completion of high school (81% and 87%). Disability and education are closely linked phenomena; increasing education attainment in states with low education levels would help reduce rates of work disability.

Persons with disabilities account for 13.4% of all employed persons. Caucasians with disabilities outearn Hispanics with disabilities, who in turn outearn their African American counterparts. African Americans with disabilities are the group with the highest proportion of those with incomes less than $5,000. Persons with disabilities are less likely to hold executive, administrative, or management jobs or to be doctors, scientists, lawyers or teachers.

Summary of Disability Statistics

1. More boys have disabilities than girls, but more women have disabilities than men.
2. African Americans and Hispanics are overrepresented among persons with chronic health conditions, except in the older (over 65) age group.
3. African Americans are overrepresented for disorders of the central nervous system (CNS) (e.g., mental retardation, CP, and epilepsy). It appears that African American children with these types of physical disorders are less likely to be mainstreamed and more likely to be placed in special education.
4. Ethnic minority persons with disabilities are more likely to have lower education levels, which has a disastrous effect on employment and income. Factors of increased import to persons with disabilities are health, life, and disability insurance, medical care, durable medical products, and personal assistance; as income decreases the ability to procure these assets also decreases, which in turn heightens the handicap associated with the disability.
5. Accessibility (ramps, elevators, braille signage, etc.) may be less prevalent in poorer areas and rural areas, thereby having a disproportionate impact on minorities with disabilities.
6. The importance of education for persons with disabilities cannot be overemphasized. As the U.S. workplace moves to one of service, technology, and information, education and training will take on inflated importance for persons with disabilities.
7. By the year 2000 there will be about 96.3 million Americans over age 44.[3] Older workers are less likely to become reemployed postdisability; they often find themselves over- or underqualified for jobs, and have a 20% rate of being below the poverty level. Older workers with disabilities also may be forced into early

---

[3]Note that the ADA (1990) considers a worker "older" at age 40.

retirement. The median income for persons over 65 is about $12,075 for Caucasians, $7,400 for Hispanics, and under $7,000 for African Americans. Thus, older minority workers are likely to work out of necessity.

8. There are synergistic effects of dual or triple minority status (disabled, racial or ethnic minority, female, elderly) which too often result in unemployment, poverty, and isolation. As America's safety nets are tattered by budget cuts, this sector of the population is going to need more aid.

IMPLICATIONS

"To the extent that the ADA achieves its goals and people with severe disabilities join the labor force, rates of severe work disability should decline over time" (U.S. Department of Education, 1993, p. 20). This statement carries a vital implication, namely, that disability is a social construct, a chronic condition that imposes limitations in some contexts and not in others. We see this in the relationship between work disability and education; as education increases, work disability decreases. If all persons with physical disabilities were well educated and worked in white-collar jobs, there would be less effect of disability on employment. Thus disability is not an entity that can be considered in isolation. Attention to other factors in a person's life (e.g., low education level) reduces the effects of the disability, ameliorating its impact on work, and hence on income, while providing opportunities for socializing and purpose in life.

The clinical implications are clear: We must encourage children with disabilities to stay in school, even—and perhaps especially—in families with lower socioeconomic status. The clinical role must go beyond the armchair, to help mobilize supports for continued education. This includes finding mentors; talking with resource teachers, counselors, and principals; encouraging and supporting the family; finding practical solutions (e.g., transportation, places to study, and access to assistive technology); and locating and utilizing community resources (e.g., church, support groups, and volunteers). The effects of low education combined with a disability are especially strong for people of dual or triple minority status—women, people of color, and the elderly.

TWO

The Minority Model
of Disability

This chapter establishes the minority model of disability, beginning with an overview of three predominant models (moral, medical, and minority). I examine the ways in which disability is like and unlike minority groups based on other characteristics (e.g., ethnicity, gender) and discuss the impact of multiple minority status. Models of disability are reflected in the words we use; thus, the second section of this chapter considers the language of disability—euphemisms, politically correct terminology, preferred and forbidden words—and how this language frames our perspectives. I give special attention to two concepts prevalent in the empirical literature on disability: "burden" and "adjustment." This attention leads to a discussion of how language promotes a pathologizing perspective and suggests a framework for a nonpathological orientation. The chapter concludes with the clinical implications of models of disability, language usage, and a nonpathology orientation.

THE MORAL, MEDICAL, AND MINORITY
MODELS OF DISABILITY

Disability is often called a social construct, meaning that the disability is best understood in terms of how society perceives disability. Historically, there have been three predominant social constructions of disability: the moral, medical, and minority models. Each has a perspective on what "the problem" of disability is, who holds the problem, and avenues that best address the problem.

The first and oldest is the *moral model*. In this view disability is a defect caused by moral lapse or sins. It brings shame to the person with the disability. In cultures that emphasize family and group over individuals, the shame spreads to the group. The person and/or the family carries the blame for causing the disability. Disability is seen as "divine retribution for sinful deeds, as retribution and preparation for the hereafter, as a warning to one who strays from the path of the devout, or as a test of a person's faith" (Florian, 1982, p. 292). Thus a disability represents the reification of sin, failure of faith, moral lapse, or evil. For example, I recently received a mail-order catalogue (*Wireless*, 1998) offering a "Gaelic blessing plaque" which had the following message: "May those who love us, love us. And those that don't love us, may God turn their hearts; and if he doesn't turn their hearts may he turn their ankles so we'll know them by their limping" (p. 5). We see in this saying the moral model view that outward manifestation of disability reflects inner maleficence.

The moral model posits disability as a test of faith, the notion that "God gives us only that which we can bear." In this view the family of the person with the disability somehow has been selected for its various attributes (faith or strength, or a test thereof). The disability tests not only the person with the disability but his or her family as well. Although the moral model is the oldest view of disability it is still very much extant and pervades our language, culture, and ideology. In some cultures the moral model is the more prevalent view (Chan, Lam, Wong, Leung, & Fang, 1988; Florian, 1982; Jaques, Linkowski, & Seika, 1970; Jordan & Friesen, 1967; Schneider & Anderson, 1980). The recent possibility of prenatal testing has resurfaced the link between genetic conditions and cultural connotations. Genetic disorders "are commonly perceived as permanent, irreversible, chronic, family-linked, stigmatizing, complex, and evocative of strong emotions, such as fear, pity, and guilt for passing the defect to offspring" (Shiloh, 1996, p. 476). The transmission of a defective gene becomes imbued with moral implications—the passing of bad seed.

The moral model of disability often contains within it the myth of disability as mysticism. In this view, as disability impairs one sense, it heightens another, often to mythic proportions. The prototype for this figure is the Greek blind seer who spouts oracles. This image is legion in fiction, films, and medicine. For example, following is a description of the book *Close to the Bone* by Jean Shinoda Bolen, MD: "Offers compelling evidence that life-threatening illnesses can illuminate the essential truths of life—often rendering the survivor stronger both spiritually and mentally" (Barnes & Noble ad, October 13, 1996). In this quote we see our need to impose order and purposefulness on random events such as incurring a life-threatening illness—from physical adversity comes increased emotional and spiritual strength. In the professional literature we find phrases such as "disability as a growth experience" and "transcending disability" (Vash, 1981, pp. 124, 131). These phrases promulgate the idea that disability imbues one with special abilities to perceive, reflect, transcend, be spiritual.

The *medical model* gained momentum in the mid-1800s with the advent of more enlightened and humanistic medicine. This perspective takes the moral or sin aspect out and replaces it with a more paternalistic view. Disability is seen as a medical problem that resides in the individual. It is a defect in or failure of a bodily system and as such is inherently abnormal and pathological. The goals of intervention are cure, amelioration of the physical condition to the greatest extent possible, and rehabilitation (i.e., the adjustment of the person with the disability to the condition and to the environment). Persons with disabilities are expected to avail themselves of the variety of services offered to them and to spend time in the role of patient or learner being helped by trained professionals. In the United States, the medical model predominates. The main contribution of the medical model is its repudiation of the view of disability as a lesion on the soul. Further, the medical model has spurred medical and technological advances that have improved the lives of people with disabilities.

The *minority model* (also called the "social model") is a new paradigm from which to view disability. It posits that disability is a social construction, that the problems lie not within the persons with disabilities but in the environment that fails to accommodate persons with disabilities and in the negative attitudes of people without disabilities. Persons with disabilities are seen as a minority group—in the same way that persons of color are a minority group—that has been denied its civil rights, equal access, and protection. The definition of a minority group includes "identifiability, differential power, differential and pejorative treatment, and group awareness" (Dworkin & Dworkin, 1976, p. viii). Key impediments for any minority group are prejudice and discrimination, social isolation, unequal treatment, economic dependence, high unemployment and underemployment, inferior housing, and a higher rate of institutionalization (Biklen, 1988). Yet when people without disabilities are asked what they think will be the major problems for persons with disabilities, they cite the impairment (i.e., the physical limitations). When persons with disabilities are asked the same question they tend to point to social barriers and the pervasive negative attitudes of others toward persons with disabilities as their main impediments. Negative attitudes are a major obstacle in rehabilitation; they impose an additional requirement of coping for the person with the disability (Florian, 1982).

The minority model developed in the early 1900s but then mostly disappeared until it reemerged in the early 1970s. The impetus for its renaissance was the Rehabilitation Act of 1973. The Act had been passed by Congress in 1973 but could not be implemented, as is true for any law, until the regulations outlining implementation procedures and guidelines were published. These regulations were awaiting the signature of (then) Secretary of Health, Education and Welfare Joseph Califano, but 4 years had transpired since the Act was passed, and still the regulations were not signed. This led to a protest by persons with disabilities at the steps of the Capitol and in cities around the country (most notably San Francisco). Although the 1960s saw a great many protests throughout the country, the sight of a group of persons in wheelchairs, with ventilators, signing, and with canes or guide dogs was novel and highly unusual in that persons with disabilities did not have a unified organizational umbrella to pull them together as one voice. Shortly after the protests began Secretary Califano began negotiations with disability groups until satisfactory regulations were developed and signed, thereby activating the Rehabilitation Act. This Act ushered in a new era of laws and civil rights for persons with disabilities and cemented a firm entrenchment of the minority model in a significant sector of the disability community. Many participants in those protests went on to become leaders in the disability community, providing leadership not just *for* but *by* persons with disabilities.

The search for any solution is directed and constrained by how the problem is framed. The *moral* model frames the problem as one of sin and moral lapse and puts the onus on the individual or family. In this model, solutions to the "curse" of disability are to be found in the realms of faith, forbearance, exorcism, ostracism, and even death. The *medical* model posits the problem as residing in the individual, and the solutions are medical intervention, aid in "adjustment" to disability, modifications of the disabled person's lifestyle. The *minority* model takes the problem out of the realm of the person with a disability and places it in the social, political, and economic world. Solutions are universal design, education of those without disabilities about persons with disabilities, laws ensuring equal access and protection, and better enforcement of such laws. It also maintains that decision making *about* persons with disabilities should be *by* persons with disabilities; indeed, the disability rights movement has adopted the slogan of South African blacks in the time of apartheid: "Nothing about us without us."

Let me give an example of how the minority model reframes the question and hence offers different solutions. Often at work I've been asked whether I will be attending specific events. The unasked question behind the overt one is, "Do we need to pick a place that's physically accessible?" My response is that it doesn't matter whether or not I will be attending—in either case the site must be accessible. Putting aside the issue of the law (as an educational institution we must ensure that all functions of the school are equally accessible to persons with disabilities) there is a compelling moral reason why, irrespective of my attendance, a site must be accessible. To bring this point home to faculty I have asked them this question: "Would you hold this function at a site that didn't allow Jews? Would it be relevant to that decision whether someone Jewish was actually in attendance or not?" This reframes the problem as what it really is, namely, a civil rights issue. When we reframe the question in this way, an immediate shift of perspective occurs. We now focus not on me, the person with the disability—"Will *you* be attending? Can *you* manage two stairs? Do *you* need an extra wide parking space?"—but on the environment. It now becomes incumbent upon the external world to make itself accessible. We reframe "I can't climb stairs" to "Why isn't there a ramp?" We might focus on the immediate larger social group, namely, the faculty, and ask a different question: "Why is the faculty holding its meeting in a place that is not accessible?" We then might go up one level to focus on the community and ask, "Why was this building erected without due consideration of accessibility for persons with disabilities?" And going up another level, to the sociopolitical arena, we then ask, "Why do we tolerate discrimination against our citizens?" and "At what cost do we do so?" This is the crux of the minority model, this shift in focus from personal, individual, and problem in isolation, to group, environment, attitudes, discrimination—from individual pathology to social oppression.

Similarities and Differences with Other Minority Groups

Calling persons with disabilities a minority group implies that there are some essential features of minority experience shared by all out-groups (Goffman, 1963). What are the similarities between persons with disabilities and other minority groups? (See Tables 2.1 and 2.2, listing similarities and differences, some of which are discussed here.)

The previous section discussed the core similarity, which is the experience of prejudice, discrimination, and stigma. These are the essence of what it means to be a minority group member. These issues are always present to some degree and necessitate explicit laws for protection of rights. Thus the minority person is burdened with the extra and constant task of paying attention to these factors; only majority persons can escape without giving these factors due consideration. If minorities are unrepresented in professional and political arenas, then minority issues are less

TABLE 2.1. Similarities between Disability and Other Minority Groups

Issue	Comments
Minority-group status	The core experience of a minority group is generally prejudice, discrimination, and stigma. Being a minority means having to think about being a minority; only the majority group has the luxury of avoiding this.
Assimilation	Pressure to assimilate, emulate the majority culture.
Inferior status attributed to inherent traits	Confusion of biology with the results of social oppression, positing of genetic inferiority.
Concerns about procreation	Subjects of eugenics movements, forced sterilization, and social Darwinism.
Intermarriage	Issues around marriage (intermarriage, validity of marriage, different marriage patterns).
Hate crimes	Targets of organized brutality (e.g., Klu Klux Klan and skinheads); targets of hate crimes and violence (however, disabled only group excluded from hate crimes act).
Standardized testing	Lack of representation in groups used to norm a wide variety of assessment instruments; inappropriate use of tests.
Representative from own group	Have to be better to be thought of as being as good as majority group. Successes and mistakes interpreted as representative of the minority group. Conspicuous successes are considered exceptions that prove the rule, and person is allowed probationary entry to the majority world (i.e., we ignore their minority status, and expect assimilation and shedding of minority culture).
Role models	Fewer public role models, more negative images, and fewer positive images in media.
Lack of professionals	Underrepresentation in many professions, including those that interact most with minority group.
Mental health services	Underserved population in mental health; special training and awareness necessary for professionals. Few professionals of like minority.
Underrepresentation	Politically underrepresented in terms of both absence of minority issues raised by candidates/office holders and fewer like minorities in office.
Insurance risks	Issues of insurance risk (e.g., higher car insurance because living in certain areas, higher risk of AIDS, and seen as at risk for worker's compensation).
High risk	Higher rates of school dropouts, substance abuse, and unemployment (less true for gays/lesbians).
Affective regulation	Unacceptability of certain emotions (especially anger), and prescription of other emotions.

TABLE 2.2. Differences between Disability and Other Minority Groups

Issue	Comments
Separate but equal?	Separate is not viewed as inherently unequal. People with disabilities have separate buses, separate transportation systems (paratransit), separate entrances, separate water fountains. "Proximity is not the same as integration."
Isolation in family and community	Usually the only one in family who has disability. Usually no immediate family, friends, neighbors, with like condition. Birth of child with disabilities is usually unexpected (we generally can predict ethnicity, though not gay/lesbian). Those with disabilities generally do not reside in segregated living areas (unlike communities of like religion or ethnicity).
Becoming a member of disability minority group	Disability has open enrollment—anyone may join at any time. Minority status may be conferred after birth.
Pride	Until recently (and now only for small group within the disability community), there has been no inherent pride in the condition of disability.
Whose fault is it?	Often blamed or held responsible for disability condition.
Realm of discrimination	Discrimination occurs in all major life activities (e.g., phones, stairs, shopping, employment, movies, restaurants, bathrooms, water fountains, and sidewalks).
Developing a community	Less well-organized and less visible subculture. Most in the disability minority group do not consider themselves part of a disability community, though most say disability is a minority group.
Disadvantage	Most under- and unemployed minority group (about 70% of persons with severe disabilities are unemployed). Wages lower than for able-bodied peers.
High risk	Possibly the highest rate of substance abuse, estimated at over 25% (compare with 10–12% in general population).
Body as reflection of self	Disability often broadcasts misleading messages about the self; the body does not always emit the proper social cues (e.g., visually impaired not recognizing someone approaching; unusual body movements associated with CP; body twitch of Tourette's).
In subservient role	Disabled spend more time being helped by professionals (i.e., spend disproportionate amount of time in settings in which the person with a disability has low status or where the characteristics of the setting connote inferiority (e.g., physical therapy, special education, hospitals, and doctors' offices).
Disclosure	For hidden disabilities there may be an element of choice to disclose disability status (same for gays/lesbians).
Visibility	We don't think it strange when we don't see disabled people; we don't expect to see them, don't notice their absence. But we do notice their presence.

TABLE 2.2. *continued*

Issue	Comments
Uses valuable resources	Disability is expensive. Disability is time consuming.
Pain, fatigue, and weakness	Disability often involves *pain* (with need for pain management), *fatigue* (with need for activity monitoring and trade-offs), and *weakness* (with need for flexibility to allow for daily variations in functioning).
Prescription of affect	"Expectation of mourning" and requirement of cheerfulness.
Extra tasks	Nothing can be taken for granted; must call ahead, or get information about accessibility. Can get stuck somewhere, have power failure, become fatigued or incapacitated.

likely to be made a part of the structural system. The result is that majority persons make key social, professional, and political decisions for and about minority persons. For example, a local graduate institute utilized its personnel and human resource officers, none of whom have disability experience, to develop a policy for responding to the ADA. Similar processes occur at many organizations and institutions.

Minority persons are encouraged and coerced to look, behave, and think like the majority—to assimilate. For example, a Deaf man said to me, "I can't do my deaf walk in the hearing world or people look at me funny. I have to walk like a hearing person." Role models are mostly persons from the majority group. If a person becomes expert in some way, he or she is said to have transcended the minority status. The highest compliment people think they can say to a person with a disability is, "I never think of you as a disabled person." With one line, all your struggles are dismissed, and a core part of your identity obliterated.

Another similarity is in the area of affect, the prohibition against certain emotions (notably anger) and the prescription of other emotions (cheerfulness, in the case of persons with disabilities). (This issue is discussed more fully in Chapter 4, as it is critical to understanding the experience of being a person with a disability.) Another similarity among minorities is the increased risk of negative outcomes, such as school dropout, unemployment, substance abuse, and early death. Further, many ascribe these risks to features of the minority group itself (i.e., you are that way because *people like you* are like that). There is the confusion of social roles and forces with biology (*The Bell Curve* being only one in a long line of examples). As such, there is pressure not to procreate lest you create more people like you. In selecting partners there are two seemingly incongruent pressures, first to remain within the ghetto and marry only among one's own and, conversely, to find partners from the majority group and thus improve what is seen as the inherently inferior gene pool. Forced sterilization is one extreme outcome of this ambivalence, and one that is more current than you might think. To cite but one example in one study most of the 50 professionals surveyed (legal, medical, social welfare, developmental disabilities agencies, and education professionals) reported that they had been involved in some capacity with the sterilization of persons with disabilities (Brantlinger, 1992).

There are important differences between minority status based on disability versus that based on other factors. One difference which fundamentally affects the lives of persons with disabilities is the acceptance of the doctrine of separate but equal. Although clearly struck down by the courts regarding ethnic minorities, this principle is more than just tolerated; it is encoded into law and policy. There are separate entrances (with signs showing that the ramp is around the back), separate drinking fountains, separate buses, and even an entirely separate transit system (usually called paratransit, in a sublime linguistic pun), separate classrooms, separate seating, separate lines, and separate procedures.

A second important difference is that a person with a disability is usually the only such person in the family and the neighborhood. Thus, as is the case for gays and lesbians, there are no immediate role models, no automatic sources of support, and no mirrors of like condition to reflect back that such a condition is "normal." Further, the family cannot be counted on to view or treat disability in a positive way and, in fact, may add to the problem for the member with the disability.

The community of persons with disabilities has open enrollment—anyone can join at any time by acquiring a disability. This perhaps is exactly what contributes to the need to distance ourselves, the knowledge that this, too, could happen to *me*. And, as discussed more in Chapter 3, this knowledge may spur people to find reasons why it couldn't happen to them; holding the person with the disability at fault for the condition (echoes of the moral model) provides such a reason. Further, the inherent pride people feel for being a member of a minority group (e.g., that based on ethnicity or race) has not extended to persons with disabilities—"Say it loud, I'm blind and I'm proud" just doesn't have the right ring to it. No one is really saying it's *better* to be disabled than not (whereas one might say it's better to be Jewish or Jamaican or Peruvian). The idea of disability pride may seem oxymoronic to outsiders but has been adopted by the disability community to express the acceptance and the value of difference. Disability pride has "borrowed from other minority pride ideologies in relinquishing the goal of assimilation into the majority . . . culture" (Gill, 1994, p. 13). Further, we are saying that being a person with a disability should not be viewed as a tragedy. (Overheard at a party: "She was born with deformed arms, but she was a beautiful girl, with a lovely face, so it was a particular tragedy.") But because disability is not viewed as inherently desirable, there is less cohesiveness among persons with disabilities, less apparent reason to hang together. As a result of this and many other factors, persons with disabilities are a less organized and visible subculture, with little political clout. Policies for and about us rarely make headlines. For example, most of the articles on the ADA have focused on the impact of the law on businesses. As always, the perspective is the impact of persons with disabilities on the nondisabled, not the reverse.

Disability by definition alters the body, many times in visible ways. Some of these ways affect how that person's communications are received. For example, a woman with a visual impairment remains expressionless as she approaches you because she doesn't recognize you until you either speak or she's less than six feet away; you mistake her lack of recognition for aloofness. A young man's speech disorder makes talking for lengthy periods tiring, so he tends to keep his statements short, his answers often limited to one or two words; you mistake his reticence for being uncommunicative or shy or conclude that he isn't very bright. A middle-aged woman with Meniere's disorder (inner ear) tends to stare straight ahead to avoid sudden motions or feelings of imbalance; you mistake her stare for rudeness or inattentiveness. All these examples show that the ways in which a person's body is affected by the disability, as well as ways that the person manages symptoms of the disability, can inadvertently and adversely affect interpersonal communication.

Many cultures make jokes about that culture's sense of time (e.g., Israeli time is give or take an hour; parent time is half an hour late for every child). But "crip time" really is different; it is the extra time it takes to accomplish tasks as a person with a disability. For example, every time I stop for an errand I spend 2 minutes lowering my scooter off the lift in back of my car, then reverse the process at the end. Three errands add 12 minutes of scooter time. My children learned at a young age to wait for me on the sidewalk out of the way of cars. Accomplishing cleaning tasks requires built-in rest periods. Changing my babies often involved the following steps just to get ready to begin: (1) putting baby in an umbrella stroller; (2) wheeling baby with me to the bathroom to get a washcloth and small bowl of warm water; (3) wheeling to changing table to put down cloth and bowl; (4) sitting down on floor to get change of clothes and fresh diapers from lower drawers or shelves; (5) unbuckling baby from stroller; (6) using furniture to hoist myself back upright, all the while maintaining readiness to catch baby if he lunged forward; (7) putting baby on changing table. In addition to things just taking more time, extra disability-associated tasks are necessitated. For example, to get a new scooter, I made over 20 phone calls in 1 month, went for a mandatory evaluation by an occupational therapist 40 minutes away, and made a series of calls to the vendor (over 1 hour away). Finally, 3 months and countless phone calls after beginning the process, a scooter was delivered to my office. It was the wrong one, so they took it back.

"Crip time" means that tasks take more time. It means that there are additional tasks. It also means that time takes on a different meaning when you have a condition that may affect your time alive, or that has forced an awareness of personal vulnerability.

Multiple Minority Status

"To date almost all research on disabled men and women seems to assume the irrelevance of gender, race, ethnicity, sexual orientation, or social class. Having a disability presumedly eclipses these dimensions of social experience" (Fine & Asch, 1988, p. 3). This is not the case, and when other factors such as gender and/or ethnicity are considered, the synergistic effects of the multiple minority statuses is clearly critical. There are several factors to consider in examining multiple minority status, notably women and ethnic minorities with disabilities. First, do the rates of disability vary by gender and/or ethnicity? As discussed in Chapter 1, most rates of disability do differ across both variables. This makes certain disabilities "women's issues" or "minority issues" which may marginalize them and fail to attract major grants or researchers. Second, does the same disability affect women and/or members of ethnic minorities differentially? We know very little about differences in how disabilities affect women, and then only in very circumscribed areas (e.g., sexual responses after spinal cord injury; transmission and course of AIDS). We know even less about how the course and effects of disabilities may differ by ethnicity, especially given the confounds of socioeconomic status and differential access to health care. Third, are attitudes toward persons with disabilities affected by the gender and ethnicity of the person with the disability? In a word, yes. Fourth, how do cultural values affect persons with disabilities and their families? To cite only one example, in an article about Chinese Americans with disabilities (Chan et al., 1988) the authors give several examples. They state that the Chinese are less positive about persons with disabilities than are whites, and that, unlike for whites, male and female attitudes toward persons with disabilities do not differ. Further, the Chinese are more likely to accept traumatic events and suffering as a fact of life; it is unknown whether this might lead to faster adjustment to disability or a slower adjustment due to a more passive acceptance of the disability. This example makes apparent that so much of what we think we know about responses to disability—by the person with the disability, by his or her family, or by the community—may not hold up across cultures even within our own country.

There is surprisingly little written on ethnic minorities with disabilities, especially given that some ethnic minority groups (especially African Americans) are more likely to incur disabilities (Asbury et al., 1992; Belgrave, 1998; Cornelius, 1995). Further, the need for population-specific psychologies (Zea, Belgrave, Townsend, Jarama, & Banks, 1996) suggests that models for understanding disability may need to be formulated more specifically for subgroups. Articles that use ethnicity as an independent variable tend to compare only blacks and whites, with other ethnic groups more rarely examined. Most empirical studies fail to give ethnicity data for participants. For example, for three major studies on the aftereffects of spinal cord injury, all published in one issue of *Rehabilitation Psychology* (1993), two gave no data on ethnicity of subjects and the third reported that all participants but one were white (Hanson, Buckeleew, Hewett, & O'Neal, 1993; McShane & Karp, 1993; Tate, Forchheimer, Maynard, Davidoff, & Dijkers, 1993). Another study on this same topic (Herrick, Elliott, & Crow, 1994) reported percentages of white and black clients but did not analyze data separately or use ethnicity as a variable. Yet studies indicate that African Americans were less likely to return to work following spinal cord injury than were whites (DeVivo & Fine, 1982; DeVivo, Rutt, Stover, & Fine, 1987; James, DeVivo, & Richards, 1993). Bear in mind that this is not necessarily or even probably because African Americans with spinal cord injuries were less inclined to work or more able to garner state financial support but more likely a reflection of differential hiring practices, compounded by additive effects of holding dual minority status.

There is more literature on women with disabilities than on ethnicity and disability. Women with disabilities have taken the forefront in examining and writing about issues for women with disabilities, and it is in this literature that we see the marriage of the personal and the professional (cf. Fine & Asch, 1988; Finger, 1990; Hillyer, 1993; LeMaistre, 1993; Mairs, 1997; Rogers & Matsumura, 1991; Traustadottir, 1990). Also, there is more acknowledgment of multiple minority status among these writings (cf. Gainer, 1992; O'Toole & Bregante, 1993). However, along with multiple communities to which women with disabilities belong (e.g., disabled, female, racial, and sexual orientation) comes multiple sources of discrimination (ableism, sexism, racism, and homophobia) (O'Toole & Bregante, 1993).

Differences and Similarities among Disabilities

Most books about disability have individual chapters corresponding to types of disabilities. This book does not discuss disabilities by type but focuses on the commonality of the disability experience (see Chapters 3 and 4, in this volume, for more on the disability experience). To discuss commonalities presupposes that such exist, and it is a fundamental tenet of this book that they do. "Historical research is substantiating that, whatever the social setting and whatever the disability, people with disabilities have been, and are, subjected to a common set of prejudicial values and attitudes and share a common experience of social oppression" (Longmore, 1987, p. 142). The "disability experience" implies the experience of prejudice, stigma, and discrimination which is common to all minority groups. These can occur in *any* facet of one's life, from the mundane (crossing the street) to the profound (employment): having to go in separate entrances and sit in separate areas, getting in the building but finding the bathroom inaccessible, going to a store that's accessible only if you're the only person in the store and seasonal overstock isn't stacked in the aisles, knowing that someone you've just met is trying very hard not to look at your disability, being told how brave or determined or remarkable you are just for getting up every morning, having a stranger say "I'll pray for you," and being told how wonderful it is now that modern medicine can prevent people just like you. Experiences like these are not disability-specific; they transcend the particulars of any one type of disability and form an essential aspect of the disability experience. And this experience can be psychologically wearing: "The disability itself can be demanding, but sometimes even more exhausting are all of the everyday hassles caused by an inaccessible environment and others' attitudes" (Gill, 1997, p. 12).

How do people with disabilities manage the social and interpersonal handicaps engendered by the disability? Do those with early onset of disability respond differently than those with later onset? It might seem intuitive that people with congenital or early-onset disabilities respond differently to their condition than do people with later-onset disabilities. You might imagine that the first group is *more* "adjusted" to their disability because they've had longer to accept it, and it has been a part of their self-concept from the beginning. Or you might posit that they are *less* "adjusted" because of the early stigmatized experiences of being a child with a disability. Neither is clearly the case, though some evidence suggests that early onset promotes integration of the disability into self-concept and leads to better self-advocacy skills. One study (Silvers, 1996) indicated no differences on a measure of well-being between persons with early-onset disabilities (prior to age 10) and persons without disabilities. A recent survey of parents with disabilities (Toms-Barker & Maralani, 1997) found that those with early-onset disabilities were more likely than those with late-onset disabilities to have completed college and to be employed. They were also more likely to have a partner with a disability, suggesting that persons with early-onset disabilities are more likely to identify with the disability community. Thus early- and later-onset disability groups may have some differences, and age of onset may be an important research and clinical variable. However, for many measures, "time since disability onset" is not a significant predictor of responses.

Although I've emphasized the commonalities of experience among persons with disabilities, of course there are tremendous differences as well. As discussed in Chapter 1, disabilities can be categorized along several dimensions, and the resulting profiles correspond to differences in subjective experience. Degree of diagnostic uncertainty, length of time from symptoms to diagnosis, and number of specialists consulted before diagnosis are but a few of the factors related to diagnosis that can distinguish among disabilities. Other factors include prognosis, predictability of course of disorder, extent of physical involvement, degree and type of cognitive involvement, and extent of stigma. These issues, separately and in combination, affect the subjective experience. Yet despite these profound differences, there is a commonality that transcends them, much like differing ethnic minorities, who have important distinctions among them but also a common experience of being a member of an ethnic minority in this country. This book focuses more on the commonalities than differences among disabilities, while providing guidance on other dimensions of importance.

THE LANGUAGE OF DISABILITY

In this age of political correctness (PC) our use of language has become a political tool. It is easy to feel that this tool has lost some of its communicative power and most of its meaning. Yet in this section I cover the use of terminology related to disability. Is this just more PC talk? I think not; embedded in PC language are social constructs and ideologies that are important to understand. Perhaps using an example can illustrate this point best. Think of the tremendous social and political changes that are implied by the terms "girls," "ladies," and "women"; to give another example, "colored," "Negro," "black," and "African American." As we see in these examples, terminology both presages and mirrors important sociopolitical movements; it might even be argued that the changes in terminology reflect paradigm shifts. And, of course, any group—whether based on gender, race, ethnicity, sexual orientation, religion, and so on—should be allowed to name itself. Groups often designate a private name, what they call themselves among themselves. Such is true within the disability community. Therefore, to illuminate some key concepts, in this section I review important words and phrases related to disability, both for outsiders and insiders. (See also Table 2.3 for phrases associated with rehabilitation.)

We must remember the enormous power of words that come laden with history. A policeman's alleged use of the "N" word played prominently in the O. J. Simpson trial. We have our version of the "N" word: cripple. As with many groups, those with disabilities have taken back the offensive language used by others toward us and made it an insider term ("crip"). Such words are now experienced as highly derogatory and offensive when used by others (i.e., those without disabilities) but may be used in certain circumstances by insiders. This lifting of words out of the mouths of the outsiders into the realm of the disability community is an important demarcation of our identity; having a secret language helps foster group identification. "Crip" says "I am not ashamed of my disability, I belong with other people with disabilities, and I have pride in my group." Used by an outsider, it is simply the "C" word. It is not the same as "supercrip," which is a derogatory word for a person with a disability who achieves notable tasks usually associated with being able-bodied, such as climbing El Capitan, a tall granite rock in Yosemite.

In the United States the current preferred language is "person with a disability."[1] This terminology evolved as follows: First, disability descriptors took symptoms (e.g., difficulty with locomotion, mental retardation, and spastic movements) and elevated them to global descriptors, such as cripple, retard, or spazz. An example from this era is the "Shriner's Hospital for Crippled Children." This language evolved to "handicapped,"[2] which is a more generic term; it implies an impairment but doesn't specify locality or severity. However, there are several objections to this term. First, it was (and still is) used as a global description, as in "handicapped person," as if the handicap defines the person, or as

TABLE 2.3. Evolution of Treatment Slogans

Era	Slogan
1950s	"Use it or lose it"
1960s to mid-1980s	"No pain, no gain"
Mid-1980s to 1990s	"Conserve to preserve it"

[1]This differs in the United Kingdom, where many who are in the vanguard of disability theory have published. See, for example, Gleeson (1997), Hevey (1992), Abberley (1991).

[2]Although it is often reported that "handicapped" comes from "cap in hand" (i.e., beggar), this is not the origin of the word. Rather, it comes from the older usage of the sports term meaning an advantage or disadvantage imposed on a contestant to equalize chances of winning (the forfeits were held in a cap).

if the personhood itself was handicapped. Second, several authors (see discussion to follow) have made important distinctions among the terms "impairment," "handicap," and "disability," and if evaluated with those distinctions in mind, the term "handicapped person" is incorrect. In making the correction, the term "disabled person" was substituted, and by the early 1980s was the more common term. The current and preferred term is "person with a disability." This phrasing places the person first (i.e., the personhood is unaffected by the condition) and relegates disability to a secondary position. These changes in language can be seen in the language from the 1970s—the Education for All *Handicapped Children* Act (1975)—to 1990—the *Americans with Disabilities* Act (1990) and the *Individuals with Disabilities* Education Act (most recently reauthorized in 1997).

Several sources (World Health Organization [WHO], 1993; Wright, 1963) make important distinctions among the terms "impairment," "disability," and "handicap." It is worth considering these distinctions because these concepts are important in our understanding of clients with disabilities. An *impairment* is "concerned with abnormalities of body structure and appearance and with organ or system function, resulting from any cause . . . impairments represent disturbances at the organ level" (WHO, 1993). Thus an impairment is the medical condition. As an example, a client's impairment might be retinal myopathy. A *disability* reflects "the consequences of impairment in terms of functional performance and activity by the individual; disabilities thus represent disturbance at the level of the person" (WHO, 1980). To continue with the example of retinal myopathy, this person's disability might be legal blindness with total loss of peripheral vision but shadow vision in central field.

So far we have seen that impairments and disabilities are classified according to the attributes of the person. In contrast, *handicaps* are "concerned with the disadvantages experienced by the individual as a result of impairments and disabilities; handicaps thus reflect interaction with and adaptation to the individual's surroundings" (WHO, 1980). In our example the handicaps might include need for books in large print, print enlarger and enhancer for computer screens, books on tape, reliance on public transportation, on bus drivers to call out stops, and on voice to recognize people. To use myself as an example, my impairments are polio and postpolio syndrome. My disability is partial leg paralysis, limp, fatigue, muscle weakness, and joint pain. My handicaps are stairs, inaccessible bathrooms, buses without lifts, icy sidewalks, unavailability of appropriate shoes, the high cost of scooters, and so on.

A trend over the last 30 years has been the substitution of euphemistic words or phrases for disability. It began innocently enough with the

"Special Olympics," but then the term "special" came to mean a child with a disability, especially those children with cognitive and/or learning impairments. Other terms followed: differently abled, handicapable, otherwise abled, special needs, disABLEd, etc. What is the message of a euphemism? Why do we call people fighting in a war "troops" (as in, "forty-six troops were killed in fighting today"), if not to obfuscate meaning and palliate the impact? Euphemisms are used because the real terms are too powerful, evocative, painful. Therefore one meta-message of having a euphemism for disability is that it is a dirty word. A second message is that disability is cute, like freckles or ringlets. A third message is that disability is just another aspect of a person, like, say, having red hair. This underplays the radical psychosocial impact of having a visible disability (see next section on defining characteristics). People who identify as part of the disabled community generally detest the cute euphemisms for disability that have proliferated since the early 1970s. Should you use them with clients? The general answer—model your language after that used by the client—is helpful only when it is clear who is the client but can be perplexing in couple or family cases. For example, in a first session with two parents who were concerned about their 8-year-old son, they used such terms as "special," "slow" and "different." It was hard to know just what the son's impairment was from their terminology, but I gathered that he had mental retardation. At the second session they brought in the son and I asked him, "Do you know why you're here?" He didn't miss a beat before he responded, "Because I'm retarded."

Now that we've made distinctions among terms, an important point must be emphasized: Two people might have the same impairment but very differing disabilities and handicaps. Thus knowing the "diagnosis" of retinal myopathy tells you little about the client's visual functional level and hence adaptive needs. This is an important point, because most of the rehabilitation, medical, and financial structures that serve persons with disabilities are impairment based (i.e., decisions often are based on medical condition). It would be better for them to be based on functional level (disability) and degree of social or work handicap. In clinical practice, assessment of functional level—and any ways the therapy itself might be affected by this—is a critical initial step.

A second point raised by the different terminology is that disability does not equal handicap. A disability might remain static but the level of handicap will vary. To continue with our example, if the modifications needed—books on tape, enhanced computer screens, and so on—are available, the person is not handicapped by the environment despite the disability. In such cases the disability becomes mostly irrelevant. But as the world decreases its accessibility and equality—if books are not available in either large print or on tape, bus drivers don't call out the stops, public transportation does not have its destination marked in accessible ways, medical personnel assume that such a person shouldn't be a parent—the person's handicap is increased. It is because we do not live in a world in which structures, services, and terrain are equally accessible to persons with varying disabilities that persons with disabilities are also generally handicapped, often severely so. This point is so important that I want to give another example. In the past month, I have been handicapped in the following ways as I go about my daily routines: I was unable to take my children to a movie because the theater is upstairs with no elevator; I selected a different restaurant because the first-choice restaurant has a lovely and beautifully accessible bathroom that is up five steps; I was on the second floor of a mall and wished to go to a store just below me, so I double-backed to the middle of the mall to the only elevator and then retraced my steps to get to the desired store; every morning I rode my scooter on the street instead of the sidewalk as I accompanied my daughter to school because there were no curb cuts on part of our route, and we took the long way around because the zig-zagged opening in the fence designed to keep out bike riders also kept me out; I waited in my car for 10 minutes outside my local grocery store for a close-by open parking spot because someone had parked illegally in the handicapped spot.

This list is not intended as a "poor me" saga but, rather, as an illustration of ways in which those with disabilities are unnecessarily handicapped in daily life. In fact, it was hard for me to generate this list—I had to delay writing it until I could keep track in a notebook. This difficulty in remembering such items stems from how routine they are—I no longer take particular notice when a place is inaccessible to me. Being shut out is a way of life for persons with disabilities. This was graphically illustrated a few years ago when a man who was only temporarily disabled and using a wheelchair wrote an article in a travel magazine. He complained vociferously about hotel shuttle buses being parked in front of the only curb cut, counters being too high, and being treated in a patronizing manner. At first many people with permanent disabilities lamented that someone with a temporary disability had not earned the right to speak for us, but what became apparent is how those of us with disabilities have forgotten to notice so much of the inaccessibility in our daily worlds. It took the perspective of a man used to being mobile and upright to notice the changes in his access when he was sitting in a wheelchair.

Disability language has suffered from an affliction of emotionally laden words or phrases such as "suffered from" and "affliction." For example, one could say about me that I "was afflicted with polio" at an early age and now "suffer from postpolio syndrome." I could be described as a "polio victim." All these phrases do more than impart information, they also convey a negative perspective, not only on the disorder but on me as the embodiment of the disorder. Further, when we use such terms as "the cerebral palsied" or "the retarded" we reduce people to reifications of disorders. It isn't just that the disorder becomes the most salient characteristic but that it comes to define the totality of the person. All else is "explained" by the disorder. Another eschewed phrase is "deaf and dumb." The muteness associated with being deaf is a characteristic of prelingual deafness (i.e., it is redundant). Thus this phrase shows a lack of understanding of what it means to be deaf. Furthermore, "dumb" is not a label anyone particularly welcomes.

The guidelines from the national association of newspaper journalists calls for "people first" language (e.g., "person with a disability" or "person with mental retardation"). Nonetheless, a common term seen in news stories, books, magazines, is "wheelchair bound." The preferred term is "wheelchair user," or "person in a wheelchair." (Among ourselves we say "person in a chair"—the wheels are understood.) This may seem like a trivial distinction, but it implies a change in perspective. "Wheelchair bound" emphasizes the loss of function, the fact that the person can't/doesn't walk, the relegation of status from upright to seated. "Many people misunderstand wheelchairs, viewing them as symbols of helplessness rather than vehicles permitting mobility" (Gill, 1997, p. 12). To illustrate this point, imagine that you are a person who can't walk, your health insurance refuses to pay for a wheelchair, and you can't afford one. Then someone gives you a wheelchair. From that perspective the wheelchair represents not loss of function but restoration of mobility; the wheelchair represents wings. Locomotion is the desired action; the route to achieve this might be legs or wheels.

A frequently used term is "mainstreaming," which originally referred to the effects of the Education for All Handicapped Children Act (though the Act never used this term), namely, the placement of children with disabilities into the "least restrictive environment"; often this meant "mainstreaming" kids into regular classrooms for all or some of the day. The term has come to embrace the concept of inclusion in a broader sense, the participation of persons with disabilities in all activities, sites, and interactions in society—social, political, economic, educational, entertainment, and personal. Mainstreaming is achieved by "accessibility"—literally physical accessibility (i.e., a person in a wheelchair could get in the door and have access to all services and functions of the site) but also figurative accessibility—acceptance, equity in treatment and opportunity. This latter definition makes a distinction between integration or coexistence and true inclusion. For example, hiring a person who is blind is integration; eating lunch with that person is inclusion.

The distinctions among disability, handicap, and impairments are not academic. They are critical levels of understanding for therapy. As therapists we must learn all we can on our own about a client's *impairment*, learn from the client, who is the expert, about his or her *disability*, and focus the treatment more on the *handicap*.

Examples of Language

Following are three descriptions of the same man performing the same actions. The language used to describe him, however, also conveys information about him and how we should feel about him.

> EXAMPLE 1: After Joe drives home from work, he goes into the living room for ten minutes to rest and read the newspaper. Then he prepares dinner. The family sits down to eat together at 6, and discusses the events of the day.

In this first example we see Joe as an ordinary family man, performing daily tasks and interacting with his family. His disability is not mentioned because it is irrelevant to the tasks discussed.

> EXAMPLE 2: After Joe drives home from work in his van with hand controls, he sits in his wheelchair in the living room for 10 minutes to rest and read the newspaper. Due to difficulties from cerebral palsy with fine motor coordination Joe has trouble holding the paper, so he lays it out on a lap desk to read. After 10 minutes Joe prepares dinner, using specially shaped knives and pots with extra handles. The family sits down to eat together at 6. Joe uses a special plate with a lip to push food against and L-shaped utensils that are easier to grab. The family discusses the events of the day. The children are used to their father's speech, which has reduced enunciation, and are readily able to understand him.

In this second example the disability is mentioned but in fairly neutral language, and we learn information about modifications Joe uses. The perspective is on the availability of assistive devices; we might think how nice it is that such things are available, and it becomes clear that assistive devices increase independence. In telling about Joe's speech the focus is on the children's ability to understand as opposed to Joe's ability to speak.

> EXAMPLE 3: Joe, who is wheelchair bound since he was afflicted with cerebral palsy at birth, drives home from work in his altered van, which has specially installed hand controls and a floor lower than normal vans to accommodate his height from a wheelchair. He

parks in the garage at home and slowly lowers the van lift, then laboriously makes his way out of the van and up a ramp to the house. Then he must rest for at least 10 minutes from fatigue due to his disorder. He is able to read the paper only with the use of a lap desk on which to rest it because his deformed fingers cannot hold the pages. After his break he wheels into the kitchen to prepare dinner. Special utensils and pots with odd-shaped handles allow people like Joe to do simple daily tasks in the kitchen. The family sits down to eat together at 6. Joe must use a special plate with a lip to push food against and special utensils with altered shapes which are easier to grab. The family discusses the events of the day. Joe is able to converse with his children even though he suffers from a speech impediment that reduces his enunciation and ability to make himself understood.

In this last example, negatively laden language is used, and this language switches the focus to Joe, what he can and cannot do, how he has "special needs," how he differs from "normal." By describing what Joe has to do to accomplish simple tasks such as getting from van to house or reading the paper, we make Joe seem heroic in his perseverance, and we are primed to see him as brave and plucky. (For more on pluckiness, see Chapter 4.) All three descriptions are equally "true," yet each creates a different picture of Joe and focuses our attention on different aspects of the scene. Language reflects, but also creates, reality.

Response versus Adjustment

One term merits special consideration due to its ubiquity and what it represents. The literature repeatedly refers to "adjustment" to disability. The primary goals of rehabilitation are return to work and "adjustment" to disability. Someone who is angry or seems to have a chip on his or her shoulder might be said not to have "adjusted" to the disability.

> Why do I keep putting the term "adjustment" in quotation marks? Because: I do not believe there is such a thing as "adjustment to disability." That is, the response curve, while steeper at first, does not ever level off at some mythical stage of adjustment and acceptance. Rather, it continues to wend its way, often up, sometimes downward, throughout the life-span in a continuous process. I would call this process the "response" to disability, not the adjustment. Within this framework, "responses" are not normal or pathological per se but are to be understood in the context of an individual's overall development. (Olkin, 1993, p. 15)

"Response" does not imply any particular slope or trajectory. "Adjustment," however, does; it implies a series of steps that climb toward a plateau. These steps have been conceptualized in stage models of response to disability. Persons with disabilities (and their loved ones) are "supposed" to go through stages of responses to the disability. It is commonly assumed that people's responses to disability progress through orderly stages. Stage models assume that stages have a sequence, lead to a more adaptive state, give information about the psychological status of the person going through the stages, and are more helpful than harmful to the individual. Conceptually, stage models might be illustrated as a series of steps leading to a pinnacle, usually labeled "adjustment." Supposedly by climbing these stairs (what an irony!), persons with disabilities become "adjusted" to their disability. But where's the ramp?

Numerous authors have posited stages of responses to disability, which culminate in "adjustment," "acceptance of the disability," or reemergence of the preinjury personality. Several points require discussion. First, the methodologies of the studies supposedly demonstrating stage models are extremely flawed. They generally study only a small number of subjects, in hospital or rehabilitation settings (community samples would be expected to differ; cf. Rintala, Young, Hart, Clearman, & Fuhrer, 1992), with limited gender (usually male), ages (usually young adulthood), and ethnicity (usually white, or unspecified, which may be the same thing). Measures often are simply the observations and subjective opinions of the researchers. But "we must again remind ourselves how seriously mistaken outsiders can be when led astray and deluded by the compelling nature of their own values and perspective" (Wright, 1983, p. 159). Because their assumptions were based on a pathogenic view, their models reflected this, and they "found" data to support it. Even positive responses often get reframed as pathological: It's hard to imagine anything more dismissive than thinking of a client as exhibiting "superficial acceptance" of the disability (Gunther, 1969).

Second, the idea of reemergence of the preinjury personality is a biased and flawed concept that could only come from an outsider's position. It suggests that the person with a disability comes to feel, act, think, and behave (i.e., the components of "personality") as he or she had before the disability onset. However, in going from an able-bodied person (a valued status) to a person with a disability (a devalued status), the person must counteract any feelings of shame or inferiority. Dembo, Leviton, and Wright (1975) and Wright (1983) suggest that there are four value changes that facilitate counteracting such feelings:

1. Enlarging the scope of values. This involves shifting perspective from viewing the disability as a loss (of function and of former self) to an increased valuing of what remains, of those functions still available, and to a generally wider array of choices.

2. Subordinating physique relative to other values. It may be that the relative weight of other values increases, that the value of physique decreases, or both. Other values such as kindness, wisdom, effort and cooperation are superordinate over appearance, physical strength or athleticism.

3. Containing disability effects. This refers to containing the effects of the disability to only those areas that involve the disability, allowing the disability to remain just one of an array of factors. For persons with disabilities, the disability often is perceived as a characteristic of the person rather than as a possession (rather like the difference between "a man who owns a home" and "a homeowner"). But the more disability can be seen as a possession the more disability effects are contained. In addition disability can be seen as an "impaired tool" (Wright, 1983, p. 176). Tools (e.g., legs) for action (e.g., walking) can, if impaired, be substituted for by other tools (e.g., crutches, prostheses, and wheelchairs) to achieve the same result (e.g., mobility).

4. Transforming comparative-status values into asset values. Comparative-status values involve comparison to a standard on a scale ranging from better to worse. One's position on this scale is evaluated in comparison to others. Asset values, on the other hand, are evaluated in terms of utility or intrinsic value. For example, using a Braille writer is a useful way to achieve certain ends (e.g., taking notes). It achieves worth as an asset value. It is only as a comparative-status value that it might be judged inferior by "normal" standards. Asset values focus on achieving ends, the intrinsic values of an asset, the "what can" (vs. "what can't") be done.

"Acceptance, then, is a reorganization of . . . values in a person's value system to accommodate life changes brought on by disability. Reorganization occurs through value change" (Keany & Glueckauf, 1993, p. 207). Such change implies that there is no going back to a preinjury personality, one developed without a disability. The shifts in values and roles, and the need to respond to an acquired stigma, result in irrevocable alterations.

A third problem relates to the issue of emotions. Depression is thought to be a stage in most stage models. Thus there is the potential danger that clinicians will overlook or normalize a treatable depression (see Chapter 4 on the requirement of mourning). We should remember that DSM-IV considers bereavement to last only 2 months, after which the diagnosis switches to one of the depressive disorders if a clinical depression remains. Although we might argue with this view of "normal" bereavement, we must acknowledge the inconsistency with the view of depression in disability. It implies yet again that we expect people with disabilities to be suffering and depressed (unless they are perennially cheerful; see Chapter 4). Likewise anger, supposedly a stage to be passed through, may be misinterpreted. Anger may in fact be a healthy response to discriminatory experiences, and should not so quickly be discarded or pathologized.

The empirical literature does not support stage models of disability adjustment. Studies are inconsistent in numbers, characteristics, and sequences of stages (Woodbury & Redd, 1987) and overall do not support the model (Dunn, 1977; Rape, Bush, & Slavin, 1992; Shadish, Hickman, & Arrick, 1981; Trieschmann, 1980; Yuker, 1994). Some people who "adjust" to their disability bypass stages, others seem to retain elements of all stages. There is tremendous variation among persons who experience trauma, and little reliable evidence that individuals proceed through stages of response. Woodbury and Redd (1987) echoed this view when they reported more variability than similarity in persons who sustained a spinal cord injury. A belief in stage models of response to disability is a pernicious trap for clinicians. It invites misinterpretation of individual variation as deviant and pathological. Also, recurrence of behaviors or affect supposedly associated with earlier stages may be misconstrued as regression, maladjustment, acting out, or other manifestations of pathology. Further, it may inhibit viewing depression as treatable.

What is the goal of the ascent through stages? Most of the literature refers to it as adjustment or adaptation, which I reject, as discussed previously. Living with a disability forces continued response. At times, the disability is relegated to the background, of little significance, like a soft hum. At other times its role becomes one of many factors (a trilling flute in a quintet) and other times even more prominent (the crash of cymbals). This process of receding and advancing continues throughout the lifespan.

Why "Burden" Gets Its Own Section

When Yuker (1994) called for a moratorium on research on "the presumably horrible negative effects of a child with a disability on parents and siblings" (p. 12), he may well have been referring to "the burden literature." The word "burden" portrays a common conceptualization of disability that is from the perspective of the nondisabled persons. It is as if the disability is a terrible thing that has happened to the nondisabled. Certainly disability is a family affair, but the almost exclusive focus on the effect of the person with the disability on the family, and not the reverse, is emblematic of a pervasive perspective, that of the nondisabled looking at the disabled. The following titles, from the years 1990 on, illustrate this point, and exemplify the burden literature: "Psychiatric Morbidity and Family *Burden* among Parents of Disabled Children" (Carpiniello, Piras, Pariante, Carta, & Rudas, 1995); "Patient Predictors of Caregiver *Burden*, Optimism, and Pessimism in Rheumatoid Arthritis" (Beckham, Burker, Rice, & Talton, 1995); "Family *Burden* Following Traumatic Brain Injury" (Allen, Linn, Gutierrez, & Willer, 1994); "A Study of Social *Burden* Felt by Mothers of Handicapped Children" (Tangri & Verma, 1992); "Perceived *Burden* and Coping Styles of the Mothers of Mentally Handicapped Children" (Sequeira, Madhu, Subbakrishna, & Prabhu, 1990); "Effects of an Intervention Aimed at Memory on Perceived *Burden* and Self-Esteem after Traumatic Head Injury" (McGuire & Greenwood, 1990); "Effects of Parent Training on Families of Children with Mental Retardation: Increased *Burden* or Generalized Benefit?" (Baker, Landen, & Kashima, 1991); "Negative Symptoms in the Traumatically Brain-Injured during the First Year Post-Discharge, and Their Effect on Rehabilitation Status, Work Status and Family *Burden*" (Gray, Shepherd, McKinlay, & Robertson, 1994); "Aging Family Caregivers: Support Resources and Changes in *Burden* and Placement Desire" (Heller & Factor, 1993); Parents of Adults with Mental Retardation Living In-Home and Out-of-Home: Caregiving *Burdens* and Gratifications (McDermott, Valentine, Anderson, Gallup, & Thompson, 1997).

Even when the word "burden" is not in the title, it is often there in spirit: "Easing the Strain: Assessing the Impact of a Family Fund Grant on Mothers Caring for a Severely Disabled Child" (Beresford, 1993); "Parental Stress from Caring for Children with Disabilities" (Inanami, Ogura, Rodgers, & Nishi, 1994); "Psychosocial Problems in Families of Disabled Children" (Singhi, Goyal, Pershad, Singhi, & Walia, 1990); "Stigmatized and Perpetual Parents: Older Parents Caring for Adult Children with Life-Long Disabilities" (Kelly & Kropf, 1995); "Current Parental Stress in Maltreating and Nonmaltreating Families of Children with Multiple Disabilities" (Benedict, Wulff, & White, 1992).

In reviewing these titles, any one of them might seem completely justified in using the word "burden." Disabilities do impose new demands on families. However, the additive effect of this kind of perspective is alarming. First, the disability is infused into the personhood, to become "the disabled." Then it is not just the disability that is a burden but the person with the disability. Second, the repetition of the idea that persons with disabilities are burdens begins to permeate consciousness. For example, in a 1991 Harris poll (no. 912028) about 13% of the surveyed population specifically associated persons with disabilities with burden. Third, it perpetuates the continual bias of research from the perspective of nondisabled persons' vantage points. Fourth, we would serve better those who treat children with disabilities and their families by empirical literature that did not consider such children burdens. How can clinicians help but be influenced by this pervasive view of such families? When we as researchers consider directions for study, it is imperative that we consider not only what should be done but what must cease (see Chapter 14 for further discussion of research).

A NONPATHOLOGIZING ORIENTATION TO WORKING WITH CLIENTS WITH DISABILITIES

One could approach the study of persons with any condition (whether it be disability, homosexuality, or heart disease) by examining the effects of that condition on "normal" development. This approach looks for and finds differences and tends to pathologize those differences. This is the "pathogenic" model. This model assumes that these conditions are or create stressors, which will lead to pathological states unless warded off by guardians at the gate. The guardians most studied and discussed are coping and social supports and, to a lesser extent, certain cognitions and attributions. A contrasting model would try to identify variables that allow and promote resilience, hardiness, health, self-esteem, and "adjustment." (For example, Antonovsky, 1979, 1987, developed a "salutogenic" model that examines factors which promote well-being.) The type of model used (pathological or salutogenic) is particularly relevant in working with people with disabilities. Most such people function well and manage their lives quite adequately. Yet the literature has consistently hypothesized pathology and failed to identify and examine health and wellness factors. Therapists thus are primed to see the disability itself as the wellspring of the problems that come to clinical attention.

IMPLICATIONS OF THE MINORITY MODEL FOR THERAPISTS

A premise of this book is that the minority model best serves clients with disabilities, that ultimately "coming home" to one's own group promotes well-being and insulates one from the ravages of prejudice, discrimination, and stigma. However, we also must be attendant to the fact that the client will have his or her model, as will the family. These three models (client's, family's, therapist's) may be in concordance or com-

pletely diverse. The therapist must balance advocating the minority perspective with taking the client and his or her family where they are. (See
also Chapter 7 on assessing the client's model of disability.) Let's examine what clients might say that would give an indication of their model.
Consider a mother who calls for an appointment for her 14-year-old son
with CP. She leaves the following message on your phone: "Hi. I'd like
to make an appointment for my son, who's 14. His father and I have
some concerns about him, and the school counselor suggested we see a
therapist."

Now let's think about the meaning of the rest of her message,
depending on what is said and what is not said. Before looking at Table
2.4, try to fill in the blank table presented on the following page. Do not
be discouraged if you find this task difficult. Some of the distinctions
among models, taken out of context of a whole pattern, are subtle, especially if you are unfamiliar with disability culture.

EXAMPLE 1: "My son has left hemiplegia, but he looks mostly normal. He has a slight limp on one side and one hand doesn't work as
well as the other. But he does all right. We thought he should be
seen because, now that he's older, he doesn't seem as mature as his
peers. He makes jokes that seem very young, and I don't want him
acting like the class clown. I think his peers just tolerate him, but he
doesn't really have any friends."

EXAMPLE 2: "My son has CP from a birthing accident. I was bleed-
ing badly, and losing a lot of blood. In trying to save me there probably was a time that the baby suffered and didn't get enough oxygen. But we thought he was going to be okay. Then, when he was
about 6 months old, he still couldn't sit up, and I knew something
was wrong. When the doctor told me it was probably CP I just
knew it. God saved my life that day, but at a price. My son is suffering because of something I did."

EXAMPLE 3: "My son has CP. We've tried to help him learn how to
live with it, but it's been hard. We don't really know other parents
in this situation, and my son doesn't know other kids with disabilities. This year more than before we're seeing that his behavior is out
of synch with that of his age group, and we're afraid that he's going
to be more rejected by his peers. We know he's never going to be
like them, and we want to help him find a group where he'll fit in.
We hate to see him so lonely; the phone never rings for him."

EXAMPLE 4: "My son has CP. It has affected his right side, so he
does things with his left hand, even though he probably would have

Example	Theme(s)	Main Concern(s)	Explanation of disability	Who has the problem?	Model
1					
2					
3					
4					
5					
6					

been right-handed. He has some learning difficulties, which I understand are related to his CP. He gets extra time on tests and goes to resource room for two periods each day for help on his homework. But he doesn't really have any friends, and the phone never rings for him. My husband and I are concerned that as his peers get older, not just in age but more mature, our son will be left further behind."

EXAMPLE 5: "My son has CP from a birthing accident. I was hemorrhaging badly and he must have lost oxygen for a time. My husband and I had tried to have a baby for a long time. We were so happy when my son was born. We didn't discover he had any problems until he was about 6 months old. So I had that time with him as an infant to grow very attached to him, and the feelings got stronger after the trouble I'd had in the birth. Then when we found out he had CP, we were stronger. I know that God only gives us that which we can bear, and He knew I was strong enough then to bear this. Sometimes I wonder if I am, but mostly I just know I can help my son."

EXAMPLE 6: "My son has CP. He's walks with a limp and can go about two blocks. He can partially use his right hand, though he eats and writes with his left. He has some learning disorders and is less mature than his age group; he's more impulsive, his jokes are more grade-school level. We're concerned because as he gets older he's less tolerated by his peers. There are only two kids with a visible disability in his middle school, and next year he goes to high school which is even bigger, and he might be about the only handicapped kid there. We want to teach him how to handle the teasing and rejection but also to prepare the high school for how to help him. We'd like to find him some other kids like him, but we don't know where to look. When we asked the resource teacher she was appalled, she said we would be holding him back to try to put him with other kids like him, that we should encourage him to behave more appropriately and find normal kids to hang out with. We're not sure what's best for him, so we'd like to talk about it. I think it's really our problem, that we don't know how to help him."

In the two moral models (examples 2 and 5), the nature of the problem is most diffuse, the cause of the problem is an event involving the mother and considered to be an accident, and the focus for intervention is on the mother. However, lacking a clear presenting problem, the treatment goal seems to be a removal of mother's guilt, and/or the amelioration of mother's character. In the two medical models (examples 1 and 4), the focus is on the son, and the desired result is more friends through increased normalization of the son. In the minority model (examples 3 and 6) the problem is the interaction between son and world (peers, school), the focus of intervention is the parents and how they can help the son and the school, and the goals are to change the son's environment to make it more accepting and accommodating and to increase the resiliency of the son. Thus the model is reflected in how the problem is conceived and how it's presented, the locus of the problem, and the goals for the treatment. Rather than being some abstract theoretical perspective, the disability model permeates the clinical work from the first interaction with the family.

Nonetheless, we should make a distinction between political and clinical views. Individual clients and families are not bound to uphold the political banner. If, for example, a mother thinks that her son's CP is a test of her faith, and this helps her, and it does not result in a dysfunctional system for the son, it would be presumptuous to subordinate her clinical needs to political ideology. It is only in the ways that this is dysfunctional that the clinician should intervene. In example 2 the son will be aware of the mother's guilt and is likely to feel responsible for her suffering; his disability causes her moral pain, which is a heavy burden for

TABLE 2.4. Moral, Medical, and Minority Models

Example	Theme(s)	Main concern(s)	Explanation of disability	Who has the problem?	Model
1	He looks mostly normal	Not mature; no friends	Left hemiplegia	Son	Medical
2	Son is suffering	Unspecified	Birthing accident	Mother and son	Moral
3	Finding a group to fit in	Loneliness, rejection	CP	Son, peers, parents	Minority
4	Son left behind	Isolation; no friends	CP, LD	Son	Medical
5	Mother's strength	To help the son	Birthing accident	Mother's character	Moral
6	Finding like peers	Preparing school for son, rejection inoculation in son	CP	Parents, school	Minority

any child. In example 5, the focus of the disability story is on the mother, and this focus is keeping the story of the disability hers and not allowing it to transfer to become her son's story. The point is that, as every family therapist knows, there are an infinite number of ways that families work well, and we should not presume to know them all. However, our expertise in family systems allows us to surmise about the more limited numbers of ways that problems develop and are maintained. With regard to disability, the moral and medical models, by their emphasis on defects and pathology, offer more ways for things to go wrong.

THREE

The Disability Experience: I. Stereotypes and Attitudes

What are the commonalities of experiences across disability types? If there is a disability community, then its foundation rests on this communal experience, whose essential components are not the disability per se but the interpersonal and psychosocial experiences that result from being a person with disabilities. This chapter and the next consider several aspects. First is an examination of impression formation: how in general people's perceptions are subject to stereotyping, through central characteristics, spread, and attractiveness. Second, I discuss prevailing cognitive schemas that influence perceptions of people with disabilities. Third, this chapter synopsizes the vast literature on attitudes toward disability. These three areas (stereotyping, cognitive schemas, and attitudes) are important areas to consider because they influence therapists' perceptions of the clients with disabilities. Further, to understand clients with disabilities is to understand the prevailing experiences and attitudes toward disability that they encounter multiple times on a daily basis. The next chapter continues the examination of communal experiences and focuses on constraints on affect, cognitive schemas, and role models. Together these areas might be called "the disability experience."

IMPRESSION FORMATION

When we meet a new person we form immediate impressions in order to impose coherence on the myriad bits of information received. These impressions are subject to stereotypes. Social science has contributed to our knowledge of the process of how we stereotype, and this section reviews three key concepts from social science: central characteristics and spread, attractiveness, and prevailing cognitive schemas.

Central Characteristics and Spread

In an early and seminal series of experiments Asch (1946) examined how we form impressions of other people, particularly their personalities. He distinguished between qualities that are essential to impression formation and those that are peripheral. For example, consider the following list of attributes of a person: *a 45-year-old male mathematics professor; intelligent; warm; quick witted.* If the descriptor "warm" is replaced by "cold" in this list, the total impression of the person alters, because "warm" and "cold" are central aspects of a person. When a trait is central it carries with it a set of other assumed traits that may or may not be accurate. When a person was described as "warm" (vs. "cold") the participants in Asch's study chose other attributes for that person such as "good-natured, humorous, sociable, popular, humane, altruistic, and imaginative" more often that they did for the "cold" person (Wright, 1983, p. 53). However, not all qualities were affected by the "warm/cold" variable, and further, other qualities of a person could be described and altered that would not affect the global evaluation. In other words, central characteristics do not tell about all attributes of a person, and not all attributes are central. To further complicate matters, "warm" and "cold," which were central characteristics in one context (the above list of attributes), were shown not to be central when part of a different list of attributes (Asch, 1946).

Disability is a central characteristic. When other attributes are unknown (e.g., when first meeting) its role is profound in impression formation. The perspectives of persons with disabilities and others are divergent on the relative importance of the disability: "Data indicate that most disabled people say that their disability is not the most important thing in their lives" (Yuker, 1994, p. 9). Yet the fact of disability is perceived by others to be a defining aspect of the person, an inescapable defining characteristic.

A closely related concept to central characteristic is "spread" (first introduced by Dembo et al., 1975). Spread "refers to the power of single characteristics to evoke inferences about a person" (Wright, 1983, p. 32). In paradigmatic studies, participants were given only limited data about a person (e.g., Mussen & Barker, 1944; Ray, 1946) and asked to rate the stimulus person on numerous other personality traits. The single fact of disability (or absence of) affects ratings. Thus a known characteristic (disability) spreads to affect assumptions about unknown characteristics. This is true not only for disability but for other central characteristics, such as gender, ethnicity, or nationality. If the central characteristic has a positive valence, the spread also is likely to be positive, and the reverse is also true. There are three important points to stress about this work:

1. Subjects felt able to perform the task at all—given limited information they were able to generate characteristics; why didn't they protest that they didn't have enough information, and how were they able to derive other personality traits?
2. Subjects were able to provide ratings for groups with which they had never had any contact (e.g., Turks).
3. When subjects were asked how it is possible to generalize from only one known trait, the answers showed a coherent progression of ideas (e.g., "He has already suffered so he knows what it's like to suffer, therefore he is less selfish and more empathic").

Thus the person's beliefs about disabilities (e.g., "Disability causes suffering") led to stereotyping.

The reverse spread also occurs. That is, if a personality trait is known about a person with disabilities, that trait is ascribed to the disability (i.e., is explained by the disability) even in the absence of any corroborating evidence or causal link (e.g., a teenager with a disability is said to practice his violin assiduously because he can't participate in sports). Thus a clinician who knows that a client has a disability and that the client is depressed may explain the depression as *due to* the disability. The professional literature is replete with such titles as "The Psychology of Disability" and "Understanding the Disabled," as if persons with disabilities are psychologically different than persons without disabilities—an idea which is thoroughly discredited empirically. Such works attempt to ascribe personality formation of "the disabled" to the disability itself.

Spread explains how disabilities are perceived as more severe than they actually are. A negative value attached to the fact of disability spreads to other unrelated aspects. Thus a person in a wheelchair is assumed also to be cognitively impaired; a person with mild mental retardation is viewed as more profoundly retarded; people raise their voices to talk to a person who is blind. A deficit in one characteristic spreads such that similar deficits are ascribed to other characteristics. At its most extreme, spread occurs from the single deficit (i.e., disability) to the whole person and his or her entire life. The person is devalued, and the person's life is viewed as a tragedy, as one not worth living. (See discussion of physician-assisted suicide in Chapter 11.)

Attractiveness

A thing of beauty is a joy forever
— Keats, "Endymion"

And a thing of ugliness? Is disability ugly? Does disability in some way interfere with beauty? (For more on this, see Hahn, 1993). Physique is an attribute with a large impact on evaluations of characteristics. Even the observer who is consciously unaware of physical attributes may still be influenced by them.

An early study on attractiveness (Dion, Berscheid, & Walster, 1972) established that undergraduates in a psychology course assumed that physically attractive persons possessed "more socially desirable personalities than those of lesser attractiveness, and it is presumed that their lives will be happier and more successful" (p. 289). They rated attractive men and women (shown in photos with three gradations of attractiveness) as more likely to attain prestigious occupations and have better prospects for happy social and professional lives; to be more competent spouses; to be more likely to find an acceptable partner and have happier marriages, marry earlier, and be less likely to remain single; and to have more total happiness in their lives. This was true for male and female participants and for male and female stimuli. This study is consistent with findings from other studies on attractiveness.

Numerous authors have examined how disability is portrayed in literature and the movies. Generally it is a metaphor for underlying character flaws or undesirable traits. Picture the generic movie: All we know about the villain is that he has a club foot. He is never shown until the end when his identity is revealed. Until then, all we see is a closeup of a man's lower extremities, as one leg slowly is dragged along after the other. The deformity "explains" the villainy. In a current example, a movie critic writes of a character in *Children of the Revolution* (Lane, 1997), "Welch is a wonderful creation, a man so spineless that he is physically hunched from lack of will" (p. 104). Now, far be it for me to remove any literary device from the pens of writers. From Richard III to Mr. Rochester in *Jane Eyre* to *The Hunchback of Notre Dame* (pre-Disney), great literature has abounded with characters physically and figuratively impaired. But we must separate fiction from fact; a literary device should not necessarily be an organizing principle in real life.

The notion that the body reflects the soul is well entrenched in our society. This is a notion that traps persons with disabilities in three ways. First, persons with disabilities are judged on attractiveness, as is everyone, and it helps to be more attractive than less so, especially if you have a disability. Second, the disability itself may affect the degree of judged attractiveness. As discussed later in this chapter, some disabilities are more "acceptable" than others, which may be due in part to the change in body appearance and attractiveness attendant to some disabilities. Third, the body with an impairment may give misleading cues about itself—a grimace from muscle spasms seen as a leer, a shoulder twitch viewed as a dismissive gesture, a limp interpreted as indicating pain. As Mark O'Brien, the subject of an Academy Award—winning documentary on the poet in an iron lung (*Breathing Lessons, the Life and Work of Mark O'Brien*, 1996), said, "Disability causes me to believe more strongly in a duality between body and spirit, because I don't want to be this body, I want to be the soul." Thus, just as the field of psychology is trying to reintegrate mind and body, people with disabilities are trying to break free of the constraints of their bodies.

> Carla, a woman in her mid-30s, was by no means attractive. Her face was plain, her hair like short sticks of straw either matted down or sticking out at odd angles. She dressed in ordinary clothes—T-shirts over pleated skirts was a typical outfit. In addition, she walked slowly and with a cane, her five-foot height hunched over and halting. When seated she slumped down so her feet touched the floor. In addition, when conversing with others she minimized body movements to avoid back pain and to concentrate on speaking; she had a severe stutter. In contrast, Lila was a tall, striking woman with thick, long blonde curly hair, like Botticelli's Venus on the halfshell. She carried herself regally, and her face, hands, arms, and body were animated and energetic when she talked. She wore T-shirt and jeans, or sundresses, looking slim and feminine in either. She had a stutter more severe than Carla's. Both were studying to be teachers. People said of Lila that it was an especial "tragedy" that so vibrant a woman was marked with a stutter. They gave her great encouragement to advance in graduate training. However, almost everyone said Carla could never be a teacher and counseled her to drop the program.

COGNITIVE SCHEMAS: NEED TO BELIEVE IN A FAIR WORLD AND THE PROBLEM OF BLAME

When people hear I had polio (in 1954), they often are confused—isn't there a polio vaccine to prevent things like this (i.e., people like me) from happening? People are curious about how it happened; they begin to wonder out loud if my parents were negligent in getting me vaccinated. In fact, the Salk vaccine was not out of clinical trials and widely available until 1955. People often look visibly relieved to hear this; why?

Because it provides an explanation for my misfortune; it relieves anyone of fault; the explanation is unique to that time (prevaccine) and thus the same problem (contracting polio) cannot recur, and especially not to them or their family (they had the vaccine). The world is put right again. People prefer to have explanations for bad events, and if the bad event happened to another person, they prefer explanations that exempt themselves from the possibility of the bad event happening to them.

The seminal study on blame was by Walster (1966), in which she examined how people assigned responsibility for an accident. The hypothesis of Walster's study was that as the magnitude of the outcome of an accident increases, it becomes increasingly unpleasant to acknowledge that the same could happen to anyone; therefore, we become more likely to assign blame, and in so doing find some protection from the randomness of the event. Participants were the ever-popular undergraduate psychology majors (44 of each gender), who were asked to rate the degree of responsibility of a young man (Lennie) involved in an accident. All descriptions of this man were identical, and only the seriousness of the consequences of the accident differed: The accident resulted in a minor dent in the fender and there was no potential danger to others; the car was totaled and there was no potential danger to others; there was only minor damage to the car but there was the potential to cause injury to others; there was considerable damage to other persons. In all conditions Lennie's behavior is identical; only the actual consequences change.

Results indicate that consequences did not affect how much participants liked Lennie. However, significantly more responsibility was assigned to Lennie for severe accidents than mild ones, although they did not deem him as more careless. Lennie was viewed as having taken equal precautions in each of the four conditions, but he was judged as more responsible for the accident when consequences were severe, and the standard by which he was judged was raised as consequences were more serious.

You can do a version of this study next time a "natural" disaster strikes, whether it's flooding, a hurricane, earthquake, mudslides, or other event. Read the accounts in the newspapers. After the initial reporting of what happened, by the next day blame will begin to be placed. In my area, after the Oakland fire (1989; several people killed, thousands of houses destroyed, considerable potential for damage to property and life) newspaper articles immediately raised questions about who was at fault, the response time of the fire departments, the overgrowth of plants around houses, the possibility of arson—no one said, "It was just one of those things." Or even that California, with its four seasons (earthquake, mudslides, drought and fire), inevitably has fires flamed by the hot, early-fall winds.

What does this mean for disability and persons with disabilities? First, people are going to seek explanations for the disability. About 3 to 5 years after onset of disability, the person with the disability has stopped talking about how it happened; it's a moot point. It's other people who want to know, "How did it happen?" Second, they want the explanation to be one that precludes it from happening to them. Cognitive steps are taken to distance oneself from the cause of the disability, and hence from the person with that disability. Third, some presumed "causal" reasons for the disability may further increase the desire to distance oneself from that person. For example, if the disability is viewed as being incurred due to negligence, carelessness, or irresponsibility, these negative traits themselves engender distaste above and beyond that due to the disability per se. "Because the scientific practice of epidemiology focuses on risk groups, modes of transmission, and the direction of the spread of illnesses, this leads to an idea of the culpability of specific groups of infected individuals" (Batten, Follette, & Hayes, 1997, p. 99). Fourth, association with persons with disabilities is viewed as reflecting badly on the other person (a "courtesy stigma"; Goffman, 1963, p. 31). This contagion variable increases motivation to see the person with a disability as "other," and to avoid contagion by decreasing contact. The ultimate reduction of anxiety in facing negative events is achieved by eliminating the possibility of the events themselves (e.g., the eradication of polio). However, the signifier is often confused with the signified: eliminating the disability is confused with eliminating the person with the disability. Not only have we eradicated polio but also *people like me.* It's as if we tried to eliminate racism by eliminating races.

> Norma is a 35-year-old Caucasian woman in her third month of her first (and planned) pregnancy. She sought counseling to help her make a decision about whether to have amniocentesis. She has "quiggle disorder,"[1] which is genetically transmitted. Amniocentesis can test for quiggle, along with over 150 other genetic conditions. Norma complained that "everyone just assumes that I'm going to have amnio. They just assume that I'll want to test for quiggle. But what if the test is positive? They just assume I'd terminate the pregnancy. But would I? Why would I? And if I wouldn't, why bother to have amnio. in the first place?" Bob, Norma's husband of 4 years, wanted her to have the test: "It just seems like we should find out." Norma was bothered by this, feeling that her husband's request said something negative about his acceptance of her as a person with

---

[1]Goffman (1963) made up this condition to stand for any stigmatized condition: " 'My dear girl, how did you get your quiggle'; 'My great uncle had a quiggle, so I feel I know all about your problem.' " (p. 16)

quiggle. "He wants to avoid having a child *like me*. Then how can he say he really accepts *me*?" Further, she was perturbed by the implications of testing for quiggle for her own sense of self-esteem. At the same time, she understood firsthand how difficult childhood can be for a person with quiggle, and wanted to spare her child that pain. To complicate matters, the decision had to be made in the next few weeks or the opportunity for amnio. would pass.

WHAT WE'VE LEARNED

Disability is usually a central characteristic. As such, others form impressions of the person with a disability based on the presence of the disability. Beliefs the observer holds about disability (e.g., disability causes suffering) will be instrumental in what other attributes the person ascribes to the person with the disability. Known traits are thought to emanate from the fact of having a disability, as if the disability caused those traits. The body with a disability may give misleading cues about the person.

Attractiveness is likewise a central characteristic. We prefer more over less attractive people and infer positive traits to the former. Lesser attractiveness and disability combine synergistically. Further, disability per se may be construed as unattractive. If disability is viewed as a negative occurrence, then able-bodied persons will seek to safeguard themselves from its occurrence to them. Several cognitive beliefs aid this view, including blaming the person with the disability for the disability or ascribing the disability to things that couldn't happen to them. By distancing ourselves from the disability we may also distance ourselves from the *person* with the disability.

ATTITUDES TOWARD DISABILITY

The attitudes of others are an important variable in the lives of persons with disabilities. Omitting this discussion would be like trying to teach students about ethnic minorities without mentioning prejudice, discrimination, and oppression. As discussed in Chapter 2 (in this volume), these are the sine qua non of the minority experience, and the fact of their existence for persons with disabilities constitutes the core of the minority model. Attitudes toward disability "represent important influences on persons with disabilities in behavior, social relationships, education, employment & health" (Yuker, 1994, p. 3).

This discussion presents a brief and synthesized review of the vast literature on attitudes toward disability, the bulk of which supports the contention that attitudes toward persons with disabilities are mostly negative. But we must bear in mind during this discussion the numerous studies in social science showing—counterintuitively—weak links between attitudes and behaviors. Further, "general quality of research in this area is not very high" (Yuker, 1994, p. 4).

Factors That Affect Attitudes

Attitudes toward disability are a function of several factors (see Table 3.1). In general, in the United States, women hold less negative attitudes toward disability than do men. This has led some researchers to hypothesize that women, as a minority group themselves, hold more positive attitudes toward other minority groups (in this case persons with disabil-

TABLE 3.1. Factors That Influence Attitudes toward a Person with a Disability (PWD)

Perceiver characteristics			
Previous contact with PWD Amount Type of contact	Information about the disability	General prejudice	Authoritarianism
PWD characteristics			
Social skills and attractiveness	Comfort with own disability	Perceived intelligence	Demographics Gender Age Ethnicity SES
Characteristics of the disability			
Disability Type Severity	Stigma of specific diagnosis	Perceived cause of disability	Perceived contagion or heritability
Characteristics of the milieu			
Social context and group norms	Purpose and consequences of interaction	Whether interaction is observed	Value of diversity in organization
Social context			
Mass media, ad campaign, and charity drive portrayals of PWD and that disability	Availability of role models with that disability	News reports on disability	Value of diversity in society

ities). However, this theory is not supported in several ways. First, this difference is not always found in other countries, and a few times it is reversed. Second, the gender gap in attitudes toward disability has diminished over the years. Third, examinations of attitudes toward disability by other minority groups indicates that being a member of another minority group is not predictive of more positive attitudes. There are large differences in people's attitudes toward disability and tremendous intragroup variability.

Two key factors that affect attitudes toward disability are information and beliefs. "The beliefs that a nondisabled person has about persons with disabilities is probably the major variable that influences attitudes" (Yuker, 1994, p. 5). These beliefs are affected by information about the disability, which in turn is affected by prior contact with people with disabilities, attitudes of significant others, education, and mass media. However, this does not imply that just adding more information about disability will improve attitudes. Not all information about disability or persons with disabilities has positive effects. Interestingly, information that indicates how people with and without disabilities are similar can have a negative effect, perhaps because it can increase awareness of vulnerability. As discussed in the previous section, this may lead the able-bodied person to distance him- or herself from the person with a disability. Information about the origin and cause(s) of a disability can influence attitudes. Those disabilities that are the result of external factors (e.g., war) generally are viewed more positively than are those brought about—whether directly or indirectly—by the person (e.g., car accident). Mass media is especially influential on the attitudes of persons with little prior information and contact with persons with disabilities. It can also shape attitudes toward disabilities about which there is little other information (e.g., in the early years of the AIDS epidemic). Information that helps make the person with a disability more individual and fills in other areas of knowledge about that person reduces the effects of stereotypes.

Another factor influencing attitudes toward disability is contact with persons with disabilities. Findings in this area have been quite robust. Consistently studies indicate that the type of contact is crucial. Attitudes improve when the contacts are between persons with and without disabilities who are of equal status. The able-bodied doctor–patient-with-a-disability relationship (or, for that matter, the therapist–client relationship), which is an unequal status relationship, not only fails to improve attitudes but, in some cases, seems to make them more negative. Contact involving cooperative interdependence, in which there is support from authority figures, improves attitudes. Further, as contact leads to increased nondisability information about the person with a disability, the negative effects of the disability are lessened. For example, I often teach one-day workshops on various (nondisability) topics. When I scoot into the room the audience often looks dismayed or disconcerted, but by lunchtime they have learned enough other things about me (teaching style, humor, my work as a professor, my knowledge about the topic) that the disability recedes into the background and its effects on audience members' views of me are minimized. Thus, contact improves attitudes if it is personal, mutually rewarding, cooperative, intimate on both parts and persists over time. Further, the quality of the contact is improved when it occurs between persons of equal status or in a situation in which the person with the disability holds a higher status. Such contact is facilitated by characteristics of the nondisabled person: If they hold fewer negative beliefs about persons with disabilities, and are demographically and in personality similar to the person with the disability, they are more likely to engage in contacts that encourage positive attitudes toward disability. Thus, ironically, those whose attitudes are more negative are least likely to have positive contacts, to gain information, or to experience interactions that promote more positive attitudes. The social norms and politics of an organization, agency, school, or clinic, and the attitudes of those who head them, are also influential in promoting or discouraging contact and positive attitudes and can override the tendency of a person to avoid persons with disabilities.

Another factor relates to the perceptions of the person with the disability. If he or she is perceived as competent in areas valued by the other and as socially skillful, more positive attitudes ensue. Of key importance in clinical work are several variables that promote more positive attitudes on the part of the able-bodied therapist toward the client with a disability: (1) the perception of the abilities of the person with a disability to communicate successfully, (2) the client's ability to display acceptance of the disability, and (3) the client's willingness to discuss it. Thus clients who go on job interviews, or students who go on practicum or internship placement interviews, should be encouraged to be relaxed and open about their disability and tutored in how to do it (through role-plays and mock interviews). (This is not to minimize the powerful negative effects on the applicant with a disability who encounters prejudicial treatment and illegal questions.)

How do people feel when they encounter a person with a serious disability? The majority (92%) say they often or occasionally feel admiration; 74% feel pity, 58% feel awkward or embarrassed, 16% experience anger because persons with disabilities cause inconvenience, and 9% feel resentment because persons with disabilities get special privileges (cited in Yuker, 1994). There is a self-perpetuating cycle of stigma in that people with little contact with persons with disabilities often have little knowledge and hold many myths about persons with disabilities. Because they don't have contact with persons with disabilities, they don't have opportunities for corrective experiences or increased information.

The myths about disability (as about gays and lesbians) are remarkably immune from data—that is, myths persist in the face of data that contradicts them. Only if forced experiences bring new learning do the myths subside. For example, opposition to group homes (e.g., for those with MR or other developmental disabilities) in one's community are common, but opposition usually subsides after such a facility has been established. Attitudes of the public and of neighbors toward persons with disabilities are strongly influenced by the friendliness and social skills of the person with a disability. (This is another example of the extra burden placed on persons with disabilities; attitudes toward "their people" can be negatively influenced by a grumpy mood on a bad day.)

Attitudes toward Disability and Demographic Variables

Education

The demographic variable that accounts for the most variance in attitudes toward disability is education; higher levels of education are associated with more positive attitudes toward persons with disabilities. Because education is part of overall socioeconomic status (SES), we would expect SES and attitudes to be positively correlated, but the data are not consistent on this point. Differences between occupational groups in attitudes toward disability have been shown, but this is mostly due to differences in education and training, and because different personal attributes are valued in different professions. Further, some professional roles promote contacts with persons with disabilities in inferior positions, which often has a deleterious effect on attitudes toward disability. Even training that might be expected to affect attitudes often doesn't; there is no correlation between number of courses in special education and attitudes toward disability. There are no data to support the contention that therapists of any discipline bear attitudes toward disability that are notably different from the general public's (Chan et al., 1988).

Culture

Persons in the United States generally show more favorable attitudes toward disability than do people in other countries (Jaques et al., 1970; Westbrook, Legge, & Pennay, 1993). Nationality is an important determinant of attitudes toward disability and suggests that broad social movements and political factors can have a substantial effect on the lives of persons with disabilities, by affecting the attitudes of the populace toward them. Ethnic differences in attitudes toward disability have been found. One early review of the literature (English, 1971) concluded that race does not influence attitudes toward persons with disabilities, but other studies refute this (Chan et al., 1988; Florian, 1982; Florian, Weisel, Kravetz, & Shurka-Zernitsky, 1989; Jaques et al., 1970; Westbrook et al., 1993). Belgrave (1998) reviews select studies indicating that African Americans hold more favorable views toward disability than do Caucasians. In contrast, two studies of attitudes among professionals (Olkin & Howson, 1994; Paris, 1993) found that mental health workers and medical students who were ethnic minorities held less positive attitudes toward disability than did their Caucasian peers. These studies suggest that kinship of minority experiences cannot explain the differences in attitudes toward disability between men and women, because the findings do not extend to other types of minorities.

Age

Age per se is not an important variable in determining attitudes toward disability, and age-related findings are mostly due to education and amount of contact. Although infants as young as 4 months can differentiate between normal and abnormal faces (cf. Kagan, Henker, Hen-Tov, Levine, & Lewis, 1966), this recognition of novel stimuli is not the same as innate prejudice. But by age 6 preferences are clearly shown for "normal" children over those with disabilities. Attitudes then seem to deteriorate over the elementary school years (Weinberg, 1978), and level off somewhere around early adulthood (18–21). The data on age at which attitudes plateau are important because they indicate that by the time adults begin specialized training, their attitudes are already well formed. This finding suggests that vigorous efforts to ameliorate negative attitudes toward disability must be undertaken in graduate schools; we cannot make the mistake of thinking that people who choose helping professions, special education, nursing, rehabilitation, and so on, have more positive attitudes than do others. An early study suggested that "training [in a specialty area] after a certain level of education does not bring radical differences in perception of exceptional children" (Panda & Bartel, 1972, p. 265). Studies of attitudes toward adults with disabilities would suggest the same thing.

Personal Attributes

Personality variables of the nondisabled person (other than prejudice and authoritarianism) are not determinants of attitudes toward disability. Yuker (1994) went so far as to call for

> a moratorium . . . on studies of the relationship of attitudes to nondisabled person demographic and/or personality characteristics. The hundreds of

prior studies clearly demonstrate that variables such as these contribute little to our understanding of attitudes toward people with disabilities. Research should focus on alterable characteristics of nondisabled people . . . rather than on demographic and/or personality characteristics which are usually not amenable to change. (p. 8)

Characteristics of the Person with a Disability That Influence Attitudes

First, it should be stated at the outset that studies indicate that there are no overall personality difference between those with disabilities and those without (Yuker, 1994). Further, the severity of physical disability is not correlated with the degree of psychological adjustment; that is, greater severity of physical disability does not equate with greater difficulty in psychological adjustment (Abroms & Kodera, 1978; Nosek, Fuhrer, & Potter, 1995; Olkin, 1981; Olkin & Howson, 1994). Thus what handicaps persons with disabilities are the attitudes of others and social difficulties more than the physical impairments themselves.

In initial contacts, superficial characteristics of persons with disabilities, such as appearance and severity of disability, are important. More positive reactions are generated by persons with disabilities who are attractive, competent, and socially skilled and whose disability is slight or invisible. The influence of these variables decreases as the person with the disability becomes more known and the nondisabled person is able to see the disability as only one facet of the person. Similarity between the disabled and nondisabled person also can positively affect attitudes. This similarity is affected by the tasks valued in the context in which interaction occurs: usually athletic skills in children, academic competence in school, work skills and ability to get along with others in the workplace, a cooperative attitude in health settings, good social skills in most settings. Continued contact with a person with a specific type of disability tends to result in that specific disability being rated as more acceptable than others.

Of great clinical importance is that a positive attitude of the person with a disability toward disability in general—as evidenced by self-acceptance, open acknowledgment of the disability, and disclosure about self—has a positive effect on others' attitudes. As the person integrates the disability into a healthy and robust sense of self, others are more likely to follow suit by relegating the disability to its proper status in the overall context of the person. This places a burden on the person with a disability to take the lead in putting others at ease, and it is one of the things persons with disabilities often object to. Further, holding a positive self-view does not fully protect one from incurring prejudice, stigma,

or discrimination, although it may lessen their frequency and, importantly, their psychological impact.

Family and Friends

Disability affects not only the person with the disability but many others
in a circle of family and friends. One Harris poll (cited in Yuker, 1994)
showed that 47% of those in a national sample "personally know"
someone with a disability—53% as friends, 24% as household members, 45% as other relatives. It cannot be assumed that the family of a
person with a disability holds positive views on disability or will promote integrating the disability into a positive self-concept. In this way
persons with disabilities are like gays or lesbians. There are other similarities. They are likely to be the only one (disabled, gay, or lesbian) in
the family. Thus they can't look to family as role models. Nor can they
necessarily rely on family for support. Family members may not help
foster a positive identity and may in fact inhibit it and be part of the
problem. Further, the child with a disability (like gays or lesbians) may
join a community of like people and attain a certain awareness and consciousness of and about issues related to that community. This can be
threatening to a family, as they perceive the person to be leaving them
behind and to be a part of a world about which they know little. After
all is said and done, the main findings are somewhat intuitive: The two
most important factors in the family's responses to a child with a disability are acceptance of that child as a full member of the family and acceptance of the disability itself.

Several areas of research are notably neglected. These areas include
the effects of families on their children, siblings, parents and spouses/
partners with disabilities, and the attitudes and responses of fathers
toward a child with a disability. Also, there is scant research on the couple relationship when a partner has or acquires a disability. Another
neglected area is the nature of families' information about the specific
disability in their family, their sources of this information, and the effects
of it. More often than not, families have little information about disability in general, or about the specific disability in their family (or worse,
incorrect information). Not surprisingly, given the lack of information
coupled with the absence of role models or normative information, families often don't know what is reasonable to expect for their child with a
disability. Not knowing what to expect can lead parents to uncertainty
and lack of confidence in their role as parents. Although their interactions within the family with the person with the disability is personal,
intimate, and sustained over time, it is also characterized by unequal status and may not be mutually rewarding. Thus it has the potential to

exacerbate awareness of the disability and negative characteristics of it and, hence, negative attitudes. (See Chapter 5, in this volume, for more on families with disabilities.)

Unlike family, friends can be chosen. As an adult with a disability we can choose as friends those whose acceptance of the disability is solid. In the Harris poll cited previously, 53% of those who "personally knew" someone with a disability knew them as friends. These people have generally positive attitudes toward disability, "often more positive than those of family members" (Yuker, 1994, p. 12). What is important is the degree of intimacy or closeness between the friends, not how many friends with disabilities someone has. Merely knowing someone with a disability as an acquaintance may increase rather than dispel prejudice. Curiously, there are virtually no studies on the characteristics of people who have friends with disabilities.

Employment and Employers

Attitudes of employers toward recruiting, hiring, retaining, and promoting persons with disabilities are crucial to the overall well-being of persons with disabilities. World War II provided a large-scale naturalistic study of work-related factors for employees with disabilities. When the able-bodied men went off to war in droves, companies at home hired people with disabilities (and women) in unprecedented numbers. Studies from that period show that such employees had at least as low, and sometimes lower, absence rates and on-the-job accidents. Nonetheless, the perception that workers with disabilities were unreliable remained, and when soldiers returned after World War II employees with disabilities were laid off and not rehired. Further studies repeatedly have confirmed that employees with disabilities are equal to or better than nondisabled employees in terms of productivity, safety, absenteeism, lateness, and turnover. In summary, studies on employment of persons with disabilities support the following:

1. Employment rates are not related to disability type, IQ, and completing preemployment training.
2. The general condition of the labor market is important. Employment of persons with disabilities increases when labor is short (e.g., during wartime), and decreases when it is not.
3. Employer characteristics affecting employment of persons with disabilities are past experiences with employees with disabilities (i.e., contact), and commitment to such employment.
4. "Good" employees with disabilities are those with a positive attitude toward work, themselves, and their disability.

Educators, Health Personnel, and Other Professionals

The most important variables affecting attitudes toward disability of educators and health personnel (as for all persons) are information about persons with disabilities and prior contacts with such persons on an equal basis. Characteristics of students with disabilities that influence attitudes are similar as for students without disabilities: academic performance, compliance, being difficult to teach, and misbehavior. Unimportant factors for educators are class size, school size, type of school, grade level, or years of teaching experience. It may surprise readers to learn that there are few significant differences in attitudes among regular or special education teachers, administrators, and other educational personnel; any differences found are accounted for by the effects of increased information, contact, and general attitudes toward people. As in the workplace, the relevant attitudinal norms prevalent in the school are important influences.

Health care workers prefer patients, including those with disabilities, who are manageable, compliant, treatable, likeable, motivated for rehabilitation, and have a favorable prognosis. Attitudes of health personnel are worth special consideration because there is an almost virulent antipathy in the disability community toward the medical profession. Further, as for teachers and mental health professionals, we expect that certain types of people will be drawn to the health field, and such types will have more positive attitudes toward those they help. This does not seem to be the case. "The attitudes of many people in helping occupations toward patients are at least somewhat negative. . . . People in health roles tend to make personalistic attributions, and may have a fundamental negative bias focusing on negative characteristics and symptoms" (Yuker, 1994, p. 15). "Virtually all helpers perceive themselves as superior to people who need help" (Yuker, 1994, p. 16). Bear in mind that health personnel have a lot of information about specific disorders but not about persons with those disorders or about persons with disabilities in general. The bottom line is that those helping professionals who children and adults with disabilities are likely to encounter most frequently are teachers, medical personnel, and employers, whose attitudes are no better than the general public's, and in many cases worse.

Stigma Hierarchies and Their Implications

Although overall attitudes toward disability are more negative than attitudes toward those without disabilities, some disabilities are viewed even less favorably (Abroms & Kodera, 1978; Asch, 1984; Jones, 1974; Miller, Armstrong, & Hagan, 1981; Olkin & Howson, 1994; Shears &

Jensema, 1969; Stainback & Stainback, 1982; Tringo, 1970; Westbrook et al., 1993; Yuker, 1994). In general, physical disabilities are ranked higher (i.e., are seen as more acceptable and have a lower degree of stigma) than are sensory impairments, which in turn are ranked higher than social, psychological, or cognitive impairments (Albrecht, Walker, & Levy, 1982; Cohen, 1986; Goodyear, 1983; Horne & Ricciardo, 1988; Miller et al., 1981; Tripp, 1988). Factors that influence attitudes are severity, visibility, treatability, effect on life expectancy, degree of contagion, or transmissability. Such conditions as asthma, diabetes, and heart disease are low on most of these dimensions and hence less negative attitudes ensue. Among the higher-ranked disabilities are conditions leading to increased difficulty with ambulation (leg braces, limps, crutches), amputation of one limb, deafness and blindness. At the lower-ranked end are conditions associated with wheelchair use (paraplegia and quadriplegia), little people, MS, CP, and facial disfigurement. These differential ranking of acceptability are masked at lower levels of intimacy (e.g., having as a coworker and living in the same neighborhood) but become quite pronounced at closer levels of intimacy (e.g., dating and marrying) (DeLoach, 1994; Olkin & Howson, 1994).

Several models have been proposed in the literature to explain these rankings, only one of which seems to hold across all studies (Olkin & Howson, 1994). Discarded theories include a medical model—that disabilities less amenable to medical amelioration and with poorer prognosis for improvement (or "normalization") will be rated lower. For example, amputation of a limb is fairly final but is in the top half of rankings. A second model used to explain rank orderings is the degree of objective impairment associated with a disability. Again, this model fails to hold up across all conditions. For example, deafness is extremely handicapping in the hearing world but is ranked well above facial disfigurement, which may have no degree of associated functional limitations. This view underscores yet again that disability does not equal handicap, and that others' responses may be the most handicapping factor in living with a disability. Another model unable fully to account for rankings includes the saliency and visibility theory, which states that conditions more readily discernible to others are more stigmatized. This model flies in the face of cancer and AIDS, which are highly stigmatized conditions that may have few outward manifestations (at least initially). Others have suggested that placement of the disability is important, such that disabilities are ranked lower as they approach the face. This model only explains the low rankings of facial disfigurement but would predict that an arm amputation is more devalued than a leg amputation, which is not empirically supported. A closely related hypothesis is that the more a disability interferes with the communication process the greater the stigma. Certainly communication disorders, especially those that substantially alter the communication process (e.g., severely decreased fluency) are stigmatized, but this model can't account for all rankings. In keeping with the idea that disability and handicap are not synonymous, a possible explanation for rankings is the degree of impact on daily living, but again it fails to be demonstrated fully in studies of disability acceptability.

The most adequate model that has been proposed in the literature to explain rankings is the notion of esthetics (Hahn, 1993; Livneh, 1982; Olkin, 1981; Tringo, 1970). As later amended (Olkin & Howson, 1994), this model seems to account best for rankings, and incorporates some of the features of other models. The term "esthetic model," however, implies only a visual pleasingness, which is too limited. I call it a *total body Gestalt model*: We hold notions of a total body in how it should appear, move, function, think, behave, and communicate. In these notions some aspects are weighed more heavily than others, such as the role of the face in determining attractiveness, of speech in assessing interpersonal skills and communication, of intellect in assessing value. "All of these factors are evaluated (and differentially weighted) to derive what might be called a 'deviation score.' The greater the deviation the greater the stigma" (Olkin & Howson, 1994, p. 93).

Attitude Change

Attitudes toward disability are difficult to change. There are hundreds of studies on this issue and overall the results are not encouraging. Effect sizes are small and almost a quarter of the studies trying to improve attitudes toward disability had the reverse effect of making attitudes worse. Information alone is insufficient to improve attitudes but may still be a necessary first step. Some information, however, such as the problems of persons with disabilities, or how to manage children with disabilities, may promote an us–them mentality, and worsen attitudes.

Summary and Conclusions about Attitudes toward Disability

Attitudes toward disability and persons with disabilities by those who are able-bodied are a significant factor in the lives of persons with disabilities. Overall, such attitudes still are quite negative. Some disabilities are more stigmatized than others, and there is a remarkably stable hierarchy of acceptability of various physical disabilities. A total body Gestalt model has been proffered to explain this hierarchy (Olkin, 1981; Olkin & Howson, 1994). Improving attitudes toward those disabilities on the lower end of the hierarchy would be expected to generalize up, but improving attitudes toward those higher on the hierarchy would not be expected to generalize to the more stigmatized conditions. Although virtually all people don't mind having people with disabilities in more peripheral roles (e.g., living in the same country and working in the same building), when levels of intimacy are increased (e.g., being romantically involved or having your daughter marry one), attitudes become more negative. Most attitudes research has examined attitudes toward disability out of context of other demographic factors (notably ethnicity and increased age). Attitudes bear only a weak link to behaviors.

In general, it is hard to change negative attitudes. We know that in some circumstances some attitudes can be changed in some people, but we really don't know much beyond this. A "science" of attitude change is far from a reality. A change in attitudes may be conceptualized better by positing it as a result, rather than a cause, of other cognitive or behavioral changes. We should focus more on changing behaviors toward persons with disabilities than on attitudes toward them. The most dangerous class of ABs are those who have some minimal and tangential experience with disability (e.g., dating a woman who works in a medical practice that employs a man in a wheelchair) and who therefore think they know and understand about the disability experience. A little knowledge is a dangerous thing when it inhibits further learning.

I would argue that more research on either attitudes toward the generic notion of "disability" or on relative differences in attitudes toward specific disabilities (e.g., hierarchy of acceptability literature, to which I myself have contributed) is counterproductive. Such research at this time in disability history conveys a troubling meta-message, that what persons with disabilities need to improve their lives is simply a function of improving attitudes toward "the disabled." This is a blind alley (you should pardon the expression). By focusing for so long on attitudes the field has neglected more basic issues. These include enforcement of the ADA, increased participation in the work force, accessibility of substance abuse programs and more training of rehabilitation personnel in substance abuse among persons with disabilities, more resources for independent living and personal attendant services, less enforced institutionalization in nursing homes, less relative focus on finding cures at the expense of improving care—in short, our civil rights. To give a concrete example, I am less interested in why ablebodied people park illegally in handicapped spots than I am in getting them to stop doing so. If imposing $500 fines and vigilant enforcement achieve this goal, then I no longer care about people's attitudes toward handicapped parking.

As I reflect on my own growth as a person with a disability, I see my research on disability reflecting the changes I went through. I focused for a long time on attitudes and relative positions of stigma for differing disabilities. I look back on the findings from this phase of my research with a profound "so what?" My focus and energy has significantly shifted. I've come more to agree with the notion that "attitude change is the . . . dream of social change without political action . . . which asks disabled and non-disabled people to disengage from the physical world of inaccessible construction and enter the mapless world of hope" (Hevey, 1992, p. 36). Yet the stigma hierarchies—the relative position of different disabilities on the scale of acceptability—hold an important message. My error, perhaps, was in thinking that this message was for the AB world when, in fact, it's a signal to those of us in the disability community. We are so thrilled to *have* a community, to have found a united voice in our press for civil rights, that we are naturally reluctant to tackle issues that divide us. We avoid many of the distinctions among our disabilities and our functioning, in a desire to help move the whole group ahead. Thus we insist with equal vigor on the rights of a woman with a severe communication disorder to be an elementary school teacher, of a person who uses attendant services 18 hours a day to raise an infant, of a graduate student with learning disabilities that significantly impede organizational and writing skills to complete a doctoral thesis. I am not saying we shouldn't; I am saying we must think and talk about it amongst ourselves, so that we can be the main architects of policy— nothing about us without us.

Clinical Implications of Research from Social Science and Attitudes Studies

As clinicians, we are subject to all the same factors that influence others, and are not immune to prejudice. Worse, we believe ourselves to be above all that, to be universally empathic by training and skill. But our beliefs about disability, our responses to the fact of disability, to attractiveness, to loss of health, and so on, affect how we view the client, the role we think the disability plays in the client's character and presenting problems, the case formulation, and ultimately the treatment. We might err in the direction of overinflating the role of the disability in shaping personality, while perhaps simultaneously underestimating the effects of stigma and discrimination. In considering the presenting problems we might assign the disability a starring role because we've confused disability per se with the effects of having a stigmatized condition. Another error might be to focus unduly on the onset and cause of the disability when these are no longer issues of relevance for the client, or worse, to refuse to believe that they are not, and to mislabel the client's disinclination to discuss them as resistance, repression, or denial. There is no "disabled personality"; do not seek to address who the client would be without the disability. It is at best fruitless and at worst a discourteous display of misunderstanding that will cause the client to leave.

Whose attitudes should we be concerned with? Of first concern are our own attitudes and behaviors toward our clients inasmuch as these profoundly affect our conceptualizations about and stances toward clients. As discussed in this chapter, we are not superhumans redolent with benevolence and devoid of prejudices (see Chapter 13, in this volume, for more on countertransference issues with clients with disabilities). Second, we should be concerned with the attitudes of our clients with disabilities not just toward their own disability but toward other persons with disabilities. Our clients live in a world monopolized by ABs, and as such are prone to internalize the pervasive bombardment of negative messages (we just don't have a good word for it, like "homophobia"—perhaps it should be "cripophobia"). The next sphere of clinical attention should be the family of the person with the disability. Families of young children with disabilities will be the major source of influence on their child's development and self-acceptance, but their stance cannot be assumed to be positive or facilitative, and as such families are important targets for intervention. The next level of focus might be the disability community itself, as here is where the young adult with disabilities may find a home. Finally, we must not neglect a critical means of improving the lives of persons with disabilities, which is to make the AB world a more tolerant and accepting one. As mental health professionals with some expertise in understanding human psychology, this might be our most lasting legacy.

FOUR

The Disability Experience: II. Affect and Everyday Experiences

This chapter continues the exploration of commonalities in the disability experience. The intent is for readers to feel as if they've had a good look around a usually sealed room. This inside look includes a discussion of the ways in which society prescribes and prohibits how people with disabilities are to behave and feel. Furthermore, if there is a "disability experience," how might this experience shape cognitions and world views? Finally, to whom can people with disabilities look as role models, and who chooses them? Clinicians will find that both their clients with disabilities and they themselves are hard pressed to find guidance from healthy and functioning role models with disabilities. This absence contributes to the isolation that is part of the disability experience.

PRESCRIPTIONS AND PROSCRIPTIONS

The able-bodied community imposes restrictions on the behaviors and affect of persons with disabilities. These restrictions include the encouragement of pluckiness, the prohibition of anger, and the presumption of mourning. In addition, this chapter discusses the effects of having a disability on one's privacy and personal power and control.

Regulation of Affect and the Requirement of Mourning

The requirement to regulate affect is a common part of disability. There is the dual requirement of what to be and what not to be: One must be cheerful; one must not be angry. This issue of forced cheerfulness has been addressed most eloquently in Hugh Gallagher's *FDR's Splendid Deception* (1985). Franklin Delano Roosevelt, a president with a profound disability, successfully hid the extent of his disability from the world. Gallagher contends that the price for this was a bargain FDR struck with the United States: We (the nondisabled) will let you (the disabled) live and work among us, provided that you never make us unduly aware of your disability or its attendant difficulties, and provided that you at all times appear cheerful. We have been stuck with this bargain ever since, and as yet have been unable to break free.

The FDR legacy is evidenced in a 1993 obituary taken from the *San Francisco Chronicle* (August 3, 1993). At the top of the obituary is a picture of an attractive young woman. The caption has her name, and in smaller letters it says, "She was paralyzed in 1985." This is her main identity. The title of the obituary is "Radio career cut by gunman's bullet": this model and disk jockey had to switch careers when she became paralyzed by "a gunman's bullet on a deserted highway in 1985" (Hallissy, 1993). She died of breathing problems related to double pneumonia, but this 28-year-old woman will be remembered "as a fighter who overcame the obstacles that paralysis put in her way and managed to live a happy and full life." A quote from a friend takes this theme over the top: "She never complained. She'd always have this big smile." And now we come full circle. Think of FDR. You probably envision him sitting behind a desk, his head thrown back, a huge grin on his face, and in one hand the cigarette in its long holder. Now, 40 years later, we have this young woman who "always" had this big smile. Disabled people are supposed to smile. In case we missed this point, the latest reminder comes from, of all places, Mattel toys. In May 1997 Mattel issued the first Barbie (actually, friend of Barbie, or FOB) in a wheelchair. Her name is "Share a Smile Becky."[1]

The flip side of this requirement of cheerfulness is the interdiction against anger. I strongly believe that for persons with disabilities, anger is rarely tolerated, accepted, or understood. The problem is one of decontextualized rage (i.e., rage seen as response to a single event rather

---

[1]Barbie's "dream house" turned out not to be accessible: The doorways were too narrow for Becky's wheelchair. Mattel has pledged to make the house accessible. Life imitates Barbie.

than to a greater social history and context), viewing rage as a violation of the desired (cheerful) norm set for the group, and the assumption that rage for persons with disabilities indicates individual pathology, lack of adjustment, and failure to be appropriately socialized. Yet to understand persons with disabilities it is necessary to examine and understand the issue of their rage.

Anger among the disabled is a complex issue. First, we are mindful of the bargain struck by FDR that the disabled must remain cheerful and never be despondent, despairing, or angry. Second, in the same way that impairment is viewed as residing within the person and not in the environment or in society, so too the anger is seen as a reflection of the person, and of the person's disability. It is said to be either a stage of "adjustment," and patronizingly tolerated by others, or as a failure to appropriately go through the stages to reach the final plateau of "adjustment," and thus pathologized.

Third, anger suggests that we are not grateful enough. We, who depend to some extent on the assistance of others, cannot express anger because to do so would jeopardize our continued care. We "should" be grateful not only for others' assistance but also because we are so much better off than others with worse disabilities (able-bodied people can look me in the eye and say this, unaware of the irony). Like the big fish eating the littler fish eating the littler fish, we are always supposed to compare ourselves to the smaller fish, not to the next larger fish in the chain. By keeping us grateful not to be an even smaller fish (i.e., more disabled), those without disabilities protect themselves from our envy and resentment. We collude because we want "people to do things for me because they liked me rather than because they pitied me" (Zola, 1982b, p. 220).

Fourth, in addition to the prohibition of expressions of anger *by* persons with disabilities, we are faced with the unseemliness of anger *toward* persons with disabilities. "People are very wary about being openly angry or critical of someone with a chronic disease or physical handicap" (Zola, 1982b, p. 223). Perhaps the visible manifestation of disability is seen as implying a deeper characterological weakness, a basic flaw, such that anger toward us would destroy us.

To these two regulations (you must be cheerful, you may not be angry) we add a third: the requirement of mourning. Most of psychology views disability as a loss—a loss of the healthy or undamaged body, loss of function, loss of the wished-for perfect child. As such, the loss "must" be mourned before the process of "adjustment" to the real body, function, child can be negotiated. The possibility of mourning becomes the requirement of mourning. This does not mean that mourning does not or should not occur. Wright (1983) makes a useful distinction between the "requirement of mourning" and the "period of mourning." In many instances persons who sustain a disability may well experience a period of mourning, with its components of sadness, loss, and grieving. But this is not inevitable or universal. Nonetheless, the requirement of mourning persists, and is particularly strong within the mental health community. The logic goes as follows: "You have a disability. Having a disability is awful. Therefore you must be suffering. I see you as suffering. Ah, but you are not suffering, in a situation in which suffering should occur. Why not? It must be because you are brave, courageous, plucky, extraordinary, superhuman." Thus the requirement of mourning is coupled with the requirement of cheerfulness. Those are the choices: suffering, loss and mourning, or continual pluckiness. Virtually all persons with disabilities I know have been told how brave they were, sometimes for *simply getting up in the morning.*

Wright (1983) cites several motives for the requirement of mourning. One is the need to see others as devalued in order to maintain one's own position of status or value. This is similar to the notion of cognitive dissonance. If I do/am X, then X must be valuable. You are not X, so to maintain my belief in the value of X the condition of Not-X must be devalued. A second motive "arises when the perceiver becomes threatened by the apparent adjustment of a person with a disability because one's own ego is found wanting by contrast" (p. 81). To avoid acknowledging one's own weaker ego, the perceiver needs for the person with a disability not to be coping well or living a life of quality and fulfillment. The thought arises: "If a person with a disability can do it even though he or she has a disability, why can't I do it without the disability?" A third motive is to force compliance with codes of proper conduct, with the way one ought to act and feel, much like certain behaviors are seen as appropriate at a funeral. This idea is closely allied with the moral model of disability, the idea that the disability is a punishment for a sin. If it's a punishment, then one "should" suffer, or what good is a punishment? These two aspects—the requirements of mourning and cheerfulness-comprise the essential paradox of disability.

The person with a disability who fails to conform to these requirements has "a bad attitude" or is "in denial." Rehabilitation patients must simultaneously mourn their disablement and enter enthusiastically into their rehabilitation regimen. Hostility toward the staff is unacceptable. For the person with a disability the latitude for a normal range of emotions is curtailed. We are expected never to let the disability get us down. At the same time, people underestimate some of the effects of disability while overestimating the misfortune and suffering of persons with disabilities. Even family overestimate the degree of suffering from the disability. It often is assumed that there are higher levels of distress, anxiety and depression among persons with disabilities. It is vital for us as clinicians not to interpret the discrepancy between others' views and those of the client with a disability as denial on the latter's part. We must be mindful of the fact that persons with disabilities are more like than unlike persons without disabilities. Similarly, we should not underestimate the debilitating power of daily prejudice, stigma, and discrimination.

Privacy and Control

Being a person with a visible disability is to be stripped of many of the usual boundaries of self. Because a part of oneself (one's disability status) is apparent to others, one becomes "a person who can be approached at will" (Goffman, 1963, p. 16). A somewhat analogous situation occurs when a woman is in the third trimester of pregnancy. Acquaintances feel free to ask personal questions ("Was this a planned pregnancy?"). Indeed, perfect strangers come up and pat your belly, as if your stomach had pushed through and broken that invisible shield around your personal space. Something about the state of visible pregnancy invites such intrusions. This is what happens with disability as well—the personal questions, the intrusive touching. The exposure makes one subject to "the conversations strangers may feel free to strike up . . . conversations in which they express . . . morbid curiosity about [your] condition" (Goffman, 1963, p. 16). These invasions happen unpredictably, intruding into your day unbidden. One example: I get off my scooter in a shoe store to examine something more closely. A man nearby says to me, "Good for you!" and punches the air in front of him enthusiastically. Another example: I get to the checkout counter at the grocery store. The clerk, seeing me on crutches, asks, "What did you do to yourself?" (As if it were my fault.) I answer, "I had polio" and, as I knew they would, the people in line behind me go rigid with tension. My answer has made them uncomfortable. They identify with being in the position of the clerk who has asked a question that now is seen as thoughtless. Suddenly I stand there not as a mother buying fruit but as a "polio victim," the fact of my disablement a blinking neon sign. This can happen anytime, anywhere. It can happen once a week or twice in 10 minutes. It can happen in front of my children, who will learn through repetitions of this scenario that something is wrong with having a mother with a disability.

With this blinking neon sign on me it's hard to be invisible, or just one of the crowd. When I come late to a meeting *everyone* knows it. As another woman said, "being three feet tall and using a power wheelchair makes me stand out more than any rational person would ever care to do" (Collins, 1997, p. 12). Having a visible disability means always being noticed, standing out, being different, *everywhere you go*. People will respond to your differentness. Some people will want to soothe you (and assume you need soothing); some will want to heal you (embrace their religion and you could throw away your crutches); some offer redemption (Jesus loves you); and some need to tell you how really okay they are with you as you are, and in the telling prove the opposite ("Some of my best friends have quiggles"). But you just want to be left alone, anonymous, invisible, just once: "Sometimes we just want to fade into the woodwork and be anonymous—be not even a crip . . . " (Milam, 1993, p. 106).

Paradoxically, given how visible I generally am, sometimes I am completely invisible. For example, sometimes when people meet me for the first time I'm on my scooter. If at the second meeting I am walking (either on crutches or unaided), many times people simply don't recognize me. They think we've never met. I got encoded in their memories as a scooter, and they sure would remember a scooter if they saw it again. But they don't see *me*. One year my son's teacher, having met me on my scooter, kept trying to clarify at our second meeting (I was on foot) exactly what my relationship to my son was. I finally understood her confusion, and said "I'm his mother." Not the scooter; me. The reverse can also happen. I received a traffic ticket, and the officer saw me seated behind a steering wheel (and not on my scooter). I went to court to fight the ticket, and sat on my scooter through an hour of this officer citing details from each ticket he'd written. I thought I was doomed. However, when my name was called and I scooted to the front of the room, the officer looked confused, and told the judge he had no recollection of me (and thus the ticket was dismissed).

Often people make comments about the nature of the disability itself. Someone might say to me, "I saw you walking in the store the other day; you seem to be doing better" (honey, the "better" train left long ago). I could explain—that one doesn't get better, and in fact one gets worse from the combined effects of age and polio; that I always walk in that particular store because it's too crowded for my scooter; that sometimes I walk, sometimes I use crutches, sometimes I use a scooter, and the choice is often unconscious as I negotiate my way through the physical world. But I don't. You don't know me that well. I don't want to have this conversation with you. But I will take all the time needed to answer the questions of a child. If you are a friend of mine, ask me anything. It's not that I'm "oversensitive" about my disability. It's just that I don't want to share personal information with strangers any more than you do.

People want to let you know that you're not the first of "your kind" they've met. Just as the pregnant woman incurs stories of others' childbirth experiences, the person with a disability engenders stories of other persons with disabilities known to their interlocutor ("My uncle had a quiggle"). How is one to respond to this? Here the issues of privacy and regulation of affect collide. Get angry, and you confuse the other person; are seen as maladjusted, with a chip on your shoulder, stuck in one stage of "adjustment" to your disability; and are seen as representing your group, giving a worse name to persons with disabilities. Blow it off and it can be like an insidious bacterium invading your immune system. You could explain to the other person the effect of the remark on you, but really, when did you sign up for this career of disability educator to the world? You don't even remember this job having a booth on career day! So you say, "Oh really," in as disinterested a voice as you can muster, or try to joke ("Funny, you don't look like the nephew of a person with a quiggle"). No matter how you respond you are likely to enter the next encounter just a little more warily and be a little "overreactive" to the next person who has an uncle with a quiggle.

With the high degree of visibility associated with disability, a person with a disability is seen as a representative of the group. When attaining a high position, "a new career is likely to be thrust upon him, that of representing his category" (Goffman, 1963, p. 26). Conversely, one's failings or mistakes also can be misinterpreted as representative of the group. Thus the person with a visible disability is always an ambassador from the disablility community on assignment to the AB world.

All these incursions into one's privacy contribute to a sense of loss of control. The invasions of privacy occur at others' whims. They affect not only the person with a disability but also his or her family. Another factor in loss of control affects the person with a hidden disability, or with hidden aspects of the disability. This person has control over knowledge of the fact of the disability only as long as he or she tells no one. Once the information is divulged, the person loses control of the information, which then may be shared, misrepresented, recorded, gossiped about, and so on. A further factor in loss of control is that disability often involves living with a future course that is unpredictable. Persons with disabilities will respond to all of these demands of disability in myriad ways. In a testament to human resiliency and resourcefulness, there are many versions of making it work. This is the primary clinical mantra—do not insist on the response you think should be, or what you think it would be like if you had a disability.

EVERYDAY EXPERIENCES OF PERSONS WITH DISABILITIES

Okay, let's not be ridiculous—I can't really tell you about what it's like to have a disability on a day-to-day basis. But I can show how disability leads to certain kinds of experiences, and how those experiences in turn influence and shape the world view of the person with a disability. A pervasive part of the disability experience is dealing with others' attitudes toward disability. Negative attitudes toward persons with disabilities constitute a major obstacle to successful adjustment and rehabilitation (Asch, 1984; Schneider & Anderson, 1980; Tringo, 1970; Wertlieb, 1985; Wright, 1983).

Effects on Cognitions and Schemas

If there is a disability culture, that presumes some commonality of disability experience. These experiences are partly personal (i.e., the things that happen to oneself) but also events that happen to others with disabilities, events to which one resonates. This disability experience shapes one's perceptions of and stance toward the world. Let's approach this issue of how having a disability creates a different world view by analogy. Imagine you are from some small country far away, and you've come to visit and study the United States. You are interested in race relations, particularly between blacks and whites. Your research unearths two events: the Tuskegee study on syphilis and the Rodney King incident and subsequent trial resulting in acquittal of the white policemen. You might conclude that there is much racial tension in the United States, to put it mildly. If you, the visitor, were black, you might feel wary. And if you had a personal experience of racism here, these three events together—Tuskegee, King, and personal experience—would probably create in you a conceptual framework for thinking about race in this country. In other words, it doesn't take that many events or experiences to form your view, provided these events are emotionally powerful and personally meaningful. Then, even if most of your interactions with whites were positive, the overall effect comes more from those powerful negative events, which overshadow the positive experiences.

Let me use myself as an example to show how disability, like race, can frame one's world view. One day I came back to my car with my infant son and a cart full of groceries. I took my son up into my arms, and as I was opening the trunk a woman stopped and said, "May I help you?" I gratefully accepted. To my amazement, instead of helping me load the groceries she forcefully took my son out of my arms. Both he and I freaked, and I took my crying son back. The woman turned to walk away, saying, "I know, I know, you people like to do it all yourselves." This emotionally powerful incident might have remained an isolated one, but within the next few years I read about Tiffany Callo (which, whether accurate or not, I remember as the case of a mother with a disability losing custody of her baby in large part because of her disability) and then read a newspaper account of a Michigan case of two parents with disabilities who used personal attendants (they lost custody of their son because they were unable to care for him without assistance). I read in a scholarly journal that "disabled women are at risk for a range of undesirable outcomes, including . . . loss of child custody" (Kallianes & Rubenfeld, 1997, p. 203). Thus four events helped shape my view—one personal experience and three I read about that had personal meaning for me—that I, as a mother with a disability, could lose my child more easily than a mother without a disability.

This example shows how my perspective was shaped in one area. Suppose this process were repeated over many areas, as indeed it has been. Soon much of my perspective is influenced by my experiences as a person with a disability. In other words, it doesn't take many experiences or events to heavily shape my world view. Even if 99% of my experiences are positive, the 1% of negative experiences can have a greater impact if they are emotionally evocative, personally meaningful, powerful, and I have reason to believe that they are not isolated instances (e.g., by reading that they have happened to others). Over time my "reality" becomes discrepant with the AB one. Think of how many African Americans and Caucasians seemed to have such different responses to O. J. Simpson's acquittal. This gives the flavor of how two separate sets of realities coexist. Each side thinks the other side "just doesn't get it."

There is a second way that disability shapes perspective. Again, an example: I contracted polio in 1954, one of two isolated cases in the state of Michigan. A random event had happened to me. The occurrence of this event, the fact of its having happened, was a lesson to me: I learned that lightning can strike and having learned that could not unlearn it. This knowledge influenced how I viewed subsequent events. For instance, I was worried about having amniocentesis during pregnancy because of the risk of miscarriage (never mind the implications of doing tests for disabilities on my yet unborn child!). I was assured that the risk was very low and was cited statistics, which I didn't find in the least bit reassuring. Why not? Because in 1954 only two people in the state of Michigan contracted polio, and I was one of them—those odds were minuscule, but they happened. It was a lesson to me in another way: I knew that many other people had not learned that lightening could strike them, and I both envied and disliked them for this. And in an odd way I felt I had special knowledge and prized this specialness.

I feel "special" in other ways as well. Throughout my week I do things differently from nondisabled people. I park in designated areas. I enter through different doors to avoid stairs or heavy doors. I can't use the bathroom in one store because it's inaccessible but get to use the restroom next door because the owner makes an exception for me. I call a restaurant for a reservation and ask about their accessibility and then don't believe their answer so I go downtown to check it out for myself. Salesclerks in my local stores all remember me—I'm the lady on the scooter. I have a card in my wallet that identifies me as the proper owner of my handicapped parking placard. I avoid the art fair in my city's downtown because the crowds on the sidewalk make it hard to negotiate my way. I have some special skills related to my disability. First, I can identify fine gradations of pain, knowing when the pain crosses the line from nuisance to warning signal. From about 10 paces away from a curb I can tell if my right or left foot will be the one to go up (or down) the step and change the length of my pace accordingly so I go up (or down) the step with my "good" foot (I cannot do this consciously; if I stop and think about it, I lose this ability). I have well-honed skills in sensing non-verbal responses of others, sharpened by a lifetime of figuring out how people react to my disability. I have developed methods of managing stigma. And I know from the pain in my right ankle when the barometer drops and it's likely to rain.

I am not like everyone else. I am the exception. Things don't apply to me. This is a form of narcissism I sense in myself and others with disabilities. We are so used to pushing and shoving our way in, being our own advocates, being on the outskirts, being the exception, being different, that we start to think we are the exception in ways and situations other than those related to the disability. Clinicians must understand this process and not mislabel it as a personality disorder.

In this section on cognitive schemas we've seen that the world view of a person with a disability can be shaped by that experience in several ways. First, events important to the lives of persons with disabilities take on accentuated meaning, and it doesn't take many of them to have a profound impact on the person's organizing structures through which the world is viewed. Second, the fact of disability often forces an admission of personal vulnerability, an appreciation of how random events can happen to a person, and an altered relationship to probabilities. Third, having a disability means being the exception so often that it becomes a modus operandi. Fourth, being a person with a stigmatized condition hones skills in detecting nuances of nonverbal responses in others, and in stigma management. Finally, if you're lucky, you can "feel it in your bones" when it's going to rain.

But one thing people assume is an important and salient cognition for me turns out not to be. Many people who hear when I had polio are struck with the irony of my contracting it so soon before the polio vaccine was available. People assume I feel some bitterness about this timing when in fact the issues of "why me" or how narrowly I missed were never mine. I believe this attitude generalizes to other persons with disabilities. Issues of how close one came to not having a disability, "if only" I had done this, not done that, been in this place and not in that place—I don't believe these are common themes among persons with disabilities, at least not beyond the first year post-onset (but I can't be sure—no one's ever asked us, as a group, about this issue). I think it's able-bodied persons who are struck with this issue, in part because of their need to explain how such things happen (and hence couldn't happen to them, as discussed earlier). But as a person with a disability, getting deeply into the "if only"—therein lies madness.

Role Models, Mentors, and Heroes: Living in a Nondisabled World

If a child is the only one with a disability in the family, to whom does he or she look as a model? What are the norms for children with disabilities? Where are the role models for parenting with a disability? Who are our icons, our heroes? As it happens, this is a subject under great debate in the disability community. At issue is who gets to choose, "us" (i.e., persons with disabilities) or "them"—ABs?

This debate has become embodied in Christopher Reeve. The actor who portrayed Superman on film became quadriplegic in a riding accident in 1995. In an irony not lost on anyone, the embodiment of superhuman strength of heroic proportions became one of us. But then a certain uneasiness set in. Part of it was the typical perception that the rich really are different from us (the not rich). Whoever says you can't throw money at a problem doesn't have a disability. Disability is a problem that money can ameliorate tremendously: Wheelchair breaks? Buy a new one. Fatigue interfering with family life? Hire a cook. Can't drive? Hire a driver. House inaccessible? Work with an architect to design an accessible one. Money does wonders. Mr. Reeve has two full-time attendants and commands enormous fees for speaking engagements. The second stirrings of uneasiness came with the article about him in *Newsweek,* called "To stand and raise a glass." This was a quote from him, and his focus on *cure*, on eventually standing, on eventually holding a glass, is a message anathema to many people with para- or quadriplegia. The rallying cry of the disability community is "care, not cure," which means redirect funding to provide help with independent living now, for people who already have disabilities, and put less emphasis on fixing or preventing people like us. So when our most high-profile member called for cure, indeed, started raising money for a cure, we became wary. Then he appeared at the Academy Awards, and without speaking a word, his mere presence alone on a stage in his wheelchair brought thunderous applause. Frankly, it brought tears to my eyes. Why? I admired his courage *just for being there*, for having survived. (You see, those with disabilities are not immune to any of the same messages exerting pressure on us all.) And then all hell broke loose. Christopher Reeve was chosen (by ABs) to speak at the Democratic National Convention in 1994. Suddenly the Internet was awash with the topic. I received as many as 40 e-mails a day about this for several weeks. Debate centered on whether he was "our" spokesman, who gets to decide who speaks for us, and whether he was or he was not entitled to his views on living with a disability and the hope for a cure, and whether we were being harsh and judgmental. But we don't have a lot of spokespeople, people with disabilities who command much attention, so we have to be careful about who is in that role. If you only get 15 minutes in the spotlight, you want to use them well.

Air time—the medium of TV—is a powerful source of role models. There are four predominant roles for persons with disabilities on TV. The first and most ubiquitous is the role of villain, whose disability explains the villainy—the psychopathic killer with a club foot. The second and increasing role is a nonrecurring character on a sitcom whose raison d'etre is to be a person with a disability; the point of the character is the disablement, which serves as convenient metaphor. For example, in June 1997, the Nanny (played by Fran Drescher) dates a blind man (played by Jason Alexander) because she doesn't want guys to like her only for her looks. The role is played by a sighted man (you could tell; he had sighted mannerisms) and his function in the show is to make a point about seeing beyond appearances. His blindness is a symbol for inner vision. Fran realizes she has been using him, and returns to the sighted man. The function of the blind man is no longer needed. The third role is a relatively new one on TV. It began, as far as I can tell, with the sitcom *Murphy Brown,* which takes place in a TV newsroom. One of the employees of the newsroom is a man in a wheelchair, and he can be seen in the background going about his business, as would any employee. He has no lines, but the role is groundbreaking—just a regular guy doing regular work. There is a fourth role, though it is a rarity. It is a character with depth and multifacets, only one of which is the disability. The first such role was Lenny, a man with mental retardation, on *LA Law.* Another is a boy with Down syndrome who appears on *Picket Fences.* Thus we see four roles: villain, disability as symbol, background character, and well-rounded characters. The latter, by far the most important in creating positive models for persons with disabilities, is the newest and fewest.

Where else can we look for role models? Another example of a role model chosen for, but not by, us was Mark Wellman. (I don't know Mark Wellman. Nothing I say here is intended to be against him personally, only against the symbolism with which he was imbued.) Mark Wellman was a rock climber who became paraplegic in a fall. He continued to use his rock climbing skills and climbed El Capitan (a relatively sheer face of granite in Yosemite). San Francisco Bay Area news shows sent cameras to Yosemite to catalogue his ascent. Then, having spent the money to send crews there, they made a continuing story out of it. For a week we got Mark Wellman updates along with panoramic shots of El Capitan with two ant-looking creatures on it. Here's how he climbed: He had a partner who carried all the gear. The partner climbed up some, making a trail and carrying the supplies. He climbed back down for Mark, and helped him up to the next level. In other words, the partner climbed the rock twice and did so carrying all his own and Mark's gear. This is a pretty remarkable climbing feat. What was his name? I don't remember. And that's the point. No matter what that guy did, the media ensured that this was a Mark Wellman story. Nothing he did could compete with the crip on the rock.

So what's wrong with that? If a guy with paraplegia wants to climb a rock, isn't that his right? Of course it is. But do I need to climb a rock? As a matter of fact, I thought I did. When I was about 20 I climbed on crutches 3½ miles up to the top of Nevada Falls (Yosemite again). Being at the top was exhilarating. Climbing down the shorter but steeper route, however, it became clear that there had been a recent rock slide and the trail was obliterated, covered in rocks of various sizes. When using crutches, there is a moment of faith in which you raise your feet off the ground and put all your weight on the crutches. As I did this, the crutches would turn out to be on unsteady rocks, and I'd begin to slide down the mountainside. The descent was exhausting and nerve wracking, but I continued, having been convinced that there was no other choice. By midafternoon my energy was spent, and I still had the steepest part ahead of me and had to negotiate my way down past the falls on "the mist trail"—over 100 very steep, narrow, wet and slippery steps, between a wall of rock, covered with slippery and wet moss, and a waterfall rushing past in a crescendo of water and noise. I made a slow, treacherous, careful descent, while behind me a line of people backed up. I could hear them: "What's the hold up?" "I don't know, something seems to be holding up the line." "There's a girl there on crutches." "What's she doing here?" Well, what a good question. What *was* I doing there? My goodness, I was the crip on the rock.

That trip to Nevada Falls was a watershed (sorry) event for me. Raised to think I could do anything I set my mind to, I tested the boundaries of "anything" and found that there were limits. Wellman and Reeve (not coincidentally two very good looking white guys), chosen as spokesmen for our group, are what we call "supercrips" or "overcomers." We hate that overcomer crap. Because most of us are just regular people. Itzak Perlman (one of my early heroes, in part because he always insisted that his TV appearances show him walking out on stage with his crutches) said that when he began playing violin professionally all the stories about him described him as a man who had polio and who also played the violin. It was only after he became one of the four premier violinists in the world did the stories switch to describing him as a premier violinist who also happened to have had polio. Most of us are not premier violinists. Most of us will never climb a rock. But we would still like to be thought of as people first, not as a disability. When we talk about using "people first" language ("person with a disability" as opposed to "disabled person"), this is what we mean. It's not semantics. It's a way of looking at us and seeing *us*, not the disability.

Roosevelt was a hero, one with tremendous resonance in the disability community. The debate over his memorial, over whether he would be depicted in at least one statue in his wheelchair (he wasn't) cut deep. As my friend (who had polio) said to me, "FDR delivered this nation from the depression and won a world war; what have *you* done for us lately?" FDR was a man of convictions, a leader, and a visionary, all during a time in which he had to hide his disability from public view. We're not likely to get another FDR anytime soon, and we hate to see his memorial robbed of its significance for people with disabilities. It isn't only the absence of his wheelchair (remember, Roosevelt *could not walk*) but the way in which the memorial ignores current issues of disability. The Braille on the memorial is as high as eight feet off the ground and is so large that the spacing of dots within a letter and between letters is nonsensical. Robbed of our past hero and robbed of our present participation, just what will the FDR memorial come to symbolize for us?

If we don't want ABs to choose our heroes for us, who would we choose? My first role model (I was about 7) was a colleague of my father who also had polio, which left him with considerable weakness and paralysis. I most vividly remember that he didn't have sufficient stomach muscles to produce a decent sneeze. He lived in a two-story house with an inclinator chair-a chair that travels on a rail up and down the stairs. He was married, had children, and had a career. He lived a "normal" life. It was my first example that people like me could be normal.

The disability community is full of heroes, people of enormous courage. My husband, who was diagnosed with MS just as he was hitting his professional stride, has continually altered his career path as increasing symptoms change his functioning, always doing what has to be done to remain a gainfully employed individual. He is not a hero in the conventional sense, yet he is a positive role model for others with disabilities. We must not focus so much attention on the rock climbers that we lose sight of the "profoundly ordinary" (Kirshbaum, 1994) persons with disabilities who are not premier violinists.

FIVE

Families with Disabilities

"Families with disabilities" is an imprecise term, failing to denote who has the disability or the nature of the relationships of the other people to that person. The person with the disability may be a grandparent, a parent, a spouse or partner, a teenager, an infant, a sibling. Nonetheless, the literature leads us to believe that "families with disabilities" is code for "children with disabilities and their families." Much of the literature equates *families* with disabilities with families of *children* with disabilities. (See, e.g., Hansen & Coppersmith, 1984; Hersen & Van Hasselt, 1990; Saddler, Hillman, & Darling, 1993; Singer & Powers, 1993.) For example, "Disability and the Family: Research, Theory and Practice," a special issue of *Counseling Psychology Quarterly* (1991), had seven out of nine articles on children with disabilities (the remaining two were on adults with brain injuries). The vast majority of work on disability in the family is in the area of children with disabilities. And then there is silence, as if these children have no future (Kirshbaum, 1984).

Earlier chapters tried to place disability in the context of the totality of an individual (age, gender, ethnicity, etc.). Now we take that disability in that person and place the total into a larger context, the family. And in so doing we see that it is impossible to understand one without the other. Therefore, what I mean by "families with disabilities" is that the disability of an individual has meaning and ramifications for the entire family. It may be a cliche to say that disability is a family affair, but it is also true. We say in family therapy that "the relationship is the client"; that is, the relationship is something synergistic and encompassing of the total family. Similarly, treatment of families with disabilities means that the disability is a family member, belonging simultaneously to everyone and to no one.

A current positive trend in therapy with families with disabilities is to "empower" such families. This concept presumes a disenfranchised group that is bolstered, through understanding, support, and advocacy, to become active and involved in self-determination. Empowerment has become the philosophy of services in the 1990s (Bolton & Brookings, 1998; Blotzer & Ruth, 1995; Condeluci, 1989; Hahn, 1991; Koren, DeChillo, & Friesen, 1992; Singer, & Powers, 1993; Vash, 1991; Zimmerman, 1990). "Empowerment entails the acquisition of values and attitudes that are incorporated into the individual's personal worldview and thus constitutes a foundation for action" (Bolton & Brookings, 1998, p. 132). Koren et al. (1992) see empowerment as a common value across many disciplines, and they credit several factors for the development of the empowerment model, including the consumer movement and its emphasis on self-help and self-reliance, clinical models with families that emphasize strengths over deficits, services to increase self-efficacy, and values commensurate with empowerment in public policies and programs. Gutierrez and Ortega (1991) describe three levels of empowerment: the personal (incorporating feelings of personal power and self-efficacy), the interpersonal (ability to influence others), and the political (social action and social change, and the transfer of power among groups in society). These should not be thought of as stages of empowerment, although they have been discussed that way (cited in Koren et al., 1992). If these were stages, then personal empowerment would have to precede political empowerment. As discussed earlier, this is not the case in the disability community. Time and again we see examples of people with disabilities taking leadership roles and being vocal and forceful advocates for social and political changes for persons with disabilities, while their sense of personal power is limited and the advocacy skills are not applied in their own lives. This is one of the paradoxes of disability. Another paradox is posed by the juxtaposition of the philosophy of empowerment in treatment models with the assumptions driving most of the research on families with disabilities. As we shall see, the research literature is not making the kinds of assumptions or asking the kinds of questions that lead to practice models of empowerment.

In discussing families with disabilities it is important to reiterate a distinction made in Chapter 1 (in this volume) about the difference between disability and health. Disability does not inevitably imply poor health. Nor does it imply dying. The death of a child or a parent during one's childhood is indeed a tragedy. A disability is not.

CHILDREN WITH DISABILITIES

In the waiting room was a Caucasian man in his late 30s. On his lap was a girl who looked to be around 6. She was severely disabled—her limbs lacked muscle tone and were limp, her weight was entirely supported by her dad, her head flopped to the side until it rested against his upper arm. Her eyes wandered and were somewhat vacant, and her mouth hung open. The father held a book in front of them and was reading aloud.

In imagining this tableau, simultaneously both familiar and foreign, what thoughts or images go through your mind? Probably many people would focus on the daughter, perhaps thinking how sad, and how horrible it would be if they personally had such a child. The word "vegetable" may have crossed some minds. You might have wondered whether the birth of this child could have been prevented through prenatal testing and abortion, or whether some medical malpractice was responsible. You focus on the daughter. But focus for a moment on the father. The look on his face as he performed a common parental activity of reading to a child was a look of love—it was the profoundly ordinary face of any dad reading to his little girl.

How can we call such a daughter a "burden"? On what basis do textbooks repeatedly claim that parents of children with disabilities "cannot make an honest attachment to their real child until they have withdrawn their affection for the normal, wished-for child"? (Lindemann, 1981, p. 123). "The parents must end the psychological attachment for the child that was idealized during the pregnancy and accept a child who has an imperfection" (Ziolko, 1993, p. 185). "When a young child is developmentally disabled or has a congenital or inherited defect, the parents feel injured. The sad, resentful, discouraged reactions of the parents, which have been referred to as mourning reactions for the healthy child that was expected . . . require that time and support be given to the parents to enable them to prepare for the care of the child they did not expect" (Solnit, 1989, p. 30). It is in the context of such statements that Yuker (1994) implores us to "stop studying the presumably horrible negative effects of a child with a disability on parents and siblings" (p. 12). Contrast these statements with those of 12 mothers of children with severe impairments: "Some [of the mothers] described a special kind of bonding that occurred with their infants who were handicapped" (Wickham-Searl, 1992, p. 256). Research has focused too exclusively on understanding the parents' loss or burden of a child with a disability and negligible amounts on understanding the kinds of experiences these 12 mothers have.

The literature on families of children with disabilities or chronic conditions is voluminous. As discussed in Chapter 2 (in this volume), much of it can be characterized as investigations of the "burden" of the child with a disability on the family. Most of these studies share a set of assumptions: (1) Having and caring for a child with a disability is a burden; (2) this burden will tax and strain the family's resources in every respect; (3) we need to understand more about how families cope with this burden. As Quittner, Opipari, Regoli, Jacobsen, and Eigen (1992) note,

> over the past two decades, most research examining the impact of childhood disability on the family has focused on identifying the problems or deficits in these families compared to those in families raising children without disabilities. Typically, this research has been characterized by the assumption that *all* areas of individual and family functioning will be negatively affected, painting a picture of generalized stress and emotional distress in these families. (p. 275; emphasis in original)

What if we were to make totally different assumptions? "If families could view disabled loved ones as members of a legitimate social minority community instead of victims of medical tragedy, would it lead to an easier adjustment and outcome for all?" (Gill, 1994, p. 15). How can the burden literature help us understand the father in the previous example? With the predominant focus on negative attitudes toward disability there is less understanding of positive, caring, loving, intimate relationships between an able-bodied person and a person with a disability.

An excellent article on caring relationships explored the question of how nondisabled people who are in caring and accepting relationships with persons with severe disabilities define them (Bogdan & Taylor, 1989). The persons with severe disabilities all had profound or severe mental retardation, were in or from long-term institutional care, and could be typified by the following description:

> Twenty-year-old Jean cannot walk or talk. Her clinical records describe her as having cerebral palsy and being profoundly retarded. Her thin, short—4 feet long, 40 pound—body, atrophied legs, and disproportionately large head make her a very unusual sight. Her behavior is equally strange. She drools, rolls her head, and makes seemingly incomprehensible high pitched sounds. (p. 138)

As the authors point out, this is how an outsider might describe Jean. "Jean and the other severely and profoundly retarded people in our study have often been called 'vegetables' " (p. 138). In seeking to understand persons in relationships with these partners[1] they constructed a "sociology of acceptance" (p. 136). These authors discussed four dimensions of acceptance.

1. *Attributing thinking to the other.* The nondisabled people in these relationships held the view that thinking is not the same as communication, and although communication was limited in the partners that did not mean the partners did not think. They saw the partners as more intelligent than they appeared and viewed the partners' physiology as keeping them from revealing their thoughts. Thus the nondisabled persons became adept at reading subtler clues of internal states and would empathically take the role of the partner and think about what they themselves might want, feel, or think were they in the partner's situation. A key factor was that they discounted the pronouncements of professionals on two grounds. First, professionals had been wrong before (e.g., in declaring that the partner would not live or ever be able to leave the hospital). Second, the professionals had too limited a sample of partners' behaviors and thus didn't know them as well as the nondisabled persons did.

2. *Seeing individuality in the other.* The nondisabled persons saw "distinct, unique individuals with particular and specific characteristics that set them apart from others" (p. 141). Personalities were described in mostly positive terms, they gave the partners nicknames and noted their likes and dislikes (sometimes through subtle communications such as the speed at which one young man thrust his tongue in and out). They eschewed technical and medical terms (e.g., profoundly mentally retarded). A bond was formed, and "normal" motives and feelings were attributed to the partners. They paid attention to the appearance of the partners, giving them haircuts, keeping them clean, dressing them in nice, age- and gender-appropriate clothes. The partners were accepted and included in daily life.

3. *Viewing the other as reciprocating.* Most research on relationships subscribes to the notion that satisfactory relationships are ones in which there is reciprocity—one receives as much as one gives—and that disequilibrium leads to relationship stress. These nondisabled people did not view the relationship with the partner as one in which the partner needed to give as much as he or she received. They also perceived that they were gaining from the relationship. In general, they saw two benefits: companionship, and new social relationships they would not other-

---

[1]Bodgan and Taylor (1989) use the term "partner" to denote the person with the disability in the relationship; I have adopted that terminology here.

wise have had. They felt that they were better people because of the relationship (e.g., they had learned to be more accepting, more caring, more at ease with persons with disabilities); they felt special and had a sense of accomplishment and self-worth.

4. *Defining a social place for the other.* The partners were included in the definition of the family, had a role in the family, and were part of its rituals and routines. The nondisabled people stated that the group would not be the same without the partner.

Now look back at the vignette of the father and daughter that opened this section. Applying the notions of Bogdan and Taylor, we notice how the father loves this daughter, thinks she hears and enjoys his reading, views her as special in his life, chooses books according to what he believes his daughter would like to hear, identifies with other parents of children with disabilities, and sees his daughter as integral to the family. In other words, he behaves like an ordinary dad. Why does this seem so surprising?

Parents set the tone for the role of the disability in the family. When parents hold more positive perceptions of their children with disabilities, their attributions and behaviors are more positive, as are the effects on the child. The reverse is also true: When parental perceptions are negative, effects are negative. When the effect of a child with a disability on the family is negative, the problem is often more due to a low level of marital satisfaction than to the disability itself. Although initial reactions to the birth of a child with a disability may be stressful and negative, parents often quickly exhibit coping behaviors. Not surprisingly, families that cope better are those with more resources (competence, skills, family and community resources and supports) and tend to hold an internal locus of control. Marital satisfaction is a key factor distinguishing distressed families; thus clinicians should not confuse the effects of a child's disability with those of a distressed marriage.

A child with a disability is usually the only family member with a disability, or at least with that particular disability. Thus the stigma of the disability may be experienced both from outside and within the family. That this is so makes the experience of childhood disability fundamentally unlike that of ethnic minorities. In addition, in most families with children with disabilities, the birth of that child or the onset of his or her disability is usually the family's first experience with disability. It also may be their first experience with minority status or a stigmatized difference.[2]

---

[2]It is also possible that the child has seen others in the family with the same disability, and that person may have deteriorated and possibly died. Thus issues of vulnerability and mortality must be raised earlier than is usually considered developmentally appropriate.

In the early years of a child with a disability, the family often is pre-occupied with physical, medical, and schooling implications of the disability. This forces the disability into a prominent position, making it hard to see it in perspective. As the family is learning about the disability the child may be an infant or very young and hence is not included in this knowledge acquisition. It is not uncommon for children with disabilities to lack basic factual information about their own disabilities and their physical effects. For a variety of reasons, families may not discuss the disability, or limit discussions only to specific aspects of it (such as the need for a new assistive device, or whether a bus stop is too far). This "conspiracy of silence" (Rousso, 1982, p. 80) about disability can lead the child to the conclusion that disability is a bad thing if it is unmentionable. Children may cope with this by either denying the disability (wanting it to "go away") or overinflating its role in the self-image. If the child denies the disability he or she is ill prepared for others' negative reactions, may fail to gain critical information about the disability, and does not incorporate it into the self-concept, and the disability occupies an ego-dystonic role that circles the outskirts of the identity. At the other extreme, the disability becomes the "central characteristic" and "spreads" to envelope the identity.

Added to the family's struggles with the role of disability are societal attitudes. Public attitudes and media put the emphasis in disability on incapacity, abnormality, and victim or childlike status. It can be hard for the family not to internalize at least some of these negative views, and the child with the disability is especially vulnerable if the family fails to teach coping skills, alternate models of thinking about disability, or how to incorporate the disability into the self-image.

In adolescence, issues of independence, sexuality, and peer relationships take a paramount role. Establishing a first sexual relationship usually occurs in the context of increased independence from parents. For the teen with a disability, physical dependence may continue, hampering emotional and psychological independence. Most teens "take" independence; adolescents with disabilities may have to be "given" independence deliberatively. Independence from parents usually leads to increased questions and independent exploration about sexuality. If the independence is hindered, this type of questioning and exploration may not develop. Thus the teen with a disability may lack adequate and accurate information about sex and may not know what "normal" functioning is. He or she may even associate sexual feelings or feelings of alienation and differentness with the disability, not knowing that this is typical of adolescence. The social isolation that can accompany the stigma of disability in adolescence can seriously curtail opportunities for socialization, exploration, questioning, and discussion.

Children with disabilities have certain rights guaranteed by law. These laws focus mostly on education. But what about the social and emotional development, the human rights of children with disabilities? These human rights are discussed below in terms of the issue for the child, the accompanying issues for the family, and the therapeutic tasks. In any discussion of human rights, the other "two Rs" must also be considered: responsibilities and risks (McCarthy & Thompson, 1993). First I provide a brief context, beginning with some statistics on children with disabilities, then consideration of increased risks for these children.

Recall from Chapter 1 that there are more than 4 million children and adolescents with disabilities in the United States—more than 6% of those under age 18 (Wenger, Kaye, & LaPlante, 1996). Boys are significantly more likely than girls to attend special schools or classes and to have a school-related disability (6.3% of boys, 4.5% of girls). According to one national survey (Wenger et al., 1996), African American and Caucasian children attend special schools or classes at about the same rate, but Hispanic children show a significantly lower rate of such attendance. Children from poor families (below the poverty line) attend special schools or classes at nearly twice the rate of other children (5.2% vs. 2.8%); this is not surprising, because poorer pre- and perinatal care increases the rates of many types of disabilities.

Children with disabilities incur increased risks, including a rate of substance abuse at least twice as high as for those without disabilities (Helwig & Holicky, 1994; Moore & Polsgrove, 1991; National Institute on Disability and Rehabilitation Research, 1990), greater dropout rates and more under- and unemployment (Center for the Future of Children, 1996). There is significant evidence that children with disabilities are at higher risk for sexual and physical abuse (Finkelhor, 1984; Krents, Schulman, & Brenner, 1987; Morgan, 1987; Zirpoli, 1986), particularly children with cognitive and mental disorders (Buchanan & Wilkins, 1991; Dunne & Power, 1990; Sobsey, 1994).

Human Rights of Children with Disabilities

This discussion of the human rights of children with disabilities focuses on the psychosocial and interpersonal aspects of living in this world as a child with a stigmatized condition. Table 5.1 summarizes the 13 rights that are discussed next, the accompanying family issues, and the therapeutic tasks.

Right 1: To be told the truth about their medical condition and to have ownership of the story of their disability. The first part of this right is concerned with how we label our children. We may be politically correct ("person with mental retardation"), use medical/psychiatric terminology ("developmentally delayed"), or adopt euphemisms ("intellectually challenged"). Part of our search for "correct" terms comes from our steadfast but erroneous belief that children don't know much more than we tell them. But children with leukemia know they're dying, and children with developmental delays know they're mentally retarded and can probably tell you three derogatory words for it. If we don't tell the truth to our children they learn it anyway; do we really want them to hear it first on the playground? The family's task is to be straightforward and matter-of-fact about the nature of the impairment. It is certainly imperative that the therapist adopt this stance. As therapists we often adopt the language of our patients as a way of joining with them, but this can be counterproductive if the family persists in using evasive terms for the disability.

Being told the truth is part of helping children have ownership of their own disability. Ownership means that the disability belongs to and is happening to the child. If the mother says, "Why is God doing this to me?" she must gently be reminded that the disability did not happen to her but to her child. An important part of transferring ownership of the disability from the parents to the child is the disability story. This is the story the family tells itself about the events unfolding to the discovery of the disability. For example, the family may have a story about a pregnant mother being rushed to the hospital with preeclampsia. An emergency caesarian section is done, and out of the tumult and crisis emerges a seemingly health baby. Seven months later when the baby still can't sit up the doctors suspect cerebral palsy. As the family tells the birth story the vantage point is of the crisis as it happened to the couple (he was afraid of losing her, she fainted in the bathroom). But the story has to evolve into one from the perspective of the child (his Apgar score was 7, he seemed to make developmental milestones for the first few months, etc.). The story is not a static one; it gets told and retold, each time in a new way that incorporates the cognitive and emotional developmental level of the child. Families tend to get stuck in the story they tell, and assume that the child already knows the story, understands the story, and doesn't need more information. It is useful if the therapist, early in treatment, elicits the disability story. Through this simple vehicle begins to emerge the possibility that there is really more than one story. This is the beginning of helping the child with the disability have his or her own views, wishes, fears, beliefs, and feelings about the disability, separate from the parents'. (For a clinical example of this process see Olkin, 1995.)

Right 2: To be in control of their own bodies. This includes (a) being as pain-free as possible, (b) being free from physical and sexual abuse, and (c) being included in making decisions about medical or prosthetic interventions.

a. Parents often worry that if children are given pain medication they will learn to use drugs "as a crutch." Medical personnel also may promote the stiff-upper-lip approach to pain management. A more useful technique is to realistically prepare children for medical procedures, including a frank discussion of "discomfort" and teaching coping, distraction, and management skills. Such discussions tend to make parents squeamish; little is harder than watching our children suffer. Therefore the therapist often needs to take the lead in bringing the topic up, encouraging open discussion and perhaps suggesting that the parents get more information from medical personnel so that they can better prepare their child. An initial discussion of this topic can be done without the child present, allowing the parents a chance to examine their own affect and become ready to help their child.

b. As therapists we must always be alert for signs of physical or sexual abuse. In the case of children with disabilities we must not make erroneous assumptions that "no one would hurt such a child" or that a more defenseless child makes for a less likely target. As discussed in Chapter 10 (in this volume), this is, sadly, far from the truth.

c. With "ownership" of one's disability comes greater responsibility (the third "R") for decision making. As the child increases control over his or her own body, he or she should be asked permission before being, say, a demonstration in a teaching hospital to a group of residents. Parents should be encouraged to see the transfer of ownership from them to the child as a gradual process, very much dependent on the child's biopsychosocial development. Therefore, the therapist, who is perhaps only intervening in a small cross section of the family's life, should be teaching the parents a process by which they slowly back off as primary decision makers and offer aid and assistance to their child as he or she makes more of the decisions. Problems arise when this transfer is too rapid, too early, or delayed and insufficient. The therapist will want to assess these aspects of transferring ownership as part of the evaluation of the family.

Right 3: To not be treated as part-objects or specimens. Impairments are often treated as if they are isolated body systems unrelated to the whole of the child. For example, a club foot may be held up, examined, bound, and exercised, all as if the fact that it is attached to a child at the other end is at best irrelevant and at worst a nuisance. Learning disabilities associated with cerebral palsy may be treated as an academic issue, without regard to the interpersonal and emotional context of a changing body and developing child. As therapists, one of our important tasks is to bring together all the medical, physical, developmental, academic, social, emotional, and psychological parts into one room. From this perspective we must see the child as a multifaceted person and help the family do so as well. It is unlikely that the school or medical systems will follow suit, so it is particularly important that this stance be maintained vigilantly in therapy and with the family.

Right 4: To see positive role models of adults and children with disabilities. Excellent discussions of disability images in the media are available elsewhere (cf. Kent, 1987). In general, disability is used symbolically to stand for evil, dark forces; the mere fact of its existence is used to "explain" pathology. In school, children see other children with disabilities get ostracized, stigmatized, and teased. Naturally they come up with explanations for why "I'm not like him/her." Thus the greatest source of comfort and understanding—other children with disabilities—is often the avenue children carefully eschew. Further, usually children with disabilities are the only one in the family with a disability and are isolated from like others; their access to role models with disabilities is limited. This is a serious limitation; adults with disabilities who join a group of others with disabilities often describe the experience as "coming home" (Gill, 1994). Perhaps we can help children with disabilities have this experience sooner by providing positive role models of older children and adults with disabilities, and by encouraging a view of disability as an integral but not all-encompassing aspect of self-image.

Right 5: To have a positive identity that includes and incorporates the disability. The most common statement I've heard from children and teenagers with disabilities is that they'd like the disability "to go away." This can't be good, wanting parts of our bodies to disappear! But with so few positive encounters with other persons with disabilities, children often get stuck in their early childhood responses to their own disability and don't have corrective or positive experiences to help change their initial negative mind-sets. Meeting an adult with a disability can have a powerful effect on the child. It has a tremendous impact if the therapist has a disability, both on the child (who sees a coping model) and on the parents (who see potential for their child). The danger for the therapist with a disability is the desire to deliver all one has learned about living with a disability in a neat package to the family.

Often families decide to treat their child with a disability as "normal." As therapists we may respond, "But of course!" Then we, like the family, are denying a part of the child's identity. Suppose, for example, that a Caucasian family adopts a Vietnamese orphan from birth and decides to raise her as "normal" (just like them, i.e., white). But the Vietnamese child will soon discover and be told by peers and adults that this is false. The child's conclusion can only be that being Vietnamese is a bad thing. A better approach is to foster an identity that incorporates all aspects of both the child's ethnicity and the rest of the family's. In this same way, by treating children with disabilities as "normal," we are implying a badness associated with disability. No wonder children want to excise that part of themselves. The job of the therapist is to help meld the disconnected aspects of the self-identity, discourage splitting, and foster realistic and positive appraisals of self.

Right 6: To not be made to feel that "people like them" should be prevented. Much of the financial resources, most of the charities, and now prenatal screening put the emphasis on preventing disabilities. It is psychologically hard for children to know that if their mother could have screened for and found out about the condition the child has, the pregnancy may well have been terminated and few people would have questioned the choice; it is hard to be held up as a "tragedy" to be prevented. We might well say to these children that it is not them, but the disability, we are trying to prevent, but this is a sham message when we're also trying to encourage incorporation of the disability into a self-concept.

Closely linked with the idea that such disorders (i.e., such children with such disorders) should be prevented is the notion that these children are burdens on their families. Of course, there are realistic difficulties inherent in raising a child with a disability, such as increased need for physical assistance (in dressing, feeding, etc.), greater financial demands, necessity of making adaptations in housing and environment, and living with a perhaps unpredictable disease and prognosis. But it seems counterproductive to harmonious living to think of our children as burdens. Therapists can help reframe this pervasive message of burden that families with disabilities hear. Consider how the words "child care" and "childrearing" connote normal and positive activities of parenting whereas "burden" connotes additional and unwanted tasks. For example, a mother of a child with right hemiplegia was concerned that her son could not tie his shoes (a difficult task using only one hand). But the therapist talked about teaching the son this skill as a way of maximizing the son's sense of independence and self-reliance (i.e., as a move toward health) rather than concentrating on removing the necessity of the mother having to tie his shoes for him (i.e., taking away a burden). All parents do "negative" child-care tasks, such as worrying, sacrificing, and compromising, and when these are done for a child with a disability parents often need to be reminded that these are also things they would do for a child without a disability.

Right 7: To be allowed to experience a full range of emotions. As Lollar (1994) said, "professionals must be aware of the power we have to undermine families by suggesting that normal responses are dysfunctional or pathological" (p. 23). Perhaps most important we must set aside two cherished notions: (1) that emotions go in stages—stages that are necessary, desirable, invariant, or definable; and (2) that there is such a thing as "adaptation" to a disability, which implies a hierarchy of responses with adaptation or acceptance at the pinnacle. There is only "response."

The regulation of affect for persons with disabilities is a social requirement (Gallagher, 1985), particularly the prohibition against anger and the prescription of pluckiness (Olkin, 1993). The requirements extend to the family of the child with the disability as well, especially to the expectation of mourning (see Chapter 3, in this volume). Therapists must guard against thinking that the family that is not grieving is therefore in denial. Families often are more resilient than we give them credit for. Consider the following example: A mother had a third child who was born with a rare congenital disorder, who had undergone about a dozen surgeries in his first 2 years of life. Yet this mother said that she never thought of her son as disabled: "I have three kids. My oldest daughter is a picky eater, and I always have to think about whether she's getting enough protein, a balanced diet. My middle son is a slow starter, a bit shy, and I have to take extra time to help him join other kids, to transition him to new teachers. My youngest son has operations, and I have to help him feel safe and secure in the hospital." Almost all the literature on disability will tell us that this woman is denying her grief over the substitution of a "damaged" child for the unborn perfect child. I would suggest that this is a pathological perspective that is based on theory but not on empirical evidence. When we ask different questions, such as "how do families respond?" instead of "what burdens do they carry?" we will notice the tremendous resources families bring to raising children with disabilities.

Right 8: To gain a realistic view of (a) others' reactions to them, and (b) their future. Disability is a highly stigmatized condition, subject to profound prejudice and discrimination in all aspects of life, and often ostracism from childhood peers. This stigmatization can be heartbreaking for parents, who must nonetheless resist the temptation to shield and spare their child. Conversely, I find that some parents support outrageously unrealistic future goals for their child because they don't want to discourage him or her—I'm reminded of the boy with cerebral palsy who wanted to become a pro-football player; everyone knew this was a really bad idea, but no one wanted to tell him. As the therapist it was not my role to tell him either but to encourage his parents to do so. The trick here is to support the child with a disability to be all she or he can be yet also to be realistic about limitations placed by the disability and not to foster their feeling that the child has to be better than everyone else to be thought of as good. Parents get concerned when I say the word "limitations" and seem to find it helpful when I demonstrate that everyone has limitations. For example, could the father have become a basketball player? Could the mother have been a ballerina? Probably not, yet they didn't dwell on these "limitations." We all get what we get and then cope with what we've got. The therapeutic task is to help parents inoculate their child to the inevitable negative responses engendered by their disability.

Right 9: To have expectations of sexuality, romantic love, and parenthood. The first question teens with disabilities always ask me is if I'm married, and then if I have children. This is not surprising; people with disabilities are often treated as asexual beings, and these teens are trying to collect data on me to refute the stereotype. Neither sexuality nor parenting are Activities of Daily Living; that is, these are not considered "rights," and there seems to be the assumption that these are not activities associated with people with disabilities. When a disability includes cognitive or intellectual impairments this issue of sexuality becomes quite difficult for many families as the child's body becomes that of a teenager but the social and interpersonal skills lag behind. Families seem to handle sexuality by ignoring it. The therapist may have to actively and repeatedly raise the issue before the parents can accept its inevitability. But this is an important discussion, because it is enhancing the child's journey toward greater emancipation. Often I have found that discussion of sexuality with the young teenager with a disability is the first time that there has been something private from the parents for that child. This is a good therapeutic maneuver, provided that you have already discussed with the parents ahead of time that there will be privileged communication between therapist and child.

Right 10: To affiliate with peers both with and without disabilities. Children with disabilities are bicultural; that is, they live in a mostly nondisabled world, but also belong to a minority group of people with disabilities. They can learn to move easily between these two worlds. As a person of any minority group knows, there are different expectations, behaviors, and norms in the two worlds, and varying aspects of oneself are differentially manifest in the two arenas. Having an affiliation with a group of persons with disabilities helps teach the commonalities of the disability experience, reduce isolation, and provide practical and social tips for improved living. It also helps break down the denial of disability found when families try to raise their child as "normal" (Gill, 1994). As discussed in Chapter 10, wanting to affiliate with persons with disabilities or with ABs can represent health psychological functioning ("I can choose freely") or negative self-image ("I'd never want to be with people with disabilities; I'm not like them," or "why would someone want to be with me?").

Right 11: To be assessed with appropriate measures against appropriate standards, by professionals skilled in assessing this population. There are too few therapists with disabilities (approximately 2% of members of the American Psychological Association, according to the APA Office of Demographics, Employment, and Educational Research, personal communication, August, 1994) to assume that many children with disabilities will be seen by therapists with disabilities. Although it is not necessary to be of like condition to see clients, it is mandatory to possess certain knowledge, skills, and attitudes in working with this population. Some of what we need to know we learn from clients, but it is unfair to expect them to teach us all that is necessary. Clients are the experts on what living with a particular disability is like. In this we must let them guide us. We must be careful not to trivialize or disbelieve clients' accounts of prejudice and stigma. It is useful to read some of the writings that view disability as a minority group (e.g., Nagler, 1993; Oliver, 1996; Shakespeare, 1998; Wright, 1983).

As in all therapy involving children, it is important to talk to the pediatrician. For children with disabilities there often are others involved in different aspects of care or treatment that can offer valuable perspectives—resource room specialists, physical therapists, school counselors and psychologists, neuropsychologists. Bear in mind that you, the therapist, are probably the only one collecting all these perspectives into one place. That, by itself, is an important therapeutic maneuver.

Kids often have been assessed using tests that are not appropriate given their disability, and that have not been normed on children with disabilities (see also Chapter 9). Many tests have items that are positive for such children because of the disability per se, skewing results to false positives. (Examples include questions about physical symptoms, such as tingling in fingers, or activities, such as listening to music, that are not available to a child with a particular disability.) But even using appropriate tests doesn't guard against misinterpretation. For example, I saw a 14-year-old boy with spina bifida who received a neuropsychological battery that included projective tests. His themes were full of sexual aggression. He interpreted one TAT (Thematic Apperception Test) card as being about a boy who made obscene phone calls. The neuro-psychologist interpreted these themes as indicating an incipient antiso-cial personality disorder despite the absence of any family history of this disorder, or any other signs of antisocial traits in the boy. An alternate explanation is that this boy, who had been quite ostracized and friend-less throughout his childhood, was simply insufficiently socialized, received little corrective feedback, had limited opportunity for learning about sex or exploring sexuality, and no romantic encounters with girls, and hence he gave responses in testing reflecting these socially imposed limitations.

Perhaps the most fundamental skill of a therapist working with chil-dren with disabilities is the ability to work in a nonpathologizing way. Such work focuses more on increasing resiliency than on correcting defi-cits. This core aspect of the treatment conveys an important overall mes-sage about disability to the parents and the child—a message of health and possibility, intimacy, coping and quality of living.

Right 12: To live in a barrier-free, accommodating, and tolerant physical and social environment. We can do three things related to this issue. First, we can ensure that all parts of our own offices and services are readily accessible to children with disabilities. We can do this now, before it becomes a need, so that children with disabilities are not made to feel, yet again, that their mere existence is inconvenient for others; it doesn't feel good to wheel into a room, say, and have everyone scramble around rearranging furniture to accommodate you. The second thing we can do is to become knowledgeable about the laws related to disability. Only in this way can we help families protect their children, get the ser-vices to which they are entitled, and know their legal rights. The third thing we can do is work toward social change, by trying to affect what-ever social arena we live in. Also, as we contact collaterals in the child's life we can influence the lens through which they see disability. In many ways we all can work daily to make more accommodations for persons with disabilities and in so doing help our clients in a fundamental way.

Right 13: To be a child. The phrase "special needs," often used about children with disabilities, should not be taken to imply that all the needs of these children are "special"—many of their needs are perfectly ordinary, the needs of any child. The needs of love, safety, security, attachment, sexuality, affiliation, separation and individuation, produc-tivity, meaningfulness—these are shared by all children. In most ways children with disabilities are ordinary children.

TABLE 5.1. Rights of Children with Disabilities, and the Accompanying Family and Therapy Tasks

Right	Family task	Therapy task
1. To be told the truth and to "own" the story of their disability.	To allow for separateness in views of disability; to increasingly turn tasks over to the child.	To help family titrate parents' versus child's responsibilities; to monitor the pace of transitions.
2. To be in control of own body.	To be respectful of child's boundaries; to include child in making choices.	To be alert to increased risk of abuse; to support child in taking increased charge of self; to teach parents how to help increase child's coping.
3. To not be treated as a specimen or part-object.	To see child as whole; to remember that the physical includes the psychological.	To collect data on child from disparate sources into one place; to help family view child, not disability.
4. To see positive role models of adults and children with disabilities.	To foster contact without patronizing; to locate appropriate models.	To encourage family to depathologize association with others with disabilities.
5. To have a positive identity that includes and incorporates the disability.	To think about the disability as one of many facets of the child; to incorporate the disability into the family's concept of the child.	To foster positive images of persons with disabilities; to not allow fragmentation of self-identity into disabled and nondisabled parts.
6. To not be made to feel that people like them should be prevented.	To focus on improvement of quality of life; to deemphasize cure.	To help the child not feel responsibility for the family stresses; to relieve parents of guilt.
7. To be allowed to experience the full range of emotions.	To view the child as a child first, and not to view all facets of the child through a disability lens; to allow separation of child's emotions about disability from those of the parents.	To elicit many versions of the disability story; to tolerate and not pathologize the full range of responses.
8. To gain a realistic view of others' responses to their type of disability, and of the future.	To tell the often painful truths, to speak unspeakable things, to admit realistically to prejudice and discrimination.	To foster a coping model; to teach self-advocacy skills.
9. To have expectations of sexuality, romantic love, and parenthood.	To have faith that child is and will be lovable to others; to talk about love and sex.	To bring the topic up; to talk with teens and preteens without parents present.

TABLE 5.1. *continued*

Right	Family task	Therapy task
10. To affiliate freely with peers both with and without disabilities.	To allow the child to have a (disability) world of which the parents are not a part.	To foster a bicultural model; to help parents tolerate the separation from the child.
11. To be assessed with appropriate measures against appropriate standards, using a salutogenic lens.	To accept that parents know their child best; to be advocates on behalf of their child.	To help families negotiate the medical and mental health worlds; to recommend appropriate resources; to support the parents as experts about their children.
12. To live in a barrier-free, accommodating, and tolerant physical and social environment.	To externalize barriers to accessibility; to be advocates for disability rights.	To adopt a nonpathologizing perspective on disability; to make office accessible.

Conclusions about Children with Disabilities

Children with disabilities are more likely to experience a host of negative life events, including separations from caregivers, decreased attachment, increased neglect or abuse, decreased socialization, intrusive medical procedures, pain, and negative labeling. Most of these negative events are not occasioned by the disability per se but by families' and society's responses to the disability. Our interventions may address more appropriately these familial and social obstacles. As Huebner and Thomas (1995) suggest, parents are asked to become informed and make decisions about medical, educational, or therapeutic interventions for their child. These tasks may deplete the parents at the expense of the relationship and attachment with the child. Thus the therapy may be better focused on the relationship between parent and child than on fixing the child.

A child with a disability in the family results "in *specific* rather than *global* alterations in activity patterns" (Quittner et al., 1992, p. 285; emphasis in original). We must stop telling parents that their children with disabilities represent tragedies. Although no one can deny the relief all parents feel in hearing that a newborn is "normal," this does not imply that children with disabilities are "abnormal." So much of what constitutes a "child" is common to all children. Focusing on the disability as if it altered that essence is a mistake. This is not to suggest that parents or therapists should adopt the opposite extreme, which is to downplay the disability as just another human difference or deny it altogether. To do so fails to help the child learn to live with a stigmatized condition, cope with discrimination, and become inoculated against oppression, all tasks that are fundamental to successful living with a disability.

SIBLINGS OF CHILDREN WITH DISABILITIES

So many of the comments about children or parents with disabilities apply to siblings of children with disabilities that this section runs the risk of being excessively redundant. But there are four main ideas that bear repeating. First, if it is the case that disability occurs to the family and affects all members of the family, this includes siblings, yet their role is often overlooked. Like any siblings who can grow up to have a deep identification with one another, siblings of children with disabilities can develop strong identification with disability issues. Second, siblings are subject to the same misconceptions, stereotypes, stigmas, and discrimination due to the disability as is the child with the disability. Third, the literature on siblings of children with disabilities presumes that disability must have a negative impact, and studies seek to confirm the burden of the disability on the siblings. Furthermore, studies are more likely to examine the effects of disabled children on siblings than the effects of siblings on the disabled children (Yuker, 1994). Some researchers are so intent in finding problems that seemingly positive behaviors are reframed as pathological. For example, suppose a sibling has experienced life-threatening emergencies with the child with a disability. The sibling might then develop an increased tolerance for minor daily problems, which pale in comparison (Baldwin, 1997). Clinicians and researchers might mistakenly think of this as "denial," or lack of freedom to voice negative emotions. Finally, some positive effects on siblings of children with disabilities have been consistently noted, most notably an increase in empathy and tolerance for differences. Such siblings often feel special, and take pride in knowledge or skills related to the specific disability. Such skills can range from simple tasks such as finding curb cuts or spotting accessible entrances to more complicated tasks such as administering a shot or cleaning a tracheostomy. Siblings get used to long hours in waiting rooms, or at hospitals, doctors' or therapists' offices. The disability may take precedence when there are conflicting needs in the family (say, a picnic that is canceled due to a pressing medical need). Siblings see the child with a disability teased and they may incur teasing themselves. They have to decide whether to defend the child with a disability, or protect him or her from teasing or bullying. They may feel ambivalent or negative emotions about the disability, and experience embarrassment, shame, guilt, and anger, with no available outlets to vent these feelings. Siblings are not immune to feelings of difference, unacceptability, and stigma. Children may not know that their sibling rivalries, conflicts, or teasing are normal, and may mistakenly ascribe these to the disability, or feel they are unacceptable because of it.

Siblings require varying information and assistance as they develop. As preschoolers they are just becoming aware of differences and will not yet have attached a positive or negative valence to the differences. But they may be exposed earlier than are many children to medical emergencies, hospital visits, surgeries, recovery periods, and other events that are beyond their comprehension and can raise fears for them. Children often don't articulate their fears or questions, so adults have to anticipate and divine their issues. (My younger sister, for example, thought that when she got older then she would have polio too. It never occurred to any of us in the family to tell her this wouldn't happen.) As siblings enter school they will be exposed to more negative attitudes, comments, and behaviors toward the child with the disability. Their first inkling that their sibling is different may come from questions or negative comments of teachers, other children, or other children's parents. As teenagers the opinions of peers take on an inflated role, and dating increases the desire to fit in. Siblings will be forced to make decisions about affiliating with other people who view the child with a disability negatively, who put him or her down, who imitate him or her, or who otherwise indicate stigma. As young adults siblings will have questions about genetics and whether the disability is inheritable. They may have increased responsibilities for the child with the disability, as their parents age and try to transfer some of the care and responsibility over to them. Siblings are called on repeatedly to answer "What is wrong with . . . ?" or "What happened to . . . ?" Like persons with disabilities, they may come to resent questions from strangers or passers-by but welcome questions from more intimate friends.

Siblings are an important resource for the child with the disability. They carry a credibility that parents don't always have, because they know what it's like to be a child. It was my sister who had utter faith that as I got older peers would be less rejecting, and more importantly that the ones who did mind my disability had something wrong with *them*, not me. I'm sure my parents thought this as well, but what did they know, they were parents. They *had* to be positive; my sister didn't.

Despite the common refrain to say that disabilities happen to families, not individuals, siblings are routinely overlooked in the treatment of children with disabilities. They are not consulted about treatment decisions, and they may not even be informed of them. They are excluded from discussions and not consulted about their opinions. Clinicians should not duplicate this exclusion and should inquire early about siblings and consider ways to incorporate them into treatment, as appropriate to their age and roles in the family. Instead of asking about the terrible effects of disability on the siblings, we should think about the myriad ways in which siblings with and without disabilities interact with and learn from each other, and the benefits that accrue to each.

CHILDREN WITH DISABILITIES BECOME ADULTS WITH DISABILITIES

In treating children with disabilities and their families it is especially important to use a life-span approach. There are so few role models of adults-especially parents-with disabilities that parents of children with disabilities often have no vision of what their children can become. They need examples of adults with disabilities who work, are married, have families and friends, go to restaurants and movies, and lead contented lives. When professionals who work with these families likewise do not have models of well-functioning and fulfilled adults with disabilities, this reinforces the parents' own doubts and fears for their children. Professionals can present a more positive view of disability only if they are familiar with the disability community outside the clinical populations that are more familiar to them.

When I began family therapy with a preteen daughter with CP and her parents, the parents tended to scrutinize me intently, evaluating the similarities and differences between me and their daughter. They saw in front of them an adult who functioned well, had a husband and children, and who also had a visible physical disability. For the first time they were able to begin to visualize their daughter as an adult. This modeling, more perhaps than any of the content of the therapy, was a powerful turning point for these parents and underlies the importance of professionals who have personal experience with disability. It further highlights the need for access to role models not only for children with disabilities but for their families as well. Only in this way can parents develop visions of their children's futures. Yet in the literature about disability, with its focus on children, it is as if these children will never grow up.

To understand adults with disabilities it is necessary to consider some of the experiences of children with disabilities that will be relevant to them as adults. Adults who were once children with disabilities may have developmental trajectories that differ from those of children without disabilities. Their own parents may have greeted their birth (with disabilities) with insecurity, grief, depression, anxiety, sorrow, protectiveness, or even rejection. These emotions on the part of the parents could be expected to affect the parent–child relationship. However, this should not lead to the conclusion that the bond between children with disabilities and their parents is any less robust than for other families. Nor should we conclude that there is a "disabled personality"; "personality is too complex to be accounted for by one characteristic, even one with the global implications of deafness, blindness, or mobility limitation" (Meadow-Orlans, 1995, p. 65).

Nevertheless, there are some features of childhood with a disability that differ, starting at birth. For example, blind babies become unusually attentive to sound. Although they may initially lag in acquisition of language and fine and gross motor skills, this lag does not persist. Blindness affects those behaviors that are dependent on visual feedback, such as eye contact and facial expression of emotions. These alterations in non-verbal behaviors may make the person with blindness less attractive socially and romantically, with implications for dating. Children who are blind miss the nonverbal cues that accompany, and even alter the meaning of, communication. They are particularly restricted in learning about physical differences between genders because this type of learning depends on sight. Tactile exploration of others' bodies is prohibited. Thus several factors may interact to delay early exploration and practicing of romantic relationships. Deaf babies, on the other hand, gaze intently at their mother's face. If they are exposed to sign language early, they will develop sign communication as rapidly as hearing infants develop speech. Deaf babies receive more visual and tactile stimulation from their parents than do other infants. Deaf children tend to have higher self-esteem if their parents are deaf than if the parents are hearing, perhaps due to increased identification with parents and exposure to a deaf-affirming Deaf community. Hearing mothers of deaf children have been consistently described as more directive or intrusive (Meadow-Orlans, 1995), though several explanations have been proffered for such behavior. Girls with congenital disabilities seem to have an earlier mean age for onset of menarche. Thus sex education should begin earlier (but unfortunately usually is later or dispensed with altogether). Increased directiveness and protectiveness have been observed in mothers of babies with physical or sensory disabilities, but researchers have not made careful distinctions between these traits and appropriate parenting in light of the child's increased vulnerabilities to environmental risks. Children with disabilities may be less socialized to marriage and marital intimacy because they miss some input (in case of sensory impairments) and/or have less practice because of social stigma. Despite some of these differences, the overall development of children with disabilities is more like than unlike that of other children: "Human development is, in fact, remarkably resistant to a wide range of biological insults" (Kopp & Krakow, as cited in Meadow-Orlans, 1995, p. 61).

PARTNERS WITH DISABILITIES

For better or worse, for richer or poorer, in sickness and in health, I thee wed.[3] When a partnership is joined by a disability, the disability becomes the third part of a relationship triangle, an "uninvited guest that must be incorporated into the couple's lives" (Rolland, 1994, p. 235). Such partnerships are referred to in the literature as "preinjury marriages." The issues for these couples are different from those issues in a partnership formed between an able-bodied person and one who already has a disability, or between two people with disabilities. These partnerships are referred to as "postinjury marriages." These two groups are different populations, and the marital issues quite distinct, so this section has separate discussions of these two types of marriages. But first is a discussion of all partnerships with disabilities.

Any attempt to discuss such a general topic as "partners with disabilities" is nonsensical, as such partnerships vary enormously. Clearly other factors to consider include the ages and life stage of the couple and how long they've been together, the presence and number of children, other minority statuses such as those based on sexual orientation and ethnicity, the gender of both partners, and the culture and values of the couple. Not surprisingly, the couples' responses to the disability will have the greatest impact on the responses of the children (e.g., Kotchick, Forehand, Armistead, Klein, & Wierson, 1996).

Partners of people with disabilities experience discrimination and stigma by association and the same kinds of questions and assumptions as do people with disabilities. Some will assume that the disability came after the relationship began, presuming that an able-bodied person wouldn't choose to become involved with an already-disabled partner. Others will believe that the able-bodied partner must have low self-esteem to have "settled" for a partner with a disability. If both partners have disabilities, people often assume that this was the basis of the attraction, as if the shared characteristic of disability is sufficient grounds for marriage. For example, Crandell and Streeter (1977) state: "The commonality of blindness between two individuals brings security and a large number of common interests" (p. 2).

The able-bodied and person-with-a-disability partnership is a cross-cultural relationship. The able-bodied partner may or may not be a minority of another sort, but it is essential for the partnership that the able-bodied person be able to identify with disability issues and culture.

---

[3]There are no studies on gay partnerships with disabilities, excluding HIV or AIDS. The terms "marriage" and "spouse" are used here when referring to specific studies and "partner" when the issue is applicable to both heterosexual and same-gender relationships.

Such identification will include an understanding of the physical effects of disability, the need for accommodations, and a sensitivity to environmental and architectural barriers. It also means an appreciation of the fact that the most troublesome aspects of disability are psychosocial. Several authors stress the need for the couple to define the disability as belonging to them jointly (McNeff, 1997; Rolland, 1994) and the problems attendant to disability as mutual.

Although in some cases the able-bodied partner may be less satisfied in the marriage than is the partner with the disability (as was found in a highly selective sample of persons with MS and their spouses; Woollett & Edelmann, 1988), generally there is a positive correlation between the two partners' adjustment to disability (Feigin, 1994). The disabled person's self-concept, image, and integration of the disability may place a ceiling on the acceptability and integration of the disability in the partnership. Possibly the partnership cannot be more accepting of the disability than is the person with the disability him- or herself. This does not mean that people with disabilities must receive individual therapy prior to conjoint therapy. In fact, the partnership provides support and is a catalyst for integration of the disability into the self- and couple-concept.

Both McNeff (1997) and Rolland (1994) write that a couple is at risk if the chronic condition becomes a key aspect of the relationship, or if it invades the relationship. For example, Rolland writes: "Clinicians can help couples redirect their anger from the partner to the illness. Externalization is helpful in this regard" (p. 240). I disagree, perhaps due to the differences between "disability" and "illness or chronic condition." Recall the discussion in previous chapters about how there is not some essence of "you-ness" that is joined by a disability; disability becomes a part of the "you." Similarly, I believe a disability must be firmly entrenched as part of the couple's self-definition, and that externalizing the disability interferes with acceptance of the disability as a part of the person and the relationship. In the words of a woman with CP speaking on how to make a marriage work: "Be together; face up to the fact you're disabled and *live within it*" (cited in Miller & Morgan, 1980, p. 211; emphasis added). I agree with McNeff and Rolland that neither the person nor the partnership is equated with the disability, and that not allowing the disability to totally define the relationship is important. Rolland (1994) describes several useful ways of keeping a boundary between the relationship and the disorder, which he refers to as "establishing viable caregiving boundaries" (p. 245), and I would call containing the "spread" of the disability within the relationship.

Curiously, although society puts pressure on individuals with disabilities to take the lead in making others comfortable with that disability, in family relationships this seems to be reversed: The literature focuses almost exclusively on the role of the family helping the adult member to adjust to disability, and not the other way around. The individual partners, however, may experience very different pacing of response to the disability, creating what Rolland (1994) calls a "recovery skew" (p. 250). Thus clinicians should evaluate each *individual's* relationship to the disability, as well as the gestalt of the *family's* responses.

When Disability Joins a Marriage (Preinjury Marriages)

The partnership relationship is obviously a key variable in the recovery and rehabilitation of persons who incur a disability after the union is formed. A person's marital status is the most powerful predictor of independent living outcomes for persons with spinal cord injury (SCI) (McNeff, 1997) and the marital status and emotional quality of the relationship is an important factor in recovery of men with serious cardiac problems (Waltz, 1986). Yet there is scant information about such partnerships, and most of the work is on males who acquire an SCI and their wives. (For an exception, related to women who marry men with SCI, see Milligan & Neufeldt, 1998.)

A review of more than 13,000 publications from 1980 to 1990 on family support in rehabilitation (Kelly & Lambert, 1992) found only 40 that were data based, and only 4 on personal and family adjustment to disability. None of the articles examined family adjustment by studying both partners. A later study of married persons with MS found that degree of disability was unrelated to emotional or marital adjustment, but that overall the marriages were less well-adjusted, compared to a normative sample, on one measure of marital assessment (Rodgers & Calder, 1990). And a more recent study that did collect data from both partners after one had a stroke found that both partners were vulnerable to depression; 73% of the stroke patients (78% of whom were male) were depressed, as were 44% of the spouses (Stein, Gordon, Hibbard, & Sliwinski, 1992). Thus clinically it would seem that greater attention to the partnership dyad is critical to successful rehabilitation.

In addition to the scantiness of the data, there is a problem with the pervasive paradigm in which this work is conducted. The overriding model is that of stress (e.g., disability) leading to outcome (e.g., depression), as mediated by social support and coping. "Much previous research undertaken under the influence of the stress-coping paradigm has been focused on depression and dysphoric emotional states; too little work has focused on adaptive processes associated with positive feeling states" (Waltz, 1986; p. 792). As an alternative, Waltz (1986) suggested a two-factor model which focuses on both negative and positive affect domains. The latter includes daily uplifts, pleasant social interactions, and gratifying aspects of life. Being satisfactorily married is a robust determinant of happiness and life satisfaction, whereas the absence of close social bonds and intimacy are correlates of loneliness and emotional isolation. These two domains influence the outcome of disability response.

Assumptions of pathology are being increasingly challenged in the disability community. Furthermore, it is essential that studies of couples with disabilities incorporate information from the couples themselves (Turnbull & Turnbull, 1985). "The shift from the highly objective, scientific approach to families of disabled persons to a subjective, interpretivist approach is regarded . . . as a shift in paradigms of thought" (Wickham-Searl, 1992, p. 251). This shift must occur clinically as well.

The separation of partners when one incurs an injury or disability unwittingly begins with the disability onset. The medical staff, intensive-care nurses, physical therapists, rehabilitation team—all ignore the spouse (and especially partners of the same sex). Although the able-bodied partner is often in shock, exhausted, eating and sleeping poorly, and anxious or upset, he or she is made extraneous to the rehabilitation process; "these sacrifices are viewed as minimal compared to the suffering of the spouse who is newly disabled" (Miller, Houston, & Goodman, 1994, p. 47). The partner is usually told to go home. Yet soon the partner is expected to assume the role of treatment provider, caregiver, and social support for the person with the disability. Thus begins a process of defining the disability as belonging to the individual, a process that must be overcome for the partnership to be successful (Knight, 1989; Rolland, 1994) and to remain intact. But from the framework of family systems, the disability has happened to a partnership, not to an individual. We can no longer segregate the effects of the disability on the individual, the partner, or the relationship; they are inextricably entwined.

The role of the partnership cannot be overstated: "The marital dyad constitutes perhaps the most important social context within which the psychological aspects of chronic illness are managed" (Rodgers & Calder, 1990, p. 25). Pressure is put on the able-bodied partner—by society, family, and by him- or herself—to provide support, care, love, and affection for the partner with the new disability. This is not to say that the partner does not wish to provide these assets, just that doing so may strain personal and dyadic resources. Many people, including professionals, will reassure the able-bodied partner that there is much to be grateful for, that he or she is "lucky," that others are worse off. As Crewe (1993) points out, these are outsider observations. These exhortations, however well meaning, can serve to make the able-bodied partner feel more isolated, guilty about his or her emotions, and unsupported in the new roles taken on.

The early experiences with the disability onset can set up patterns that are hard to break. The able-bodied partner becomes a caregiver in the immediate aftermath of the disability yet may be excluded from informational meetings and decision making. Couples are emotionally vulnerable at this time, and the power differential between families and professionals has the potential to incur trauma for the family. Couples need direct and honest information in simple language. They may need this information repeated several times, as they are bombarded with stimuli. Professionals should avoid sweeping pronouncements (e.g., one female client with MS was told at diagnosis in her 30s that her sex life was over). The couple should be considered a team, not a patient and caregiver, and treated as such. They will require information about community and other resources, to know what is available and how to procure assistance. Simple acts such as giving a phone number along with a referral may mean the difference between a couple reaching out for help or not making the call.

There are conflicting reports about the correlation between disability and divorce, but married women who become disabled may be particularly vulnerable to divorce (Crewe, Athelstan, & Krumberger, 1979; Crewe & Krause, 1988). Women with polio were more likely than men with polio to be divorced (Nagi & Clark, cited in Peterson, 1979), and at least one study suggests that African Americans were also more vulnerable to postdisability divorce (Crewe, 1993). Persons with disabilities are less likely to be married if they are at lower SES levels (this is also true of persons without disabilities), making this group more vulnerable to institutionalization and other less positive rehabilitative outcomes (McNeff, 1997). Parker (1993) found that in one-third of the marriages that had survived at least 4 years after disability onset, one or both partners had considered ending the marriage. Rodgers & Calder (1990) found that 59% of married persons with MS had considered divorce. They also observed that if the marriage had declined since the MS onset, the decline was attributed to the MS, but if it got stronger, it was not attributed to MS. Disability imposes powerful restraints against divorce: finances, finding adequate care for the partner with the disability, social condemnation of the caregiver for the "abandonment." Not surprisingly, the quality of the marriage prior to the disability onset is probably the most potent predictor of separation and divorce. But the psychosocial sequelae of disability are considerable stressors, and these, plus a problematic rehabilitation and care delivery system, can topple precarious unions.

When disability joins a couple, predisability marital issues will be reflected in and accentuated by the disability issues. Marital happiness in couples with a disability is related to satisfaction with the exchange of positive behaviors and affect, positive communication patterns, and absence of hostility in the same way that it is for couples without disabilities. Positive aspects of a disability onset may include a drawing together of the partners, personal growth, positive changes in values, and greater emphasis on family and personal relationships. Negative effects may include stress, compromises to the well partner's health, financial upheaval and uncertainty, loss of shared activities, and assumption of unwanted tasks and responsibilities (Crewe, 1993).

Onset of disability in a partner causes disequilibrium in the relationship. Partners have to adjust to role reversals or take on new and additional roles. A rebalancing of the partnership is necessary. This rebalancing includes issues such as the amount of time together and apart, the closeness and distance in the relationship, the role of social activities, and the degree to which one is a caregiver versus a partner (see discussion later). The couple may need to develop new areas of mutual interest as old ones are rendered more difficult or impossible. Relationships that survive a disability onset have a higher degree of reciprocity in the relational adjustment than do those that dissolve (McNeff, 1997). In intimate relationships that are functional and satisfying, the tally of exchanges and reciprocity is invisible. But when the relationship becomes unbalanced these issues take a more prominent role, and one or both partners are likely to try to redress the imbalance. However, the options for redress may be limited by the physical aspects of the disability and by the demands of the caregiving role. One study (Rodgers & Calder, 1990) of married persons with MS found that 82% of the 104 respondents rated the ability to make major decisions as the most important variable (of 15 choices) in a successful marriage.

Disability makes more prominent and immediate the issues of vulnerability, mortality, loss, trust, roles, and values. For example, several authors have addressed participants' process of clarification or change in values related to the meaning of marriage (McNeff, 1997; Miller et al., 1994; Orona, 1989; Parker, 1993; Rodgers & Calder, 1990; Rolland, 1994; Vargo, 1983). A disability onset may cause partners to lose confidence in their ability for self-determination and control over the future. Couples may cling together or push apart. "In general, couples adapt best when they revise their closeness to include rather than avoid issues of incapacitation and threatened loss" (Rolland, 1994, p. 237).

Caregiving

As the number of physical tasks performed by the person with the disability decreases, the partner may pick up these tasks. This can create inequity, conflict, blame, guilt, dependence, resentment—all of which are anathema to intimacy and a sexual relationship (Knight, 1989). The partner as caregiver can arouse feelings of ambivalence for both parties. Several authors have noted that sex and caregiving may be inversely reciprocal (Crewe, 1993; Florian & Katz, 1991; Knight, 1989; McNeff, 1997), especially when caregiving involves more intimate personal toiletry and grooming tasks that one doesn't associate with a sexual partner. The balance in the relationship between the roles of caregiver and intimate partner may differ from couple to couple, but in general "sustaining intimacy predominantly depends on creating viable caregiving boundaries" (McNeff, 1997, p. 597).

Spouses who marry before the disability onset are more likely to be providing personal care than are spouses married after the disability onset, even holding the level of impairment constant (McNeff, 1997). Yet government systems that provide financial support of personal attendant care (PCA) will not pay spouses to provide help. Thus spouses may do double duty of maintaining a household income and providing care to the partner (Crewe, 1993).

Both carers and partners with disabilities have to come to some understanding within themselves of this new type of relationship. In a study of 21 couples that had one partner with a disability (Parker, 1993), the caregivers had several means of coming to terms with their role. They valued how the partner coped with the disability and with pain and felt that this cost to the partner partially redressed imbalance in the relationship. However, if this feeling tipped over into pity for the spouse, the pity changed the relationship in fundamental and negative ways. Couples also compared themselves favorably to other, hypothetical relationships ("Other couples might not have survived what we've been through"), allowing a self-valuing, seeing the self as special. Caregivers told themselves that the spouse would do the same for them, were the tables turned. Over half the caregivers, men and women similarly, spoke of their duty or responsibility to be a caregiver. It is not clear if or how these findings translate into clinical guidelines. Perhaps we should be helping partners define their roles as important and of value (i.e., concentrating on the macro level of definition of the relationship rather than on the micro level of tasks).

Gender Differences

Gender differences in response to disability in self or partner are pronounced and hence are critical to an understanding of the issues for any couple (Crewe, 1993; McNeff, 1997; Parker, 1993; Rolland, 1994). Men and women have different skills and preferences regarding dealing with loss, coping, use of social supports, role flexibility, meaning of illness, rights and privileges of being sick, relationship to family, notions of equity and fairness, propensity for anxiety or depressive disorders, and willingness to hire outside help. For example, husbands are more likely than wives to hire someone to pick up the tasks vacated by the impaired spouse, and hence they experience less role strain (Beckham & Giordano, 1986). Wives, when impaired, have more contact with children and higher involvement with relatives than do men with impairments. Moreover, wives performing caregiving tasks for husbands are not seen to be taking on an additional role, as caregiving is thought of as a female role (Parker, 1993). Thus, the wife's enormous contributions to her husband's care, and the role strain, may not be observed by others as much as it would be if the roles were reversed. Women with disabilities are more likely to express sadness or guilt about the "burden" they feel they impose on their husbands.

Aging

A high percentage of aging couples live independently as two-person families, and more than a third of older people are married and living with spouses (Beckham & Giordano, 1986). These statistics, coupled with more recent increases in longevity, mean that many older couples will experience onset of illness or impairment in their relationship. Often the more well partner will take on caregiving tasks, and the presence of a partner is a major factor in preventing institutionalization. The caregiver is more likely to be female, as women tend to marry older men and men have higher rates of activity limitations at all ages compared to women. One author (cited in Beckham & Giordano, 1986) suggested that "the main effect of health on older marriages is to turn wives into part-time nurses" (p. 258). This may happen just at the time the couple was looking forward to enjoying increased leisure, greater financial security, perhaps travel, and release from childrearing.

Cognitive Disabilities

Many conditions can cause alterations in cognitive abilities and in personality. Traumatic brain injury (TBI) is one such cause, and one that is more likely to occur to men, usually leaving wives in the caregiving role. One of the difficulties with cognitive impairments is a paradox: To adapt, the person has to make cognitive and behavioral changes and alter coping mechanisms, yet the impairments affect the cognitive resources to make these changes. Thus the function disruption is greater than might be expected from a list of specific deficits. When the cognitive executive function is impaired, the total impact is greater than the cumulative effects of the separate deficits. Families, especially wives, report the greatest degree of disturbance when disability causes changes to cognitive functioning and personality.

There is widespread agreement about the difficulties of cognitive impairments for the partnership: "The impact of cognitive and personality changes on spousal relationships is almost certainly more troublesome than physical disability alone" (Crewe, 1993, p. 148). "I'm married, but I really don't have a husband" (Mauss-Clum & Ryan, as cited in Jackson & Haverkamp, 1991, p. 357). "Conditions involving permanent cognitive impairment are among the most challenging for couples to face" (McNeff, 1997, p. 598). "Losses suffered by the debilitating effects of head injuries, stroke, or central nervous system dysfunction can be conceptualized as partial death" (Miller, Houston, & Goodman, 1994, p. 50). "The very essence of the person with whom one has shared a life gradually begins to fade" (Orona, 1989, p. 60).

Under these circumstances, wives emotionally disengage from the marriage, feel less marital vulnerability (dependency and fear of abandonment by spouse), and redefine their role as caregiver rather than wife (Florian & Katz, 1991). Yet they are in a state of marital limbo: "Spouses cannot honourably get divorced with a clear conscience" (Lezak, as cited in Florian & Katz, 1991, p. 272). Florian and Katz (1991) cite this as an ethical dilemma for the clinician—who is the client (the couple, or one of the spouses?), and whose best interests are they to serve?

In a study by Rosenbaum and Najenson (cited in Crewe, 1993), wives in Israel whose husbands had either brain injury or SCI, it was the brain injury, not injury per se, that led wives to describe husbands as more childlike, self-oriented, and dependent. Husbands with brain injury played a reduced role in raising children. There was a drastic decrease in sexual activity, and the wives of husbands with TBI reported disliking sexual contact with their husbands. Of interest was the finding that wives reported increased contact with in-laws yet did not feel close or supported. This study may highlight one of the troublesome aspects of relationships in which disability incurs cognitive or personality changes. Parents are likely to be more tolerant of regressive behavior in their adult child, they have a smaller sampling of behaviors compared to the spouse, and they more comfortably fall back into old patterns of parent–child relating. Thus their relationship with the adult child is not as fundamentally altered. Interestingly, however, mothers, compared with wives, were more unrealistic in their expectations for the adult child with TBI; mothers may be used to the role of holding hope and encouragement for their children.

Florian and Katz (1991) recommend treatment that includes accurate information and support, establishment of realistic goals, behavioral management techniques, coping skills, sexual counseling, and functional and practical assistance (e.g., respite care, referrals, advocacy, legal and financial assistance, medical care, evaluation for appropriate assistive technology, and help in procuring it). In addition, families need help relabeling the problems (e.g., inattention may be due to distractibility and may not connote rejection). They advocate strongly for attendant care: "This care should be provided by paid attendants and not by family members. This is extremely important in the case of wives" (p. 276).

In an interesting and refreshing take on the topic of caregiving for partners, Orona (1989) discusses the moral implications of one's actions as the caregiver and the process by which one makes a moral commitment to provide care for the partner with AIDS or Alzheimer's. This includes how one enters that role: (1) by entrapment or coercion, (2) by explicit agreement or consent, or (3) by assumption of the role without questioning it (the most usual way). Although other social supports can bolster the caregiver, "fulfilling the moral commitment is ultimately an individual act" (p. 61). What is being asked of the caregiver is a practical translation of moral values: "Each caregiver has to encounter him- or herself in the process and ask, 'What kind of person am I in this situation?'" (p. 61). Then, "once the mantle of moral responsibility is accepted, it permeates the everyday world . . . with each act of care, the caregiver is faced, day in and day out, with the moral choice of reaffirming commitment" (p. 62). Under times of chronic stress, people sink or swim. What is amazing is that so many people stay afloat.

Therapeutic Tasks

The task of the therapist is to walk a fine line: The therapist must have "respect for those unique coping mechanisms" of the couple while simultaneously "confront[ing] and chang[ing] aspects of the adjustment that are not working or are dysfunctional" (McNeff, 1997, p. 611). Competence in this area requires training and skills in couple therapy plus expertise in disability, pronounced affective states (e.g., anger, loss, grief), and sexuality. Group counseling or support groups can provide empathy, support, advocacy, and exchange of ideas and information in a way that individual or conjoint therapy cannot. But other issues may require more intensive therapeutic intervention. Reestablishing emotional intimacy, romance, and sexuality postdisability onset demands honest, open, and clear communication and incorporation of the disability into the concept of the self and the couple. Couples need (but seldom receive) information about the effects of the disability on sexuality in matter-of-fact but simple language, with a focus on the remaining, rather than lost, functions. The transformed sexuality must incorporate the new lifestyle accompanying the disability, possibly including bowel and bladder training, grooming habits, and body image. Without sufficient attention to these multiple factors, a mutually satisfying sexual relationship is less likely to be reestablished. And as is often the case in our society, when sexuality is lessened, other aspects of physical closeness, such as cuddling, kissing, or holding hands, also decline, resulting in less emotional intimacy in the relationship. Loss of sexuality is less devastating to a relationship than is loss of these other types of physical gestures (Parker, 1993; Rodgers & Calder, 1990).

When a Person with a Disability Gets Married (Postinjury Marriages)

A study on hierarchy of acceptability of 13 specific disabilities (Olkin & Howson, 1994) inquired about the willingness to be in various levels of social distance from persons with disabilities (e.g., live next door to or marry). Many respondents wrote in the margin that they would not choose to marry someone with a disability, but if they were already married to someone who incurred a disability that would be all right. This is curious because there are hints that postinjury marriages are stronger, and rated as more satisfying, than are marriages that have already taken place prior to the onset of the disability (preinjury marriages).

Work status is a robust predictor of marriage for persons with SCI. Those working are much more likely to get married (about 50% at 11-year follow-up) than those who are not (about 20%). Those who subsequently married also went out more often socially, rated their own overall adjustment as higher, and were more satisfied with their social and sexual lives, living arrangements, control over their lives, and general health (Crewe & Krause, 1988, 1990, 1992).

Couples who get together after the onset of a disability in one partner may have certain attributes that make them different from other couples with and without disabilities. Compared to couples in preinjury marriages, those in postinjury marriages are more likely to be inner-directed and have better marital adjustment, to be more socially active, to have higher levels of educational achievement, and to be working (Crewe & Krause, 1988). Spouses in postinjury marriages probably "have unusual qualities or values that contribute to the success of these unions" (Crewe & Krause, 1988, p. 438). These qualities may include independence, maturity, ability to see beyond society's stereotypes and look beyond stigma, and better communication skills.

A neglected area of research is how persons with disabilities meet potential romantic partners, their dating experiences, and selection of significant others. Most of the research in this area has been conducted by persons without disabilities (Yoshida, 1994). Selection of a partner who can deal with the life of someone with a disability is essential for a happy relationship, yet we know so little about how this process occurs from the vantage point of either the person with or the person without the disability. Parents and family may disapprove of their able-bodied adult child dating someone with a disability, but the parents of the person with the disability may also be disapproving (Miller & Morgan, 1980). (For more discussion of dating and romance, see Chapter 10, in this volume.)

Gay and Lesbian Partners with Disabilities

Disability is often studied out of context of other variables in a relationship. One such variable is the sexual orientation of the partners. Gay and lesbian couples experience a cumulative effect of dual stigmatized conditions. It is possible for such couples to feel isolated or ostracized in both the gay and the disability communities. And if the disability is not one visible to others, there are two conditions about which the couple must make a choice to be "out."

The onset of a disabling condition in a gay or lesbian partner may force the relationship to be more public than it had been. At a time of potential crisis, the couple may be faced with new arenas in which they are identified as a couple. One of these may be the families of origin, which may not have had direct dealings with their child as part of a gay partnership. Health professionals and care providers cannot be relied on to be accepting of a gay relationship, and the tendency to exclude spouses from discussions, decisions, and treatment planning is even more pronounced for same-gender partners.

Logistical concerns may be more pronounced in this population. The newly disabled partner may not be covered under the other person's insurance, and the able-bodied partner may not be eligible for family leave policies or survivor benefits. Concerns about confidentiality, especially from insurance and employers, may be paramount. Policies on hospital visits and who can make critical medical decisions may not recognize gay partnerships. And families of origin may contest custody of children and try to block visitation. In short, such couples have, in addition to all the issues attendant to disability acquisition, another layer of potentially complicating and difficult factors, all converging at a time of great vulnerability. On a positive note, such couples also may have access to growing gay and disability communities to provide social, emotional, and practical support.

Conclusions about Partners with Disabilities

The severity of impairment is not the predominant factor in either individual or couple response. Other factors are much more salient in determining how a couple handles a disability. There are some hints that more pronounced manifestations of impairment can be easier to accommodate than those that are less visible or tangible. In the former case, the roles are better defined, being cared for becomes more acceptable, and humanitarian responses more likely. However, severity of disability is not directly related to marital satisfaction, whether the disability occurs prior to or after the marriage.

The needs and readiness for change of any couple wax and wane over time. Points of particular stress— and hence need—are at disability onset and at times of disability exacerbation (Rodgers & Calder, 1990). The type of interventions must be appropriate to the family's stage of development and their responses to the disability. Practitioners should be prepared to be available on the couple's timetable, to repeat sessions as needs change, and to provide references and other information when requested. Providing services in a consolidated setting, avoiding fragmentation among agencies and providers (such as medical, rehabilitative, legal, financial, and family counseling) should be a treatment goal. The ultimate treatment goal is to enhance individual and family functioning while maintaining an appropriate level of suitable interventions and care for the person with the disability. At least one study (Parker, 1993) indicates the importance of talking about the disability, and even joking. We don't often think of joking as a therapeutic intervention, but it is one that can play an important part in the lives of people during stress. And we would also do well to remember, as Rolland (1994) says, that "not all thoughts need to be communicated" (p. 239). As Parker (1993) points out, one cannot legislate happiness in a marriage, but it is possible to ensure that couples encountering impairment have adequate and appropriate supports available.

In reviewing the literature about disability and family functioning I felt a nagging worry about the coping literature and its impact on helping professionals. We are developing a perspective entrenched in labeling coping "good" (active) or "bad" (avoidant). For example, Kotchick et al. (1996) state that families should be made aware of the adverse effects of using avoidant coping strategies, such as denial, eating or sleeping more, or using alcohol or other drugs. The pressure we put on couples not only to cope but to cope correctly too easily pathologizes people who are doing the best they know how under trying circumstances. This is not to argue with findings that some types of coping are more likely to lead to positive health outcomes than are others. But our research findings are becoming dogma by which we judge our clients.

PARENTS WITH DISABILITIES

There are approximately 8 million families with children under 18 who have one or more parent with a disability—just under 11% of all families in the United States (La Plante et al., 1992; Toms-Barker & Maralani, 1997). The percentages are higher for African American (over 18%) and Hispanic (over 16%) families. Yet these families seem invisible. Parenting services ignore disability needs; disability services neglect parenting needs. One has only to look at the array of assistive devices available for persons with disabilities to see that such persons are not expected to be parents. I had to invent an infant carrier for my electric scooter. In searching for a van to accommodate my scooter and my family it was clear that manufacturers had considered only the former need; to fit the scooter in I had to give up too much seating for family needs. At day care the accessible entrance goes into a classroom; the front entrance where parents enter and sign their children in and out is inaccessible. Yet clearly people with disabilities are parents, and this group is expected to grow as more general rights are accorded persons with disabilities and they enter the mainstream of society in greater numbers.

What do we know about parents with disabilities? In brief, very little. Despite thousands of studies since the 1920s on children with disabilities, "there is little research on their subsequent family lives as adults" (Meadow-Orlans, 1995, p. 67). One reason is that funding is more apt to support research on children with disabilities, and if on adults, then on their vocational or rehabilitation adjustment rather than on family processes or parenting. The goals of research on parents with disabilities should be considered; studies can be used variously to confirm pathologizing hypotheses about such parents and their families, help policymakers, direct funding and other resources to where they can best be utilized, and get information into the hands of parents with disabilities. For example, a study may indicate that some percentage of mothers with visual impairments have, at some point in the first 6 years of their children's lives, given the wrong amount of medication to the child as a result of difficulties with measuring the medicine. This information could be used to justify discouraging women with visual impairments from becoming parents, set policies against adoption by blind women, prompt local governments to make poison control phone numbers more available to persons with visual impairments, provide impetus for the Food and Drug Administration to set standards for tactile markings on all bottles of medicine for children, and generate practical tips for dealing with this issue and collect these suggestions on a cassette of information for new mothers with visual impairments.

One of the main books on parents with disabilities (Thurman, 1985) is out of print, and a literature search yields relatively few articles, most based on opinions or methodologically flawed data. It is as if families have children with disabilities and then these children disappear from the face of the earth. A second problem in the literature is that reports on parents with mental retardation are often generalized to parents with physical disabilities. For example, a recent article, "Child Abuse and Neglect by Parents with Disabilities" (Greene, Norma, Searle, Daniels, & Lubeck, 1995), is in actuality about two families in which the mothers had mental retardation. This perennial pairing in the literature of "parents with disabilities" and problems in children perpetuates a widely held belief by professionals that disability in a parent inevitably negatively affects the children. "Research has tended to involve the search for the negative impact of an adult's disability on a child's growth, intelligence and adjustment" (Olsen, 1996, p. 41). Buck and Hohmann (1983) note that "the literature review reveals the widespread belief among professionals that disability severely limits parenting ability and often leads to maladjustment in children" (p. 233). They aptly critique the significant shortcomings of the literature on parents with disabilities. Among the more major flaws is the confusion between disability and illness, acute episodes (e.g., hospitalization) and chronic factors, cognitive and physical disabilities, and correlation versus causation. Further, many subjects for these studies were sampled from clinical populations.

A more well-controlled study on fathers with SCI (Buck, 1980, Buck & Hohmann, 1981, 1982), using controls matched on sex, father's age, and socioeconomic variables, failed to find any association between fathers' disability (or severity of disability, paraplegia vs. quadriplegia) and maladjustment in children. Children of fathers with SCI were no more likely to show evidence of difficulties in sex roles, body image, values, health patterns, interpersonal relationships, or interest and participation in sports. The fathers with SCI "expressed affection both verbally and physically toward their children significantly more often than did able-bodied fathers" and therefore, not surprisingly, "children with SCI fathers actually reported significantly more positive attitudes toward their fathers than did comparison children (e.g., love, respect, pride)" (Buck & Hohmann, 1983, p. 223). Disturbingly, over a dozen years later, more recent reviews of the literature on parents with disabilities (Cohen, 1998; Conley-Jung, 1996; Olsen, 1996) indicate that the state of the literature is still driven by pathologizing assumptions and seriously flawed methodologies. The children are viewed as "victims"; such a view carries the danger of "implicit and explicit criticism of disabled parents, their values, their choices and even their right to have children at all" (Olsen, 1996, p. 42). Thus it is still necessary (much like for gay and lesbian parents) to have research demonstrating that there are no ill effects of a parent's disability per se on the children. Two such studies come from my students' dissertations on latency-age children of mothers with disabilities (Cohen, 1998) and new mothers with visual impairments (Conley-Jung, 1996). Disability alone was not a predictor of problems or difficulties in the children. This is not to suggest that disability was irrelevant. The mothers cited numerous ways in which their disabilities impacted parenting, but most of the mothers thought and planned carefully such that any increased difficulties were borne by the mother and not the child. (See Table 5.2 for illustrative examples of baby-care situations affected by one type of disability—visual impairment in the mother.) Of great importance is that approximately 10% of these mostly middle- to upper-class mothers experienced active interference in their becoming mothers (e.g., steps to remove the child or pressure to have an abortion). Of course, factors that impede good parenting in all parents—such as history of physical or sexual abuse, substance use in family of origin, separation from parents—were also important predictors of parenting quality for parents with disabilities. Studies on such parents must elicit information on these family-of-origin factors to avoid ascribing all parenting difficulties to the disability.

Further data on the topic come from two sources: a national survey of parents with disabilities (Toms-Barker & Maralani, 1997) and a report from a national task force on parents with disabilities and their families (Kirshbaum & Preston, 1998). Both of these were conducted under the aegis of Through the Looking Glass (a nonprofit agency in Berkeley serving families with disabilities). Key issues for parents with disabilities are (1) their legal rights, including whether the ADA applies to parenting; (2) the effect of disability on custody and adoption hearings (e.g., the absence of disability-appropriate measures and norms); (3) transportation needs (e.g., paratransit services usually limit the number of passengers allowed to ride with the person with the disability, such that a mother could not take her two children to the pediatrician); (4) the accessibility and adequacy of services related to family planning, pregnancy, and birthing (e.g., little is known about the effects of childbirth on disabilities); (5) adaptive parenting equipment (e.g., assistive devices such as wheelchairs should have adaptations to allow accessibility for children, and general baby-care equipment such as changing tables). (See also Chapter 12, in this volume, for information on adaptive parenting equipment.)

TABLE 5.2. Activities Affected by Mother's Visual Impairment

Activity	Sample of issues	Possible solutions
Changing diapers	Noticing wetness; keeping baby on the changing table; dealing with diaper closures; finding all necessities; noticing diaper rash; getting baby sufficiently clean; getting feedback from last diaper as to better placement of diaper and tightness.	Preplan changing area with each item in its own predesignated place; prefold diapers without baby on changing table; use touch to feel for wetness and leaking; increase frequency of baby baths to ensure baby is clean and to reduce chance of diaper rash.
Monitoring baby's whereabouts	Knowing where baby is in the house once baby is mobile; ensuring baby is not in unsafe situation; keeping baby at one's side when outside.	Bells on baby; noisemakers in key areas (e.g., in front of fireplace); gates; safety latches on usual places plus on toilets; using a baby harness; have toddler hold one end of blanket and mother holds the other; hold hands.
Transportation	Using public transportation as a new mother; keeping track of baby, baby equipment, and baby bag; knowing which bus stop is correct place to get off.	Prepractice routes; count stops to correct stop; remind drivers to announce stops; take only small outings around neighborhood until comfort level and confidence increase; minimize items taken and preorganizing bag.
School	Reading myriad communications from school to home; getting phone numbers of child's friends from school directory; helping child with homework without access to teacher's instructions; reading grade reports.	Get teachers to give oral reports over the phone or in after-school meetings; save missives until friend or relative or partner can read them; develop own directory in large print or Braille, or scan directory into computer (for enlargement or voice).
Health	Taking temperature; giving medicine; getting to pediatrician's office.	Use talking thermometers; mark a bottle with tape or nail polish to indicate ounces; choose doctor near public transportation stop; use paratransit.
Feeding	Starting solid foods; feeding baby solids without knowing where baby's mouth is; cleaning baby, high chair, and surrounding area.	Touch baby's mouth for guidance; make first solids more liquidy and put them in baby bottles with enlarged nipple holes; wait until baby can guide mother's hand; use more finger foods rather than spooning foods.
Cleaning	Keeping house clean and organized.	Hire someone; designate areas for items (e.g., mail); develop system to reduce clutter and teach it to children.

In addition, the National Task Force Report identified several areas of further need among parents with disabilities: six key recommendations were to (1) increase public awareness and information ... to decrease attitudinal barriers against parents with disabilities; (2) increase options for and access to child care; (3) provide accessible and adequate housing options for parents with disabilities; (4) provide accessible and adequate transportation options for disabled parents traveling with their children; (5) alter regulations regarding the use of personal assistance services for child care (for example, currently a personal attendant could cook the mother a meal and even feed her, but not cook for nor serve the child); and (6) include parenting as an Activity of Daily Living and provide assistance with daily parenting activities.

As illustrated by these recommendations, there is a complexity and range of needs of parents with disabilities and their families. These needs interact with and are compounded by other factors such as SES, ethnicity, and whether the family lives in an urban or rural setting. A family is likely to be faced with multiple barriers which interrelate and have a cumulative impact.

In sum, there are tremendous barriers for parents with disabilities. These include attitudinal as well as physical and legal barriers. Some of the observations described here may be useful to clinicians in treating their clients with disabilities who are parents. (For a description of some specific issues for parents who are deaf or blind or who have SCI or MS, see Kirshbaum & Rinne, 1985.)

1. Everything takes longer. Whether it's a blind father diapering his infant, a mother with a physical disability dressing her toddler, or a father with paraplegia cooking a family dinner, many parenting activities take longer. Parents often joke about "crip time"—a more relaxed and leisurely pace. But this pacing may in fact have a positive benefit, which is to give added time to an intimate connection between parent and child. For example, a mother with a visual impairment who doesn't drive uses the time she spends walking her son to his destination to chat with him. This altered pace is a feature of disability culture that clinicians should recognize.

2. Parents with disabilities seem to rely on voice and words in setting limits for their children, disciplining them, and helping them with disability-related issues. For example, I taught my children from a very young age (about 2) that they must always be within voice range as I could not chase after them. Even when they tested every other limit, they obeyed this one. This seems to be a common theme among parents with disabilities—the really important potential problems (such as running away) are corrected early and fail to become difficulties. But the children

will test other limits, as do all children. For example, the son of a blind mother would turn on the TV without the sound to see if he could get away with it.

3. The role of adaptive equipment for parents with disabilities cannot be overemphasized. A mother who uses crutches must find a way to carry her baby from room to room. She can use a baby carrier, but this may throw her balance off and she may not be able to support the weight. Some use a sturdy stroller which can hold baby and support mother as she walks, or use a wheelchair and carry the baby in a pack or a baby seat. No parent should be evaluated on parenting skills until he or she has adopted successful adaptations and assistive devices (Kirshbaum, 1988). Otherwise all that is being evaluated is a physical limitation without accommodation. For some parents, finding and procuring appropriate adaptive equipment can mean the difference between keeping custody of their children or not.

4. Parents are able to design a style of parenting to accommodate their own disabilities. But their authority and competence are sorely tested and judged by schools that mostly failed to accommodate their needs as parents with disabilities. Parents, especially mothers, feel judged harshly by other parents for common and slight mistakes. Many parents feel that their child must be cleaner and better behaved than others or they will be seen as inadequate parents unable to attend to their children's daily needs. This pressure to be "super-Mom" (or Dad) is felt constantly. One coping mechanism is for a parent with a disability to go into the classroom and teach about disability. This is possible in grade school when there is one teacher and class. However, by middle school there are too many teachers for this to continue, and the practice may cease, ironically just as the peer relationships become more important to the child.

5. After-school social activities are likely to be an area affected by a parent's disability. In the case of visual impairments getting children to and from activities is a problem. For parents with physical disabilities issues of time and fatigue are prominent. Parents are forced to make hard choices about how to expend their time and energy, and the disability imposes limits. Parental fatigue is often an issue for the children; children always seem to have so much more energy than do parents, but for parents with physical disabilities the discrepancy can be pronounced and accommodations have to be made. For example, I do countless projects with my kids (candle making, decoupage, making lamps, holiday decorations) because mostly I can sit in one spot and do these with them. I was less apt to take them on outings until they were mobile on their own, could fasten and unfasten their seatbelts, and help carry the myriad stuff that seems to accompany children.

6. Children at some point imitate a parent's disability. For example,

a 5-year-old child may play a common pretend game of closing the eyes and stumbling about with arms outstretched, even though the child knows that the blind parent does not behave this way. My daughter puts her dolls in wheelchairs. But this is developmentally normal, no different than a son who imitates his father shaving, and does not imply any body image difficulties.

7. As grownups, the children of parents with disabilities may connect with other such grown children. They have become members of the disability community by association. Parents with disabilities often note that their children seem more aware of and sensitive to individual differences. For example, my son will note public places that are inaccessible, or the absence of other persons with disabilities in public.

8. It is common for the parent with a disability to note that the children seem to take the disability matter of factly. Infants learn early to accommodate to their parents' physical needs, for example, creeping up the wheelchair to assist the parent in lifting the baby. Babies as young as 1 month have been observed to make accommodations for their parents' abilities, and to make distinctions between disabled and nondisabled caretakers; with the latter they "behave less cooperatively, exhibiting fewer adaptations" (Kirshbaum, 1988, p. 10). In an analysis of videotaped interactions between mothers with disabilities and their babies (Kirshbaum, 1988), there appears to be a sequence of mutual adaptations between mothers with disabilities and their babies. For example, mothers signal an intention (e.g., intention to lift the baby signaled by tugging on the front of the baby's clothes) accompanied by an incomplete action (not actually lifting baby). This signals baby to make accommodations (curling up into a small ball), which allows the mother to complete the action (of lifting). Such sequences were observed repeatedly, and over time this adaptive reciprocity dance became more developed.

9. All parents seem to come equipped with a readiness for guilt about their children. When the parent has a disability the disability can become a convenient hook on which to hang the guilt. Thus parents themselves may not be good judges of the impact of their disabilities on their children. For example, when my son did not want to accompany me to the camp at which we had such a good time a year ago, I assumed he was getting to the age where he didn't want to be seen with a mother with a disability. It turns out he just didn't want to be seen with a mother; it was no longer cool to hang out with Mom, and the disability had nothing to do with it.

10. Although a parent with a disability may request assistance in performing some tasks, the generational hierarchy of parent and child, whereby the parent provides love, care, and guidance, remains intact.

For example, a child reading the directions on the back of a cake mix to his blind mother in no way reverses the essential family structure (see the section on "Parentification").

11. For all its difficulties, being a parent with a disability brings with it the same joys and rewards that having children brings to any parent. The essential functions of parenting—bonding, loving, nurturing, guiding—remain relatively unaffected by physical or sensory disabilities. Babies are born with a propensity to love their parents; disability does not impede this imprinting.

Parentification

There is a general image of parents with disabilities as "dependent and selfish in their needs for assistance from their children" (Olsen, 1995, p. 47). Thus one area of special interest has to do with the notion of "parentification." Parentification refers to the idea that children, in the absence of appropriate parental and adult figures, will take on psycho-emotional or caregiving tasks at inappropriately young ages. First applied to the children of alcoholic parents, this notion has been freely applied to siblings and children of persons with disabilities. For example, a Behavioral Science Book Service review of a recent book, *Lost Childhoods* (Jurkovic, 1997) says that the process of creating parentified children "is found in families experiencing such diverse crises as . . . *physical or emotional disability*" (emphasis added). In fact, virtually nothing is known about the tasks—or their nature, frequency, and intensity—that children of parents with disabilities perform because of the parent's disability, nor the gender and age of these children. Yet a pervasive assumption is that parents, limited by their physical disabilities or overwhelmed by the caregiving tasks associated with raising a child, will overrely on their able-bodied child for tasks that burden that child at too young an age. There are four problems with this assumption. First, it is a highly prejudicial assumption that leads to a pathological lens through which research and clinical work is conducted, doing a great disservice to the population it supposedly serves. The continual conflation of physical, cognitive, and psychiatric disabilities has led to generalizations across disabilities that are invalid. This conflation has resulted in an assumption that parents with physical or sensory disabilities lack the psychic structures necessary for parenting. Second, these assumptions are not supported by the literature. In fact, at least one study (Cohen, 1998) that paid more careful attention to the issue of burden found the opposite—that parents with disabilities take great care not to overburden their children because of the parent's disability, perhaps even erring in the other direction. In the Buck study on children of fathers with SCI, data on the issue of helping indicate that "although children reported helping SCI fathers more than able-bodied fathers, they did not resent providing aid to their fathers" (Buck & Hohmann, 1983, p. 223). Third, there are no normative data on how children help and what chores and tasks children do, so deciding what is overburdensome is presumptuous. Fourth, there are great cultural and socioeconomic differences in the expectations for children's helping behaviors.

However, we cannot simply dismiss the issue. Anecdotal clinical evidence (M. Kirshbaum, 1997, personal communication) certainly indicates that in some instances very young children (e.g., age 3) are performing personal caregiving tasks to parents (e.g., bathing a parent or changing a parent's diapers) in the absence of suitable levels of resources and support for getting these needs met in other ways (e.g., through personal attendant services). We need to be thoughtful in our approach to this issue. A distinction must be made between those tasks necessitated by disability and those by other factors such as poverty, unemployment, social class, or number of children in the household. Factors to be considered in evaluating the appropriateness of the child performing the task are (1) the age and developmental level of the child being asked to perform the task; (2) the nature of the task itself; (3) the symbolic meaning of the task; (4) whether the task causes any pain or discomfort to the parents; (5) the frequency the child performs the task; (6) if the child is the sole person performing the task and/or has primary responsibility for ensuring it is done; (7) the consequences of *not* performing the task; (8) the degree of support the child has in performing the task; (9) the relationship of the child to the person for whom the task is performed; (10) the roles of the other able-bodied members of the house; (11) time of day or night the task must be completed; (12) the total number of such tasks; and (13) any positive benefits to the child for performing the task. For example, in one study (Baldwin, 1997) some siblings of technology-dependent children reported performing caregiving tasks for that child. One child noted with pride that his friends are amazed that he knows how to clean and feed the sibling (through a tracheostomy). However, another child reported doing catheterization on an opposite-sex sibling. These two tasks may be quite similar on most of the dimensions listed here but differ critically on the nature and the symbolic meaning of the task in some fundamental way that substantially alters the nature of the task; hence one may be seen as appropriate and the other not. We should not decide this appropriateness only on theoretical grounds but should carefully collect data to be evaluated with open minds. If children are performing caregiving tasks inappropriately, the problem may lie with the family, but it also is likely to stem from inadequate resources to meet needs. Such a problem is probably best addressed by social policy and the service delivery system, not by pathologizing the population affected. It seems that families attempt to differentiate among the three related but quite distinct concepts of parentification, responsibility, and interdependence. The latter two are emphasized whereas the former is to be avoided. "We need to be careful of assuming that the caring tasks themselves deprive children of what would otherwise be a 'normal' childhood" (Olsen, 1996, p. 46).

Conclusions about Parents with Disabilities

It is common for able-bodied persons to view physical disability as predominantly a physical experience, that is, to focus on the interference the physical condition imposes on performing tasks and functions—a deficit model. Conversely, persons with disabilities often cite societal and interpersonal barriers as the greater challenge. This difference in perspective is apparent in the literature on parents with disabilities. This literature emphasizes functions and tasks of parents and has not made a distinction between *usual* versus *essential* functions of a parent. This distinction parallels a key issue in the independent living movement; rehabilitation has traditionally focused on increased physical functioning and ability to perform tasks independently, whereas the independent living movement maintains that one can require a full-time PCA and still be considered "independent." Independence is the ability to maintain choice, control, and decision-making over one's life (e.g., to hire, fire, and direct the PCA).

Parents with disabilities have been defined ipso facto as a "problem" requiring study. For example, the purpose of one recent study (LeClere & Kowalewski, 1994) was to "examine the impact of disability among all co-resident family members on children's severe and common behavioral problems and their probability of suffering an accident, injury, or poisoning in the previous year" (p. 457). This pathologizing focus has led to a narrow lens through which such parents and families are examined, and the purpose of most studies is to illuminate the deficits of these parents. Few have asked why these parents are worthy of study to begin with, much less why they are assumed to be problem parents. Certainly the studies are rarely done for the benefit of the families themselves (e.g., to improve service delivery or to design better assistive equipment). As Olsen (1996) says, "seeking to research the relationship between children's responsibilities and adult disability is a political activity, and should be sensitive to broader arguments about autonomy, disability, and disadvantage" (p. 47). Repeatedly studies of parents with various conditions (e.g., mental illness and learning disabilities) find that it is the existence of multiple, cumulative, and synergistic sources of stress that is the more significant factor associated with children's wellbeing, not any individual condition in a parent.

There seems to be a gap in the theoretical literature regarding parents with disabilities. In general, disability is posited as a disruption or distortion of normal developmental processes rather than a parallel or alternate, albeit perfectly "normal," life progression. For the most part persons with disabilities are more like than unlike able-bodied persons. And as with all families, there are a number of ways for families to be dysfunctional but an infinite variety of ways for families to work. "The traditional presence of other people in the lives of parents with intellectual disability suggests collective and communal aspects to parenting" (Llewellyn, 1995, p. 361). This idea can apply to parents with other disabilities as well. Families should not, in this age of such diversity, be examined from a normal–centric point of reference. The concept of "good enough" parenting must be sufficiently flexible to include parents with disabilities.

The resiliency of parents with disabilities is best described by one such parent. Erica, the mother, and her husband use wheelchairs. Erica describes the extra tasks involved in what would be a simple outing for other families, when her son is going out for the day with his soccer team.

> His soccer team is going to go to a soccer game at a university. First they are going to play soccer in the afternoon in [a distant town], then they are going to go and watch soccer at [the university—a good distance away]. So we go to [the town] and the playing field may or may not be accessible, and then he will be heartbroken if it isn't, because then we can't watch and we have driven all that way for nothing. Then they want to go out for pizza. Even if the pizza parlor is accessible the bathroom may not be. And it is hard enough going through a three hour game without having access to a bathroom. We could detour with a group of kids and find an accessible restaurant and meet them at the pizza place and hope that they don't stare at my husband while he is eating, and that I can handle the kids. Once you get everybody in the restaurant, even if it is accessible it won't be roomy for moving around. Then we get in the car and go to [the university] to view the soccer game and will the team sit next to the accessible seating, if there is any? Or will the team just march off to the high bleachers where they have a great view and ditch me, and then will I force my son to sit with me or let him sit with his team? And all the other parents are just saying, "Geez, I have to remember to bring a warm jacket." (Cohen, 1998, p. 80)

SUMMARY AND CONCLUSIONS
ABOUT FAMILIES WITH DISABILITIES

There are several problems with the literature on families with disabilities. First and foremost, the literature so consistently conflates disability with other conditions that one wonders what we truly know about disability in the family. Other events that confound studies supposedly on disability include illness, dying, hospitalizations, separations, history of pathology in family of origin, substance abuse, and premorbid functioning and personality factors. For example, one study (Kotchick et al., 1996) reports on families with a father with hemophilia, but half of the sample also were HIV positive.

A second problem is the perennial isolation of disability from other contextual factors. For example, there is insufficient attention to ethnicity and culture in exploring families with disabilities. A third problem is the predominant focus on children with disabilities and the neglect of other ages and populations. Thus a lifespan approach to families with disabilities is sorely lacking. A fourth problem is the emphasis on the impact of the person with the disability on others or on the family system, and little attention to the effects of others on the person with the disability. And even more neglected is the study of the effects of greater systems (e.g., policies and agencies) on families with disabilities. Finally, the issue of preinjury versus postinjury marriages points out the gaps in our knowledge about persons who choose partners with disabilities. Similarly, friends of persons with disabilities are seldom studied. The focus on stigma has interfered with development of an understanding of persons seemingly less affected by society's notions of outcasts.

Families with disabilities are often testaments to creativity and courage. They also are subject to repeated instances of social stigma, prejudice, discrimination, alienation, and patronization. The labyrinthine system of agency resources can be oppressive; medical and rehabilitation services are designed for the convenience of the providers rather than the consumers and remain solidly oriented toward the individual and not the family. This is the context in which families seek clinical treatment. The therapist must understand the services, agencies and community resources for families with disabilities and be able to work with them. However, the clinician also must come to the family with an open mind and an ability to find and appreciate the family's resilience while confronting those aspects of family functioning that fail them.

SIX

Laws and Social History

Why a section on laws in a clinical text? Because, in part, by our laws shall you know us. The recounting of laws relevant to persons with disabilities is a social history of disability in the United States. Changes in legislation both lead and reflect major social reconstructions of disability. Understanding the laws is a way to understand the disability community. Persons who are not members of a minority group cannot fathom the intimate relationship between laws and our lives. Laws are not some distant happenings in faraway places but, instead, represent concrete changes in our everyday lives. For example, a new law in California (as of January 1, 1998; *An act to add Section 13660 to, and to repeal Section 13412 of, the Business and Professions Code, relating to disability,* AB 1277) requires gas stations to provide service to persons with handicapped placards or license plates, at self-service prices. Stations must post signs clearly stating the hours such services are available. This law isn't just a nicety for me. Many is the tense evening I've driven the 22 miles home at a slower pace trying to conserve gas until I could get to the one station near my home that will provide me this service. As another example, when the city of Sacramento made all 210 of its buses accessible to persons with physical disabilities, ridership by persons in wheelchairs increased sevenfold; 70,000 wheelchair trips were recorded in 1 year. Laws on accessibility change lives.

With advances in medicine there has been a great increase in the number of people with disabilities, beginning with the discovery of antibiotics (sulfa and penicillin) in the mid-1930s to 1940s, allowing more people to survive infections. This advance, coupled with better trauma treatment learned in World War I, reduced deaths but left many more people with disabilities. They were a ready work force (along with

137

women) to replace the men fighting in World War II. The postwar period was one of great prosperity, with rapid social and economic expansion. In just 15 years from 1945 to 1960, this country saw the coming of skyscrapers, transcontinental highways, suspension bridges, passenger airplanes, Sputnik, television, and the transistor, the first Xerox copier. The Vocational Rehabilitation Act Amendments (Public Law 113) of 1943 increased states' vocational services and federal funds for those services. It broadened the definition of "rehabilitation" to include a bigger array of restorative services, and added persons with mental illness to the list of those eligible for rehabilitation services. These broader definitions meant a dramatic increase in the number of persons with disabilities and the number being served by rehabilitation agencies. In response, Congress authorized a nationwide system of training grants to increase the supply of rehabilitation personnel.

The 1950s saw several key events. The polio epidemic of 1952 was the first such epidemic with a large proportion of survivors, and it also was the penultimate epidemic of polio in the United States. Polio was virtually eradicated through first the Salk then the Sabine vaccines. A second turning point was *Brown v. Board of Education of Topeka, Kansas.* This doctrine of "separate is not equal" laid the foundation for subsequent disability rights, though not for many years. The Civil Rights Act (Title VI) of 1964 ended legal segregation based on ethnicity or race, underscoring a belief system of integration enacted by Congress and upheld by the courts.

If we were to think of the period of legislation from 1943 to 1990 as a piece of music, the music begins to swell in 1965, when the definition of eligibility for services was expanded, and reaches a crescendo in 1990 with the Americans with Disabilities Act. Each piece of legislation can be seen as building on the previous ones. In 1968 the Architectural Barriers Act was passed. In 1973 a major milestone was the passage of the Rehabilitation Act (enacted in 1977), notably Sections 503, which provided for nondiscrimination in employment, and 504, which provided for equal access for persons with disabilities to programs, services, and education. The Rehabilitation Act only applied to agencies receiving federal funds, but this covered a large array of institutions, including most educational facilities.

We need to pause in our musical tour of legislation to explore the years 1970 to 1977, which were key ones in the development of the disability community. The Rehabilitation Act was our "Stonewall," the turning point in the collective history of persons with disabilities. But several events created both hope and unrest among persons with disabilities, leading to the events of 1977. The first was the admission in 1970 (after a legal fight) of Ed Roberts to the University of California, Berkeley (UCB). Ed was a polio survivor, a quad, and respirator dependent. He was the first severely disabled person to attend a university. He was housed in the campus hospital, and as other persons with para- and quadriplegia were admitted to UCB, they were too. Ed organized this group of students, the "Rolling Quads," to protest and fight for the right to live alongside students without disabilities. They moved out of the hospital and into the community. (Ed went on to become the head of California's State Department of Rehabilitation and a founding member of the World Institute on Disability in Oakland.)

At the same time, Judy Heumann (now Assistant Secretary for Special Education at the U.S. Department of Education) started "Disabled in Action" at Long Island University. What united the two groups on opposite coasts was the belief that critical issues facing persons with disabilities were not medical but political, economic, and social: lack of accessible transportation and housing, and need for quality personal assistance and jobs. Judy moved to the West Coast, and she and Ed began what became known as the independent living movement (ILM). Its basic tenets are that persons with disabilities should be the service providers for other persons with disabilities; persons with disabilities should retain self-determination; independence is a goal, and assistance (both personal services and assistive devices) should be aimed at helping the person achieve maximal independence and self-determination; community integration is a goal; and separate is not equal. The catchphrases of the ILM were "care, not cure," and "civil rights, not charity." Judy and Ed started the first center for independent living (CIL; now commonly called independent living centers, or ILC). They spurned the growth of the "charitable" approach to rehabilitation, with its sheltered workshops, nursing homes, and rehabilitation facilities, instead advocating political lobbying, public education, and awareness. The ILCs and their services enabled an increase in the numbers of persons with disabilities able to live independently. Rehabilitation took on a different meaning, connoting not just—or even mostly—a physical reparation but restoration of dignity.

Back in Washington, Congress had passed the landmark Rehabilitation Act in 1973, but it languished, unsigned. Holding it up were the needed regulations (to be published in the *Federal Register*) for the implementation of the Act. The American Coalition of Citizens with Disabilities (now defunct) called for national action to spur the release of regulations so that the Rehabilitation Act could be implemented, and they announced a deadline of April 5, 1977. Talks did not proceed as hoped, and on April 5, for the first time, groups of persons with disabilities protested in Washington and San Francisco. In Washington, an attempted sit-in lasted less than 24 hours when building security denied entry of food or supplies for the demonstrators. So it was the San Francisco protest, coordinated by the Berkeley CIL, which made history—for 1 month persons with disabilities of all types and ranges of severity level occupied the San Francisco office of Health, Education and Welfare (HEW). Pictures of persons in wheelchairs were on the evening news—a rare occurrence. They garnered tremendous local support; Safeway and McDonald's donated food, then-mayor George Moscone personally delivered a portable shower to the HEW office, and the Black Panthers brought garbage cans full of food. In Washington, Joseph Califano, newly appointed Secretary of HEW, who admitted that he had never heard of Section 504 before he took office, began a series of negotiations and drafts of regulations, which flew back and forth from Washington to San Francisco, until a set of regulations were agreed on. The demonstrators rolled, crutched, and walked out of the HEW offices, and the Act was signed into law by then-President Carter. The result was more than a law but a new era of activism and the beginning of a strong disability rights movement.

Taking up our musical march of legislation, the Rehabilitation Act was joined in 1975 with another landmark piece of legislation, the Education for All Handicapped Children Act (Public Law 94-142), now reauthorized as the Individuals With Disabilities Education Act (IDEA), the first law "to assure that all handicapped children have available to them . . . a free appropriate public education and related services designed to meet their unique needs." This law provided for several features we now take for granted, including *due process* for families in classification and placement of handicapped students. It granted certain *parental rights*: to examine school records, to obtain independent evaluations of child, to appeal decisions, and to bring civil actions. It stipulated *requirements for testing*: No single psychometric instrument could be the sole determinant of a child's placement; tests must be administered in a child's native language. It also mandated a written *individualized educational plan* (IEP), to be reviewed annually, and education in the *least restrictive environment*. *Special education* was defined as "specially designed instruction, at no cost to parents or guardians, to meet the unique needs of a handicapped child." *Related services*, as defined by the Act, included "transportation, and such developmental, corrective, and other supportive services . . . as may be required to assist a handicapped child to benefit from special education, & includes the early identification & assessment of handicapping conditions in children."

It is important to examine what Public Law 94-142 is and is *not*. It is not a provision for mainstreaming; that word is never used. It does not mandate that all handicapped children be educated in the regular classroom. It does not abolish any particular educational environment (e.g., residential schools). It does specify that education with nonhandicapped children is the objective "to the maximum extent appropriate." Therefore the IEP must clearly "show cause" if a child is moved to a more restrictive environment. An assessment of "the extent to which such child will be able to participate in regular educational programs" must be included in IEPs.

Not unexpectedly, a key question related to Public Law 94-142 was, Who pays for all this? This was the crux of the problem in implementation of this law. If a state participates in this Act, the guarantee of an appropriate education is not dependent on whether the Act has been "fully funded." Unfortunately, just around this same time California, the most populous state, passed Proposition 13, which limited taxes on housing to 1% of their value. State funding for education plummeted and has never recovered, and other states have followed suit. Despite a White House Conference on Handicapped Individuals in 1977, and the "Decade of Disabled Persons" from 1982–1992 (remember that?), significant advances in legislation have come at a time of waning resources, less tolerance for America's underclass, and a rebellion against unfunded state mandates.

The next legislative act related to children and young adults with disabilities was the Education of the Handicapped Act Amendments of 1986 (Public Law 99-457), which focused on early, preschool intervention. The Act provides for states to receive federal funding to develop a variety of services for handicapped infants and children and their families, including diagnostic screening, early education programs, special equipment, transportation, and homemaking, financial and legal services for families. It brought significant changes for infants, toddlers, and preschoolers from birth to 5 with handicaps and provided early intervention services and preschool programs. For all eligible children, states must conduct multidisciplinary assessments, develop individualized family service plans (IFSPs), and make available case management services.

A cornerstone of the law is the IFSP (much as the IEP is to Public Law 94-142). The IFSP must include a statement of the child's present levels of development (cognitive, speech and language, psychosocial, motor, and self-help); the family's strengths and needs relating to enhancing child's development; major outcomes expected; criteria, procedures, and timelines for determining progress; and specific early intervention services necessary to meet the unique needs of child and family, including method, frequency, and intensity of services. Also to be included are projected dates for the initiation of services and expected duration, and procedures for transition from early intervention into the preschool program. The IFSP must be evaluated at least once a year, and reviewed no less than every 6 months where appropriate.

Several inventions of the 1970s and 1980s were important developments for persons with disabilities. First, by the end of the 1980s institutionalization had gone out of favor. Theoretically, institutions were to be replaced by a tiered, community-based system of foster families, group homes, supervised apartments, and monitored living arrangements. Disastrously, part one happened (deinstitutionalization) without adequate implementation of part two (community systems), and in a climate of increased pressure on city governments to find funding for services less supported by the state. Second, the invention of the microprocessor in the 1970s meant smaller, more portable, less expensive devices. Improvements to personal computers in the 1980s allowed computers to be responsive to head nods or puffs of breath, making it possible for persons with severely limited body movements to gain control of appliances and other applications through the computer. Synthesized speech on computers and hand-held devices gave new means of communication. These newer assistive technologies had an enhanced role in allowing persons with disabilities to do more tasks, thereby facilitating the goals of the ILM. At the same time, funding was becoming increasingly scarce. Government-sponsored programs curtailed services, and rehabilitation units discharged patients sooner in response to managed care.

The relationship between technology and persons with disabilities was codified in the Technology-Related Assistance for Individuals with Disabilities Act of 1988. (For a fuller description of this Act and discussion see Chapter 12.) The purpose of this Act was to help consumers with disabilities have information and access to appropriate technology. It provided a definition of technology that was used in all subsequent legislation. The most recent reauthorization of IDEA (1997) encourages consideration of student use of assistive technologies when developing IEPs. It also (1) requires that states reimburse localities for state-mandated services to children with disabilities; (2) allows schools to designate up to 50% of their IDEA allocation for coordination of service systems; (3) clarifies that tests and assessments can be conducted by "trained and knowledgeable personnel," thereby rejecting efforts of some professional associations to limit assessments to certain disciplines; (4) requires that the IEP team identify transitional services needed by students, no later than age 16; (5) permits states to terminate IDEA eligibility to any child with a disability who is convicted as an adult and incarcerated in an adult prison, but disallows termination of services for any other reason (e.g., expulsion); (6) requires that states provide a confidential mediation process for resolution of disputes between parents and schools or administrations (such mediation is voluntary); and (7) limits circumstances under which parents can collect lawyers' fees. IDEA expanded an opportunity for family therapists, who are, by training and practice, appropriate case managers, facilitators of transitional services, and experts in systems and interactions among them—practices mandated in this law.

THE AMERICANS WITH DISABILITIES ACT

The culmination of all the previous legislative momentum was the Americans with Disabilities Act, signed on July 26, 1990 (music swells). The signing ceremony was one of the largest ever, attended by about 2,000 people, including many with disabilities. As is usual for events surrounding the President, it was a well-orchestrated ceremony. Or it would have been if the portable toilets placed around the perimeters had been wheelchair accessible. Instead, people tried to enter the White House to use the restrooms, to the consternation of the Secret Service, which, recognizing a disastrous publicity picture in the making, kept trying to carry people up the stairs.

Toilets aside, the ADA, dubbed the "emancipation proclamation" for persons with disabilities, does for disability what the Civil Rights Act did for race, color, religion, national origin, and gender. It combines the key elements of the Civil Rights Act with Sections 503 and 504 of the Rehabilitation Act. The impetus for the ADA came from several sources. One was a Harris Poll (1985), the first national poll of the self-perceptions of persons with disabilities. That poll showed a 66% unemployment rate of persons with disabilities, despite a willingness and desire to work. It also indicated that about 70% of the respondents had not been to a restaurant or movie in the past year *because* of their disabilities and problems with accessibility. Further, consistent with other data, the respondents with disabilities felt that their biggest problems were not physical or medical but social and economic barriers, especially obstacles to employment.

The ADA begins with a section called "Findings and Purpose of ADA,"[1] in which it lays out why this law was needed. It notes the numbers of persons with disabilities (43 million), that historically "society has tended to isolate and segregate individuals with disabilities, and . . . such forms of discrimination . . . continue to be a serious and pervasive social problem," and that "discrimination against individuals with disabilities persists in such critical areas as employment, housing, public accommodations, education, transportation, communication, recreation, institutionalization, health services, voting, and access to public ser-

---

[1]All quotes in this section are from the law itself. The ADA can be found on the Internet at http://www.apta.org/ada/adalaw.html.

vices." One motivation for this law is because persons with disabilities have "often had no legal recourse to redress such discrimination" despite the documented findings that "persons with disabilities, as a group, occupy an inferior status in our society." The ADA has five titles, as follows:

Title I: Employment

This covers organizations with 15 or more employees who work at least 20 weeks out of the year. Exempted employers include the United States, Indian tribes, or private membership clubs (except labor organizations). Illegal use of drugs is not protected. Several key phrases appear in this section: They include *qualified individual with a disability*, which means "an individual with a disability who, with or without reasonable accommodations, can perform the essential functions of the employment positions . . . [C]onsideration shall be given to the employer's judgment as to what functions of a job are essential." A *reasonable accommodation* is outlined and includes such things as "job restructuring, part-time or modified work schedules; reassignment to a vacant position, acquisition or modification of equipment . . . appropriate adjustment or modifications of examinations, training materials or policies, the provision of qualified readers or interpreters, and other similar accommodations. . . ." Making such accommodations should not impose *undue hardship*, meaning significant difficulty or expense; factors to be considered in determining undue hardship are outlined. Of key import is that the finances of the total institution, not just the entity making accommodations, shall be considered (e.g., the parent company of a chain of restaurants, not just the individual finances of a single franchise), and the burden of proof to show undue hardship is on the institution, not on the employee making the request. (Almost 80% of reasonable accommodations cost under $1,000.) Preemployment medical exams may be conducted after an offer has been made but before beginning work, if such exams are required of all entering employees, and if results are kept separate from personnel records and treated confidentially; drug tests are not considered medical exams.

Title II: Public Services

This section applies to any state or local government (e.g., jury duty) and to any departments or services they conduct, the National Railroad Passenger Corporation and any commuter authority, and public school transportation. This section also discusses paratransit systems as complements to fixed route services. Of note is that paratransit services may be used by the person with the disability and one accompanying individual (and thus would not be helpful to a mother with a visual impairment taking her two children to the pediatrician). Further, national bus systems (e.g., Greyhound) have applied for and received "temporary relief" from the obligations of this section.

Title III: Public Accommodations and Services Operated by Private Entities

The definition of public accommodation includes but is not limited to hotels and other places of lodging, restaurants, bars, movie and other theaters, concert halls, stadiums, museums, libraries, parks, zoos, private schools, day care centers, homeless shelters and food banks, recreation areas, convention centers, bakeries, stores, banks, laundromats, repair shops, gas stations, terminals or other stations, testing sites, and "office of an accountant or lawyer, pharmacy, insurance office, *professional office of a health care provider,* hospital, or other service establishment" (emphasis added). This section is the clearest about encouraging equal and integrated participation by persons with disabilities.

Title IV: Telecommunications

This title amends the Communications Act of 1934 by adding new sections. It mandates that "interstate and intrastate telecommunications relay services are available . . . to the hearing-impairment and speech-impaired individuals in the United States." Telecommunication devices for the Deaf (TDDs) and services shall be provided "that enable two-way communication between an individual who uses a TDD or other nonvoice terminal device and an individual who does not use such a device." All states now have a relay service for communication between those using a TDD and those using voice (two TDDs can "talk" to each other without a relay service). To use a relay service, either the deaf or the hearing person calls the relay service, gives the telephone number of the party he or she is calling, and is connected. Then the deaf person (if he or she is the caller) types a messages on his or her TDD, and the message is conveyed to the relay service; the relay operator reads the message out loud for the hearing person. The hearing person speaks a response (more slowly than usual), the relay operator types it verbatim on a TDD, and the message is relayed to the deaf caller. To find the number in your state you can call 800 information, or look in the phone book under [State] Relay Service. Relay services run 24 hours a day, all days. Charges for phone calls made using relay services are reduced because of the extra time needed to complete such calls. Costs of relay services are shared by all phone customers. (Look on your phone bill for charges related to the deaf and hearing impaired. They are generally under 50¢ per month.)

Title IV also discusses, though in considerably less detail, closed-captioning.[2] It requires closed-captioning of all public service announcements funded by the federal government. Local stations airing such announcements are not responsible if the announcement came without the captioning. All televisions made since about 1992 are able to receive the optional captioning that comes with some programs.

Title V: Miscellaneous

After making specific provisions in Titles I through IV, several loose ends needed clarifying. These include the right of insurers, HMOs, and medical services to "administer benefit plans, or similar organizations from underwriting risks, classifying risks, or administering such risks"; the right of an individual with a disability to refuse any accommodation, aid, service, opportunity, or benefit; the prohibition against retaliation against any person who brings charges related to or who exercises any rights under this Act; provision of attorney's fees to a successful litigant; and plans for technical assistance in understanding and implementing the Act (there are 10 Disability, Business and Technical Assistance Centers serving all states in the United States; see the phone book). It encourages alternate means of dispute resolution besides courts.

In addition to these sections, the EEOC, which has responsibility for oversight of compliance with Title I, has released (June 1997) policy guidance regarding persons with psychiatric disabilities ("The Americans with Disability Act and Psychiatric Disabilities").[3] This much needed and awaited publication answers questions and discusses issues regarding persons with psychiatric disabilities; including types of reasonable accommodations that may be effective for such persons and when an employer may hold employees with psychiatric disabilities to workplace conduct standards.

Passage of the ADA was by no means an easy or unanimous process. It took a long time, incurred much debate, and went through 40

[2]Closed-captioning refers to words on the bottom of a screen which are seen only if the machine is capable of showing them *and* that option is activated. Open-captioning refers to programs or videotapes with words showing all the time to every viewer, without any special devices.

[3]Available from EEOC Publications Distribution Center, (800) 669-3362 (voice) or (800) 800-3302 (TTY), or downloaded from EEOC web site at http://www.eeoc.gov.

congressional hearings, 4 committees in the House and 1 committee in the Senate. Further, a compromise had to be reached whereby the law was phased in. There were several key stumbling blocks in gaining passage. The first was the need to balance integration with fiscal constraints and concerns of both states and businesses. (More than 70% of all accommodations in the workplace cost under $500; nonetheless, fears of high expenses in making accommodations continue to be prevalent in the business community.) A second impediment was the definition of disability. This problem was partially resolved by listing specific exclusions: bisexuals or homosexuals; people with "transvestism, transsexualism, pedophilia, exhibitionism, voyeurism, gender identity disorders not resulting from physical impairments, or other sexual behavior disorders; compulsive gambling, kleptomania, or pyromania; or psychoactive substance use disorders resulting from current illegal use of drugs" (note that alcohol abuse is treated differently from other substance abuse). The third obstacle was religious organizations, which ultimately gained exemption. Thus religious institutions do not have to be in compliance with the ADA, except for those that accept federal monies (e.g., church-affiliated colleges), or for those portions of their property that are rented or loaned to the public (e.g., a church wing used for boy scout meetings would have to be accessible, although the rest of the church would not).

BETWEEN LAWS AND IMPLEMENTATION OF LAWS

Even as technology, laws, and societal roles change, limits are imposed by stigma, prejudice, discrimination, isolation, and separation. Laws alone cannot provide equity, integration, or acceptance of persons with disabilities. There is a chasm between the laws related to disability and their implementation. One reason for this chasm is simply ignorance of the law. A year after the passage of the ADA, despite wide media coverage, only 19% of the American public were aware of its enactment (Harris Poll, 1991, no. 912028), and of those who did know about it, 15–35% could not recognize its key provisions. Also, Americans respond well to the ideal of equity but less well to making sacrifices to achieve it. Respondents were ambivalent in their feelings about various aspects of the law. Although most Americans (96%) support the ideal of nondiscrimination, they are less enthused about the provision of things that cost money, such as reasonable accommodations. Over a quarter of the respondents think that their coworkers would have problems working alongside persons with disabilities and would not support any policy to increase numbers of employees with disabilities. Most people (51%) report that they personally do not know anyone with a disability. A third reason is that people have negative responses to persons with disabilities. The most common feelings were pity (74%) because of their situation and admiration (93%) because they overcome so much. Although 69% felt they could work closely with a coworker with a disability, 46% would feel "personally concerned" if their teenager dated a "seriously disabled person." No amount of legislation can alter these feelings.

Clients with disabilities face many arenas of discrimination and will respond to these variously. Some will require additional skills in assertiveness and self advocacy. Others will be on the opposite end of the continuum, continually tilting at windmills. It is useful to remember the words of Thurgood Marshall from the days when he was a lawyer for the NAACP—when it is early in a war in which it is important to ultimately prevail, we must choose our battles wisely, picking only those we think we can win. Clinicians will need a wide array of skills and approaches to help a variety of clients choose their stances toward the discrimination they encounter. But all clinicians should be familiar with the laws related to disability and have an understanding of the rights of clients with disabilities. This is especially important when working with children and teenagers with disabilities and their families. Whereas some families are more well versed than I could ever be about their children's rights and entitlements, others are at sea and need guidance in finding supports, services, resources, and financial aid. It is vital to know the requirements of the schools vis-à-vis students with disabilities and to understand that collaboration with school personnel (e.g., resource teachers) is fundamental to a successful outcome. Early intervention laws stress multidisciplinary service teams, and mental health workers should be team players.

There will undoubtedly be clients with disabilities who would like legal assistance. When a case goes beyond advocacy skills to the legal arena, there are several sources of help. One is Disability Rights and Education Defense Fund (DREDF, commonly pronounced dread-if).[4] In addition, local ILCs can give referrals to local resources. The 10 disability and business technical assistance centers, mandated by Congress, are a resource for any questions or information about the ADA and have a wide variety of materials (printed and in alternate formats) that they will send for free or for a nominal cost. There are several national organizations fighting for disability rights, two of which are especially prominent. One is ADAPT, which is pushing for legislation to ensure choice in

[4]DREDF: 1629 K Street NW, Suite 802, Washington, DC 20006; (202) 986-0375.

living arrangements (in own home versus nursing home) and payment for appropriate attendant care services rather than (more costly) nursing home or institutional care. The second is Not Dead Yet, which is the vanguard group against state-sanctioned physician-assisted suicide (see Chapter 11 for further discussion). The best sources of information are often other persons with disabilities. If clients are not connected with the disability community they may achieve a sense of belonging and a valuable source of information from magazines. Several are listed here:

1. *Ragged Edge: The Disability Experience in America.* The Advocado Press, Box 145, Louisville, KY 40201. E-mail: circulation@ragged-edge-mag.com. Website: www.advocadopress.org. This is *the* magazine of the disability community. It assumes the minority model, and takes it from there. It is topical and tackles many of the taboos and thorny issues in disability. Recent topics included reactions to invisible disabilities ("Gee, you don't look handicapped"), freak shows, and awareness days in which nondisabled people simulate disabilities ("The wrong message"). *Ragged Edge* has a position and is not shy about it.

2. *Mouth: Voice of the Disability Nation.* 4201 SW 30th Street, Topeka, KS 66614-3023. This magazine, a member of the Independent Press Association, is constantly in danger of going under. It manages to keep afloat through small contributions from loyal readers. Its list of subscription fees gives a hint of its general irreverence ("Hardship subscription; all I have to live on is a sickly government check: $2; Recovering Professional; That's one Mouth for me and I'll sponsor 2 hardship subscribers: $48"). When they cover Christopher Reeve, it is likely to be in satiric cartoon form.

3. *New Mobility: Disability Culture and Lifestyle.* P.O. Box 15518, North Hollywood, CA 91615-5518. This is the slickest of the magazines, with the most paid advertisements. It is about, but often not by, persons with disabilities. When they cover Christopher Reeve, it is an interview with him and glossy photos of the "isn't he plucky?!" variety. It has flashes of disability consciousness (e.g., took a firm stand for depictions of FDR in a wheelchair for the memorial). You won't hear about things here first but not long after. It's a good source for finding companies that make things (e.g., kneeling vans, lifts, inclinators, and sports wheelchairs).

KEY POINTS FOR PRACTITIONERS

1. Your office must be accessible to persons with disabilities. The landlord is responsible for ensuring access up to your door, and you have

responsibility for the office itself and any waiting room. If you request changes to this area to provide accessibility and the landlord refuses, the burden reverts to the landlord.

2. You may not refuse to take a client solely because he or she has a disability. This does not mean that you have to take any client who calls you, and you are still bound to practice within your scope of expertise.

3. The definition of "disability" in the ADA includes persons with AIDS or HIV.

4. "Otherwise qualified individual" is defined as a person with a disability who is able to perform "the essential functions of the position, with or without reasonable accommodation."

5. The employer's judgment determines the "essential functions" of a job, but advertised job descriptions are one guide. The ADA spells out further ways to define these essential functions.

6. The responsibility for proving "undue hardship" or "significant difficulty or expense" in providing reasonable accommodations falls to the employer.

7. Drug testing is not considered a medical exam. Therefore, employers mostly have retained the right to test for illegal drugs and alcohol. Current use of illegal drugs is not protected by the ADA. Recovering or recovered addicts are protected by the ADA, provided they can perform their job, and are held to the same qualification standards as all others. They may be dismissed for unsatisfactory performance or behavior even if the performance is related to drug use or alcoholism.

8. Employers are prohibited from inquiring about medical conditions or disabilities on job applications, interviews, or tests. They may test for illegal drugs but not for medications taken under medical supervision. Some psychotropic drugs are detected in drug screens. Employers may offer a job conditional on passing a medical exam, if such exams are required of all persons offered that job, and if the results are kept confidential and in a file separate from the personnel file. However, supervisors may be informed of necessary job restrictions and accommodations on a "need to know" basis. Current employees may not be forced to have a medical evaluation unless it is clearly job related and "consistent with business necessity."

9. Workers "shall not pose a direct threat" to the health and safety of others, with the burden of proof on the employer, who must show direct threat by objective evidence. The notions of direct threat and reasonable accommodation are particularly tricky for those with psychiatric disabilities or alcohol abuse.

10. Therapists should not give clients blanket clearances to work, nor should they find broad determination of inability to work. Instead,

specific job functions should be individually assessed. A useful list of job functions is in the California Disability Guidelines for assessing general work functioning. They include eight areas, the first three of which are essential to most jobs and the latter five for more responsible positions. The eight areas are ability to comprehend and follow instructions; perform simple tasks; maintain an appropriate work pace; perform complex tasks; demonstrate at least minimal interpersonal skills; influence others; make independent decisions, evaluations, or generalizations; and carry responsibility for planning, direction, organization, and control. (For discussion, see Ravid, 1992; Ravid & Menon, 1993.)

11. Children with disabilities and their families are eligible for services beginning at birth. Evaluation of services needed is based on an IFSP. Services are to be coordinated by a case manager of the relevant profession, which could well be a family therapist.

CLINICAL EXAMPLE

Esteban, an able-bodied man in his mid-20s, came to therapy for mixed anxiety-depressive disorder, complicated by a 10-year history of poly-substance abuse. He had been mostly clean for about 2 years but was particularly vulnerable to relapses of cocaine and methamphetamines. Despite these problems, compounded by an abusive father and early loss of his mother to cancer, Esteban had held a job for 2 years and gained one promotion in that time. Initial therapy focused on maintaining drug abstinence, and the depression and anxiety. After about 8 months Esteban came to a session in crisis—after the first physical exam he'd had in several years, it was discovered that he had Hodgkin's Disease. His primary thoughts were that he would die young, like his mother; that now, after finally turning his life around for the better, he was going to have to pay for his years of drug abuse; and that he'd die alone. He felt flooded by affect, completely isolated in the world, and unable to process much of what the doctors had told him, much less agree to a plan for treatment. Immediately following that session I called several (800) phone numbers and quickly found a national support and information organization[5]; the organization agreed to send me two copies of its literature, and I read these thoroughly as soon as they arrived. In this way I learned that there are three stages of Hodgkin's, and the prognosis varied according to stage. At the next session I stated that I had asked

[5]If the disease is less common, a good starting source is the National Organization for Rare Disorders, 100 Route 37, P.O. Box 8923, New Fairfield, CT 06812-8923.

for and received written information about Hodgkin's and handed Esteban an envelope with materials. I made no attempt to either tell him what I'd learned or push him to read the materials—in early diagnosis, people are often overwhelmed by stimuli and need time and help to sort out data. Later in the session he asked me if I'd read the materials, and I answered that I had; again I elected not to say more unless asked. As it turned out he wanted to discuss his stage of Hodgkin's with me and didn't want to have to take time to explain it to me, so he was quite relieved that I had already learned about this on my own.

As Esteban came to terms with the reality of his diagnosis and was able to make important decisions about his treatment, it became clear that he would need considerable work accommodations. Treatment would involve on and off weeks of chemotherapy and radiation. Further, the treatment was over an hour away, and he would be staying in an apartment near the hospital during his "on" weeks. He was terrified that he'd be fired because then he'd lose his medical insurance, have to find work while undergoing treatment, and still not be covered under the new insurance because he had a preexisting condition. These thoughts caused him extreme anxiety. At this juncture it was important that I had some familiarity with disability laws. The first question was about the size of the company he worked for. He worked in a small office of only three employees; however, the parent company of which his office was a branch had more than 50 employees—thus the employer was over the threshold of 15 employees, making it responsible for complying with the ADA. However, an employer is not responsible for providing any reasonable accommodations unless the employee so requests; a disclosure of disability triggers the law. We role-played how to tell his supervisor about his situation. I explained to Esteban the key concepts of "essential functions" of the job, "reasonable accommodations," and "otherwise qualified individual."

Like many people, Esteban had been unaware of any laws related to disability, and of any specifics of such laws. He did not know that he was considered a person with a disability and therefore fell into a protected class. I, on the other hand, had to be mindful of not giving legal advice yet also being sensitive to the fact that Esteban was in no position, financially or emotionally, to seek legal counsel. I wanted to give information of importance to Esteban so that he was informed about some basics and to make it easy for him to find out more information. As it turned out, his employer did try to fire him, but Esteban was well prepared with specific information that got the employer to change his mind. This information included a list of the job duties, divided into essential and nonessential functions, showing that he was able to do all the former and most of the latter, a list of specific requests for reasonable accommodations (e.g., dates of time off for treatment, so absences were planned and not unexpected), and a timetable of treatment (indicating that this was a time-limited need for accommodation). In retrospect, it would have been better had Esteban presented this information to his supervisor before termination of employment became an issue, but that is a hard judgment call a priori.

SEVEN

Beginning Treatment

To work effectively with clients with disabilities therapists need some basic skills. This chapter addresses these issues, beginning with seven assumptions that underlie the treatment approach outlined here and some key factors to consider when beginning treatment. This chapter also provides general treatment guidelines, including when and how to ask clients about their disabilities, assessing the client's model of disability, the therapeutic alliance, and treatment goals. Although some readers may feel intimated at this point, this chapter is meant to help practitioners think through issues so that they can find their own way with each client.

SEVEN PRINCIPLES TO GUIDE CLINICAL WORK

As those who have read the book up to now will anticipate, the first step in treating people with disabilities is a reevaluation of your own assumptions about disability—before the client even walks in the door. The seven assumptions outlined here stem from the material presented earlier in this book and thus will not be surprising to those who have been following the discourse thus far. However, they may be quite startling to readers jumping straight into this chapter.

1. A framework for therapy. The clinician should be familiar with the minority model of disability, family systems theory, larger systemic theory (e.g., interface with medical service delivery systems), and an expanded biopsychosocial model that includes legal, political, economic, and cross-cultural elements as essential components of treatment.

2. *Biculturalism.* Many persons with disabilities are essentially bicultural, going back and forth between the disabled community and the nondisabled larger society. A clinician's ignorance of disability culture can be expected to have the predictable problems inherent in cross-cultural counseling, such as premature termination, insufficient rapport, or negative outcomes.

3. *A systemic model.* Disability is a family affair. A disability affects the person with the disability and his or her family, and thus the focus of treatment, even if conducted individually, is systemic.

4. *Disability as social construct.* Disability (vs. impairment) is a social construct. Therefore, treatment focused solely on the individual with a disability leaves unchanged a fundamental aspect of disability experience, and therapy with persons with disabilities is a political act. (See Chapter 13 for a fuller discussion of the intersection of the personal and the political.)

5. *The need for additional clinical skills.* In addition to the general clinical wisdom and skills developed over the years through education, training, and practice, the clinician must understand the reciprocal influences of disability and typical presenting problems. This means knowledge of how to modify the diagnosis, case formulation, and treatment to integrate the disability. Therapy with families with disabilities requires competent family therapists who obtain *additional* education, training, practice, and skills relevant to disability.

6. *Beyond deficit reduction.* In therapy, there is a choice to focus on goals related to amelioration of negative symptoms (e.g., depression, anxiety, and anger) or on goals related to optimization of functioning (e.g., health, well-being, and hardiness). For therapy with persons with disabilities, the latter should always be included, whereas the former may be included, as needed. Therapy that counteracts negative messages about disability, and conversely focuses on increasing positive aspects, is a desirable component for two reasons: (1) the need to mitigate the perennial pathologizing of persons with disabilities in our society and (2) the fact that disability is a long-term condition, and enhancement of personal resources provides long-term insurance of well-being.[1]

7. *The need to show and not just tell.* The professionals and clients with whom you work have no reason to assume expertise on your part

[1]Two models of health-proneness and well-being that may be particularly relevant for families with disabilities are Antonovsky's salutogenic model and Kabasa's construct of hardiness (Kahn, 1986; Kobasa, 1979; Kobasa, Maddi, & Courington, 1981; Kobasa, Maddi, & Kahn, 1982; Kobasa, Maddi, Puccetti, & Zola, 1985; Kobasa & Puccetti, 1983; Kravetz, Drory, & Florian, 1993).

in treating clients with disabilities and their families (unless you have personal disability experience, in which case you might be afforded the benefit of the doubt). Therefore you must be prepared to demonstrate that you can work within the minority model, have expertise in treating clients with disabilities, and most important, your work with patients and their families can make the jobs of personnel in service delivery systems easier, smoother, and better.

THERAPY SKILLS WHEN WORKING WITH FAMILIES WITH DISABILITIES

To extend treatment skills to working with clients with disabilities, we should be mindful of the skills we already have as clinicians. These generally can be divided into structuring skills (defining presenting problems, translating theory into practical applications, matching therapy techniques with needs of clients), emotion facilitation skills (eliciting affect and handling it appropriately), and process skills (fostering a therapeutic alliance, promoting positive expectations, functioning at multi-levels simultaneously, behaving professionally). Of course, none of us exemplifies all these skills. But some of the skills are especially important in working with clients with disabilities.

This book is written for clinicians who cover a wide range of disciplines and work settings. One useful model comes from the unique skills required for a medical family therapist (for an overview, see McDaniel, Hepworth, & Doherty, 1992). Key ideas are presented here, noting any differences with the approach outlined in this book ("disability-affirmative therapy").

The first skill is expertise working with families and with the medical delivery system, from a systems perspective. This is distinct from the consultation–liaison psychiatric role and from behavioral medicine, both of which are traditionally more focused on individual patients. However, medical family therapists are more likely than are disability-affirmative therapists to become a part of the medical delivery system and to have more contact with medical personnel in a variety of contexts (e.g., grand rounds and informal meetings). This alliance with medicine may potentially alienate clients with disabilities, as the disability community tends to share an antipathy toward medical services.

A second skill involves the ability to work with larger systems, notably the ability to enter the medical care delivery system—one with its own culture—and work within its parameters to achieve beneficial results for the person with the chronic condition, the family, the primary care physician, and the service delivery team. Doherty and Baird (1983) conceptualize this work as a quadrangle, the points of which represent the patient, the patient's family, the clinician (which includes the health care team), and the illness/condition (which has its own set of attributes; see Chapter 1). The disability-affirmative clinician interfaces with a wide array of personnel and systems, including educators, resource and special education teachers, rehabilitation teams, centers for independent living, the disabled community, and a host of other potential collaborators.

A third skill is the facility in working with health problems (chronic illness, disability, and health promoting behaviors). However, work with clients with disabilities will not necessarily focus on illness or chronic conditions. Such clients may have the full panoply of presenting problems (e.g., depression, anxiety, and relationships), and the relationship of these problems to the disability can range from very little to inextricable.

The fourth skill is the ability to conceptualize using a biopsychosocial model and to understand the ways in which all problems are simultaneously biological, psychological, and social. The clinician must integrate the psychosocial implications of biological problems and the biological implications of psychosocial problems. However, disability-affirmative therapy incorporates economic, legal, and political considerations as well.

These four skills are mandatory for disability-affirmative therapy. Nine specific additional clinical skills are discussed here.

Flexibility

The clinician also must be flexible enough to entertain a model (the minority model of disability) that is counter to the majority perspective on disability. Viewing the client with a disability as a member of a minority group promotes new ways of defining who and what the problem is and, hence, new goals and means of achieving those goals. It depathologizes many aspects of the client and mandates closer and more careful inspection of individual versus societal ills. The clinician must be open to the culture of disability and flexible in ways of understanding the cross-cultural client (with a disability). Without this openness, the clinician's perspective is narrowed through the lens of his or her own culture. "The clinician is likely to only elicit information that he or she would be able to understand, and, thus, the clinician may be susceptible to finding only what has been sought" (Tseng & Streltzer, 1997, pp. 247–248). For example, a therapist may not think to inquire whether the person has friends with disabilities, or about how accessible the client's environment is (and overlook the daily frustration of, say, a lack of curb cut near the client's apartment or not being able to eat with coworkers because the lunch room is inaccessible).

Flexibility requires therapists to shed old stereotypes and prejudices. For example, if a client says the disability is not a current issue or part of the presenting problem the clinician should not assume this is prevarication or denial because the disability is an issue *for the clinician.* Of course, some clients with disabilities will deny their disability, but clinicians have skills to learn the difference. For example, we ask many of our clients about their use of alcohol, and some tell us, "I'm not an alcoholic." We know to listen for *how* they tell us this so that we might form an independent evaluation. We learn that only clients who are alcoholic say "I'm not an alcoholic," can recall the last time they had a drink, and can remember a period when they went without any alcohol. So, too, we must develop empirical ways of understanding what clients mean when they say a disability is not an issue or part of the presenting problem(s).

Because the parameters of therapy may be altered by disability, therapists should be flexible about the frequency of sessions, time of day of appointments, length of sessions, and tolerable limits of cancellations. For example, Anna, who uses an electric wheelchair, called at the last minute to cancel because the lift on her van broke and paratransit requires 24-hour notice. Dawn, who has rheumatoid arthritis, can't make early-morning appointments because her muscles are stiff and sore on first rising, and she takes a long bath every day to get her going. Stan, who has a disk problem in his back, alternates between sitting and standing during sessions. Madeleine, who has Crohn's disease, sometimes gets a sudden onset of stomach problems and has to leave abruptly; she prefers more frequent appointments when she is not having difficulties and to skip several weeks or more when she is having an exacerbation. These parameters affect the treatment plan and delivery but should not derail it. Such client behaviors do not necessarily mean resistance, passive aggressiveness, or manipulation. Of course, some therapy settings allow for less flexibility of hours, length of session, layout of the room, and so on, and this may be alienating to some clients with disabilities.

Flexibility in conceptualizing what constitutes therapy is also necessary. Using and coordinating with other support services, collaborating with resource teachers, making school visits, talking to doctors, visiting clients in the hospital—all these and more may be part of therapy. For example, Dennis was a man in his early 20s who had quadriplegia for about 2 years. He was overwhelmed by the physical demands of his disability, very depressed, and mostly reclusive in his home (often not even leaving the bedroom). My first session with him was a home visit; my sole demand was that he meet with me in his living room, not the bedroom. By the sixth session I had become his one outing per week. Because he was so demoralized and unable even to imagine a better life for himself, I began by showing him role models—other men with para- or quadriplegia who were living fuller lives. We looked at the writings and cartoons of John Callahan, an author with quadriplegia (he wrote *Don't Worry, He Won't Get Far on Foot*, 1989). We spent two sessions watching and discussing the movie *My Left Foot*. At first, Dennis's response was to find ways that he was different (and therefore worse off) than these models. Over time, that defense began to erode, opening up a glimmer of the idea that "if they can do it . . . " The time spent reading and watching was a kind of pretreatment condition, a necessary step to help Dennis be ready to tackle the real and enormous tasks of living with quadriplegia. It was no less a valid treatment intervention than any other, albeit an unusual use of therapy time.

Hypothesis Generation and Case Formulation

A fundamental part of the formulation about clients with disabilities is that such clients are bi- (or tri-)cultural, living with a disability in the nondisabled world. The client may not think of him- or herself as a person with a disability and may not identify with other people with disabilities, but nevertheless he or she is a part of a minority group—persons with disabilities—and has experiences shared by all persons with disabilities (such as stereotyping, prejudice, and discrimination). But the client also belongs in another community, that of family, friends, neighborhood, and coworkers. This community is mostly or even all nondisabled. Some clients will identify and affiliate more with one group than the other (say, African Americans, or women, or Jews, or lesbians, or the disability community); some will feel torn among them; and still others will feel exclusively a part of only one camp. But if the client can remain open to all the cultures to which he or she belongs, then different options and solutions become available, with double the number of role models, support networks, influences, and assets.

Therapists need to know how to introduce clients into different communities. For example, in an analogous situation, I sent a client who was newly aware of being lesbian to sit in a low-key, casual women's coffee shop for an hour. For a client who was just starting to think about being part of a disability community, I might suggest certain magazines. The point is that if we are serious about clients' cultures as being integral to treatment, then we must know how to access those cultures, and how to help clients do so as well. It perpetuates oppression to fail to help clients find their way home.

The hallmark of cross-cultural competence may lie in the ability to generate multiple hypotheses. These hypotheses would take the cultural context of disability into account but not overinflate its role. Then the task would be to open-mindedly collect and interpret data to refute or confirm the hypotheses. The therapist who is culture blind would fail to see how disability alters or shapes experiences and their interpretations. The therapist who is hyperaware of culture would see disability issues imposed into all facets of the client's life and misinterpret the disability as causative. Somewhere in between lies a happy medium which incorporates disability but places it in its proper context.

> Shannon, a divorced woman in her late 30s, requested therapy because of "some disability issues" that were coming up for her as time went on and she became more impaired. She had a congenital disability and thought that she had put the psychological and emotional issues behind her. But new symptoms were prompting increased contact with the medical profession and raising the possibility of surgery. Her current symptoms included frequent weeping, feelings of alienation and anxiety, and sleep disturbance.

At first glance it seems that disability issues would loom large in the formulation of this case. But it would be a mistake not to entertain alternate explanations. I teach my students to observe the Rule of Five followed by the Rule of Two: Generate five hypotheses. For each hypothesis, finding two bits of disconfirming data means that you must throw out that hypothesis, no matter how attached you feel to it. Suppose you were to learn more information:

> Shannon came from a family in which her father was in the military and ran the household with zero tolerance for human foibles or frailty. He was physically abusive to the mother, who was clinically depressed throughout Shannon's childhood. Both parents were active alcoholics, and Shannon's older sister started poly-drug use in early teens.

Suddenly the disability doesn't seem like such a large issue anymore, does it? Rather, it becomes another arena in which the core issues of powerlessness, abuse, and denial of emotions were enacted. The disability has a part in the case formulation—a visible manifestation of human vulnerability, it was a narcissistic wound to the father which enraged him. But it is not the overriding factor.

Utilizing Time and Resources Outside Sessions

Clinicians working with clients with disabilities must have the motivation and curiosity to learn about the specifics of a client's disability. Some work outside sessions on the clinician's part often is necessary to find national organizations with information and resources, to read about the disability, and to preview relevant reading material in order to make more client-specific and well-timed recommendations.

> Lynette first came to see me 1 month after receiving the diagnosis of ankylosing spondylitis (AS)—a back disorder involving increased stiffening of the spine. She was overwhelmed by the new diagnosis and its implications for childrearing (her three children ranged in age from 9 to 16) and vocational considerations (she sat for long periods at a computer). She knew little about the disorder. After she left I looked up AS in one of my reference books and learned that it is a form of arthritis. This let me know how to find out more information: I called the (800) directory assistance and asked for the Arthritis Foundation (there is also an Internet support group for AS). I called that number and got the local (nearest big city) number. When I called the local number they had a brochure specifically on AS which they agreed to send me. It arrived in 2 days, and I bundled the brochure with photocopies of several pages on AS from one of my books and put them in an envelope. I gave the envelope to Lynette at the next session, simply saying, "I found some basic information from the arthritis foundation on AS and am passing it on to you. You can read it or not, as you wish." These materials served several purposes. They provided first me and then Lynette ready access to basic information and a way for me to let her know I was willing to become educated about the disorder. Obtaining these materials was a concrete demonstration of my support during her present crisis. By bundling the materials into an envelope I respected Lynette's pace of receptiveness to new information.

Relationship Skills: Openness and Empathy

When clients have disabilities, empathy may take on different shading from that with other clients. People with disabilities are so often portrayed as pitiable, weak, pathetic, suffering, and needy that therapists may find they adopt a compassionate stance too readily, or misconvey pity when intending to be empathic. For example, when a client with CP seems to be having difficulty opening the door from the waiting room into the hall, what will it mean to the client if you open the door for the client, do not open the door but watch to see if your help will be needed, or ask, "Would you like some assistance?" The therapist must be open and honest to understand his or her motivations behind each of these actions, but also open to the idea that the intent from the therapist may not be matched by the message received by the client.

People with disabilities are often recipients of services ostensibly erected on their behalf. One study (cited in Barnes, 1994) estimated that people with disabilities had up to two dozen "professional helpers" involved in their lives (e.g., special educators, school psychologists, primary care physicians, nurses, podiatrists, and orthotists). I counted 12 service providers whom I see with some regularity, from the shoemaker who alters every pair of shoes I buy to the orthotist who constructs my ankle–foot orthotic to the car facility that installs and fixes my scooter lift. These various entities mostly don't interconnect in any way, much less coordinate services. It is often the therapist who is in the role of synthesizing and coordinating many of these disparate aspects, especially for children with disabilities. Thus an essential skill is openness to the values and procedures of other professionals. This makes for smoother collaboration among service providers. Skills in collaboration and team approaches can widen and deepen treatment options. However, we must be mindful that therapy is *with*, not just *for*, the client with the disability. Professionals have a tendency to talk and make decisions among themselves. Therefore, this skill in interprofessional collaboration must be fully integrated into the treatment goal of empowerment (see section "Treatment Goals in Disability-Affirmative Therapy," elsewhere in this chapter).

Facility with Strong Affect

Facility with eliciting and handling powerful emotions is critical. Tolerance for rage at oppression, profound shame and disgust about aspects of the disability, anxiety about finances, depression over declining health within the family, irritation at inaccessibility, panic over one's future and one's children's future—all these are possible in any given family with a disability. Again, these are not *required* emotions for the clients but are more likely due to conditions imposed by the disability. And it is not only the individual with the disability and the family but also the clinician who will experience strong emotions. Work with families with disabilities raises affect. Topics of vulnerability, death, deformity, injustice, courage, and loss, all arouse powerful responses in the therapist. These effects are magnified when the person with the disability is a baby or child.

Values

Working with clients with disabilities and chronic health conditions can entail some examination of larger issues, such as the meaning of life, priorities, friendships, and the role of family. The therapist's comfort with grappling with more existential questions facilitates discussion of these issues. However, clinicians should not think these are inevitable or necessary questions. For example, in the film *Breathing Lessons* we meet poet Mark O'Brien, who spends 23 hours a day in an iron lung but who does not struggle to find meaning in living. Others might view his "quality of life" as restricted and impaired, but this is the outsider perspective. From that outsider perspective we ask, "What's on the menu for my life?" and know we wouldn't choose "iron lung." But remember the earlier discussion in which I pointed out that we don't get a menu. We get what we get and deal with it. Perhaps from the perspective of living in a healthy, able body you might think, "I'd rather be dead than live like that," but from the perspective of "someone like that" you probably wouldn't say the same thing. It is hard to judge the "quality of life" of another person, and we should be reticent to do so.

Using Positive Models of Treatment

Another skill is the ability to utilize positive models of treatment. This means viewing goals as positive outcomes rather than the absence of negative outcomes. Quality of life is not merely the absence of psychopathology. Although obviously not appropriate in all cases with all diagnoses, the knowledge and practice of this more positively oriented therapy will be a valuable expansion of treatment options when working with clients with physical disabilities.

> Robert is an unemployed man in his 30s, living alone in a one-bedroom apartment. He is paraplegic, uses an electric wheelchair, and has limited use in both hands. Despite an undergraduate degree in journalism and 5 years of job experience as a stringer on a small newspaper, he has been unable to find a job for the past 4 years.

At first glance Robert's life and future appear bleak, and the therapist may feel helpless. Robert himself may convey hopelessness, frustration, and resignation. The point here is not to convince you that Robert's life is peachy but to challenge clinicians to temper their usual focus on problems and symptoms and to think about what a more positively focused treatment might entail. We might focus on Robert's ability to be a role model for teens with disabilities, on his writing and computer skills, on his resourcefulness in finding things of interest to him, on his few but durable long-term relationships, on the capacity he's developed to persevere despite considerable barriers, and on the humor he maintains in the face of prejudice and discrimination. None of this is meant to trivialize the difficulties Robert faces, or the dissatisfaction he experiences in life. But unless clinicians can counter their own negative views of what life as a person with a severe disability must be like and see skills and assets along with the deficits and problems, they are likely to adopt too readily the pessimism clients often bring to treatment.

Understanding and Managing Countertransference

The emotions evoked in others by persons with disabilities are often strong, unconscious, negative, and many times anxiety producing. Feeling powerful negative countertransference does not necessarily doom the therapy—unless the therapist cannot understand, manage, and utilize the feelings and thoughts, and cannot distinguish those that inform about the client from those that are about the therapist. Easy, huh?

Able-bodied therapists will be called on to counter immediately the expectations (on the part of the client with a disability) of a negative response to the disability. To do so, the therapist must feel comfortable with the topic, free to bring it up or not to do so, and at ease with his or her own skill level in incorporating disability issues into the treatment. But what if you don't feel those things? What can the clinician do to address strong negative feelings regarding people with disabilities? There are no easy answers, but some suggestions may be useful. The first is to immerse yourself in the culture of disability. This can be accomplished partly through readings (see Chapter 14, in this volume, for suggested readings). Learning about disability, about specific disabilities, about famous people with disabilities, and about disability culture can all help demystify the social construct of disability. But close and prolonged contact with peers with disabilities is the essential ingredient in altering attitudes and responses. Only in this way can we come to appreciate persons with severe disabilities as people beyond their disabilities, and become more comfortable around some of the seemingly odd and distracting behaviors associated with some disabilities (altered speech, drooling, head drooping, spasmodic motions, twitches, lurches, grimaces, etc). If you had a reaction just to reading these words, it may seem impossible to appreciably increase your comfort level with the real thing. Start slow and build. Sit in a coffee shop across from the local ILC or outside the Department of Rehabilitation. Attend a disabilities exposition (see Chapter 12 for description and locations). Go to the local university's Disabled Students Services. Visit Berkeley (the weather's nice). But by all means don't go to hospitals. This further conflates disability with illness, when we are trying so hard to differentiate the two. And the most powerful and lasting effects involve contact over time and as equals with a person with a disability whom you get to know well.

Functioning at Multiple Levels

All therapists function on multiple levels continuously. We listen for both content and affect, we compare verbal content with nonverbal cues, we monitor the client's and our own processes simultaneously, we listen while we think about how to respond next, we act spontaneously while thinking out our stance, and so on. This processing of dual or triple levels is made more complex by physical manifestations of impairments. For example, if disability alters the body language and facial cues, then monitoring of nonverbal communication is different. It may mean in part attending to nonverbal cues *less* (i.e., not being distracted by extraneous movements). Or it may mean recalibrating the meanings attached to behaviors. For example, face contortions and large body movements carry different meanings in hearing or deaf clients. Or it may mean learning new methods of receiving information. For example, picture a client who uses a communication device which speaks some of the words in a sentence for him. In telling you the sentence "I was more upset this week" you have trouble understanding the word "upset" (the key word in the sentence!) so he types it on the device which then speaks the word in a machine monotone. With a more fluent client we might pick up cues that "upset" refers to anxiety, depression, or frustration. But in this case the nonverbal cues are minimized. So we have to ask directly for other information that helps us understand the client's message.

Facility at functioning on multilevels (e.g., verbal and nonverbal or content vs. process) with clients with disabilities requires an ability to fluidly enter and exit different levels. For example, a client with a physical disability affecting her back, legs, and stomach muscles suddenly grimaces as she relates an incident from the previous week. If the grimace is signaling physical pain I may want to work with her on getting more comfortable in the session, perhaps by trying a different chair, but without interrupting the content issue more than necessary and distracting her from the more salient therapeutic issues. With a client whose speech I have difficulty understanding I need to remember to signal my comprehension more frequently; otherwise the client repeats himself, having learned that others pretend to understand when they in fact do not. This awareness of the physical tasks involved in two (or more) people sitting in a room and conversing adds a new level to which the therapist must attend.

GENERAL TREATMENT CONSIDERATIONS

This section addresses four areas important in treating families with disabilities: how to ask clients about their disabilities, the problem of time management, applying the different models of disability to the treatment, and considering accessibility issues when designing treatment plans.

Asking about the Disability

One question I'm frequently asked is whether the therapist should ask a client about his or her disability even if the client doesn't raise the topic. In short, yes. Therapists must feel free to bring up any material that might be relevant in a case. While guarding against asking questions mostly to satisfy one's own prurient or keen curiosity ("So, how do you change a colostomy bag?"), there should be no bounds on acceptable topics for discussion. Yet of course we therapists, like all people, have topics we are less comfortable with, such as money, death, or sex. If the topic of disability is uncomfortable for the therapist, the therapist may be reluctant to bring it up. Although well-meaning, therapists tend to overdo in one direction or the opposite, either ignoring the disability (the proverbial elephant in the room) unless and until the client raises the issue or, conversely, assuming that all problems stem from and are related to the disability.

Asking about disability is not rude or intrusive. It would be if we were chance encounters in, say, the line at the post office, but ours is a different relationship. Remember how, in your first years of training, you were afraid to ask clients about thoughts of killing themselves? But you learned to do so; you learned that it wasn't putting ideas into clients' heads, and that they mostly appreciated the concern and expertise inherent in the question. Similarly with disability, most clients will not experience it as impolite. Further, you will be behaving unlike most new people with whom they come into contact, many of whom scrupulously avoid any direct or indirect mention of "the topic," all while carefully managing eye movements so as not to look at the affected body parts. By being different, you immediately set a tone for the therapy—"we can talk about things here"—that promotes a collaborative stance. Important for all clients, this has special importance for clients with disabilities, who perennially experience stigma, prejudice, discrimination, social ostracization, and stereotyping in everyday life (Allessi & Anthony, 1969; Alston & Daniel, 1972; Altman, 1981; Belinkoff, 1960; Byrd, Byrd, & Emener, 1977; Cohen, 1963; Fine & Asch, 1993; Yuker, 1988, 1994). Thus the therapy experience must immediately and clearly counter what may be the client's expectation of similar fare. Therapists without disabilities especially must create a positive reception as they are less likely to be given an initial benefit of the doubt.

Ask yourself how you would handle any other potentially sensitive issue, say, the death of a mother, or whether a client is having unprotected sex. Would you refrain from raising these issues unless the client did? I doubt it; I would think they'd be fairly high on any therapist's list of topics. Would you assume all problems stemmed from those incidents? As powerful as they are, they can't account for all the variables of a person's present psychoemotional functioning. Neither can disability.

There are two useful questions I ask clients with disabilities. Early in the interview I ask, "What is the nature of your disability?" This is the phrasing most used in the disability community. We often get to know each other through our disabilities, exchanging disability data early on. Alternate phrases, such as "What is wrong with you?" or "What happened to you?" are not well received. They imply fault and/ or something gone wrong. Although it may be true that "something happened" (e.g., car accident) or something did go wrong (e.g., lack of oxygen at birth), those were salient points only at the onset of the disability. After living with a disability for any amount of time, they no longer seem applicable. The focus of the questioning is not to discover "how did this happen?" but to elucidate present functioning and effects.

The second routine question is one I ask if the client has not brought up the disability (except perhaps in answering the first question). After hearing the presenting problem and the current living situation and context for the client, I'll ask, "Are there ways in which your disability is part of this (presenting problem)?" The client may say no, and I may disagree, but this is not unique to disability; clients often are unaware of connections among aspects of their lives. I then have a clinical situation like many others—how to handle denial or lack of insight, the proper timing of feedback or reframes, and empathically confronting the client's sensitive areas. When I'm going to ask about the disability, I do *not* say, "Do you mind if I ask you a personal question?" First, since when do therapists ask permission to ask personal questions? Second, persons with disabilities hear this question a lot, and it invariably means the following question will be about the disability, as if disability questions need to be announced. This seems as if the therapist is asking the client with the disability to put the therapist at ease about the disability, and it signals the therapist's discomfort. Clearly such a request is especially inappropriate in a therapy context.

Following are some questions I never ask: "How do you think your disability affected who you are?" or, "How might you have been different without your disability?" Such questions are essentially asking, "Who are you without your disability?" It's rather like asking, "Who would you be if you weren't (male, black, Jewish, etc.)?" The question assumes that there is some you-ness that can be separated into components, and then the additive effects of disability over that essential you-ness can be evaluated. It is not a useful model for trying to understand personality, character, temperament, or psychosocial functioning. Disability becomes an integral part of the person within several years of onset, or earlier if the onset is in early childhood.

A key point here is that therapy is less effective, perhaps even counterproductive, if the therapist has one hand tied behind his or her back and his or her maneuverability is hampered by negative counter-transference responses to the disability. Therapists must feel free to maneuver in the therapy such that decisions are made based on the therapist's professional judgments of what's in the best interests of the client; as that freedom is impinged upon by fears, stigma, social norms, and rules, therapeutic effectiveness necessarily decreases. Feeling free to make inquiries about the disability helps untie the therapist's hands.

The Relativity of Time

Persons with disabilities refer to "crip time." Indeed, many things really do take longer when you have a disability. Every disability is different, but tasks that may take extra time include getting ready to come to the therapy session (e.g., doing a morning bowel program or warming up muscles), talking time (e.g., stuttering or CP), writing a check, or getting situated in the office. Families of persons with disabilities often have developed a rhythm that accommodates the extra time for the disability. For example, my children use the time I'm putting the scooter in the car to squabble over seating arrangements without interference from me! Therapists should allow and plan for this extra time; failure to do so results in frustration for clients and therapists alike. Further, the therapist may need to negotiate with the client's insurance plan for longer or more sessions (good luck).

> Phil arrived for his first session in a manual wheelchair. He carried with him a transfer board—a smooth flat rectangular board about 1 by 2 feet—which he uses at work to help him slide from his wheelchair to his desk chair. However, the chairs in my office, as in most therapists' offices, are lower, cushiony, soft, designed to encourage sitting back, and swivel—all factors that made transferring to them more difficult. We spent about 10 minutes trying out different seating arrangements in the office. I encouraged this activity by stating something along the lines of, "It's worth taking the time now, for you to be comfortable here." We ultimately found that my desk chair worked best for him, and prior to his future appointments I removed one "client" chair and replaced it with my desk chair. This gesture conveyed patience, acceptance, understanding, and a collaborative stance more than words ever could.

Applying the Models (Moral, Medical, and Minority)

The three models of disability are not merely abstract ideas. They translate into concrete ways in which the person with the disability and his or her family thinks about the person, values or denigrates the disability, incorporates and integrates it into the self-concept or segregates it as a disembodied "bad" part, and feels about the disability. Yet most people with disabilities are not aware that they hold a model of disability. Therapy can help clients elucidate their own perspectives on disability, help them understand the implications of subscribing to one model over the others, and evaluate the models that others hold. (The next section makes more suggestions related to models.)

Making Therapy Accessible

For therapy to be effective, the treatment should not duplicate and perpetuate the client's difficulties. Thus therapy must be accessible to persons with disabilities. By this I am not talking about the physical access discussed in earlier chapters (see Chapter 5 for obligations for physical access under the ADA), or the arrangement of your office but, rather, about the more subtle issues. For example, in treating depression we might have a woman with MS increase her activity level while being mindful of fatigue and respectful of the client's need to manage energy expenditure. In teaching a teenager with CP social skills we should be mindful of the real ostracization he encounters daily. In helping a man with SCI seek employment we should be aware of the discrimination he or she inevitably will encounter. In teaching a new mother with rheumatoid arthritis ways to pick up and carry her infant we should know that she is going to have to find her own way for countless tasks involved in childrearing, that the world of baby products ignores mothers with disabilities. If we fail to consider these reality factors we fail the client.

TREATMENT GOALS
IN DISABILITY-AFFIRMATIVE THERAPY

Therapy goals are, of course, individualized for each client and family. However, common themes reoccur frequently with such clients, and hence we need goals that reflect these themes. These goals emerge from some of the theoretical work that has been done on disability and chronic conditions. One therapeutic goal is the often-cited but ill-defined notion of "acceptance of the disability." What might this mean? How does this goal translate into therapeutic tasks? The key conceptual underpinnings of "acceptance of disability" comes from the work of Dembo, Leviton, and Wright (1975) and Wright (1983). In their view, there are four basic changes in values that facilitate acceptance of disability. Reconsideration of values, then, may be one treatment goal.

In medical family therapy (cf. McDaniel, Hepworth, & Doherty, 1992) goals of treatment are *agency* (active participation and commitment to one's self care) and *communion* (a positive and facilitative relationship with the health care system and a sense of support in the family and community). The health, well-being, and resiliency literature offers guidance for overarching goals, such as the creation or bolstering of a sense of meaning in life. These varying perspectives have never been collated or synthesized into a coherent treatment model. What follows is an attempt to think through the goals that might be common to clients with disabilities, despite differences in types of disabilities, the presenting problems, psychological make up and levels of development. It comprises disability-affirmative therapy.

Goal 1: Models

A primary goal is to help clients with disabilities understand how their perspectives on their own disabilities are shaped by the three prevailing models of disability. Clients and their families can assess both their current model(s) and their desired model(s). As stated previously, the models of disability may seem abstract or theoretical, but in fact they have practical and quotidian implications. Some clients may be savvy about the models of disability; such clients are more likely to ascribe to the minority model, because those are the very people writing and reading about the models. Other clients will be completely unfamiliar with the concepts and need to be introduced to them.

A model can be elicited and elucidated by having the client address some questions. Table 7.1 presents questions about differing aspects of clients' disabilities experiences. Families can be given a copy of the table and instructed to ask themselves the questions associated with the various models. This can be done during therapy or as an individual or family homework assignment. I might ask family members to do the task by saying, "How you think about yourself as a person with a disability will affect greatly how you think about yourself overall. You may not even be aware that you had a model of disability. Take a few moments to ask yourself some questions that can help bring your model to light. Use the questions in this table to help you, but also feel free to think of other questions or situations that the table doesn't address."

Several outcomes are possible, and the clinician must have *no*

TABLE 7.1. Assessing the Client's Model of Disability

Model	Questions to ask yourself
Moral model	• Do you feel shame or embarrassment about your disability? • Do you feel you bring dishonor to the family? • Do you try to hide and minimize the disability as much as possible? • Do you try to make as few demands on others as possible, because it's "your problem" and hence your responsibility? • Do you try to make your disability inconspicuous? • Do you think your disability is a test of your faith, or as a way for you to prove your faith? • Do you think your disability is a punishment for your or your family's failings?
Medical model	• Compared to FDR's time, do you think that life for persons with disabilities has improved tremendously? • Do you think even FDR wouldn't have to hide his disability today? • Do you try to make as few demands on others as possible, because you think you should be able to find a way to do it yourself? • Do you dress in ways that maximize your positive features and minimize the visibility of the disability? • Do you believe that the major goals of research should be to prevent disabilities and find cures for those who already have disabilities? • Do you think that persons with disabilities do best when they are fully integrated into nondisabled community?
Minority model	• Do you identify yourself as part of a minority group of persons with disabilities? • Do you feel kinship and belonging with other persons with disabilities? • Do you think that not enough is being done to ensure rights of persons with disabilities? • When policies and legislation are new do you evaluate them in terms of their effects on persons with disabilities? • Do you think the major goals of research should be to improve the lives of persons with disabilities by changing policies, procedures, funding, and laws? • Do you think that persons with disabilities do best when they are free to associate in both the disabled and nondisabled communities, as bicultural people?

Note. From Olkin (1998). Copyright 1998 by National Rehabilitation Hospital Press. Reprinted by permission.

investment in one outcome over any others. Some persons may find themselves answering yes to questions mostly in one model. Others might find they hold beliefs from more than one model. What is important is not where the client fits but where he or she feels most at home, what works for the client, and what allows the client the greatest degree of satisfaction and contentment with self and others. However, some clients may find that they fit into one model and wish they didn't; the fit is uncomfortable, or arouses feelings of anxiety, anger, or sadness. This is not unusual but may be distressing to the client. The clinician should keep several things in mind. First, there is no such thing as complete adjustment to disability. One is never *there*, only *traveling* there. Thus the client's thoughts about disability will constantly change and evolve. Second, the disability itself changes and may increase with aging. This may mean a whole new trunkful of disability stuff to unload. Feelings the client thought were already dealt with may reemerge. However, a positive reframe is that any discomfort with the model that the client currently is experiencing is a positive sign that he or she is not sweeping disability issues under the rug. Recognizing the feelings leaves open more of an opportunity to change them. The clinician can make two suggestions to clients in this position. The first suggestion is to find ways for the client to ease up on him- or herself. The message to be conveyed is that one feel what one feels, and it can only feels worse if, on top of the undesired feeling, one feels bad about having the undesired feeling. The second suggestion is to advise the client to talk to other people with disabilities. It may be important that the disability be the same (e.g., for someone with postpolio to talk with another polio survivor about new symptoms associated with postpolio syndrome), or simply similar in some key respect (e.g., uncertain course, as in MS, or life-threatening, as in ALS). In other instances the specifics are less important than the shared aspects of the disability experience. But no other minority group is expected to achieve and maintain good mental health without contact with other members of its group, and we should not expect this of persons with disabilities.

The way that women with disabilities dress can be informative about their feelings toward the disability. You'll recall my own story of shedding pants and donning dresses as part of my own "coming out" as a person with a disability. Recently I gave a talk to a postpolio support group and was not surprised to see that the 40 or so women in attendance were all dressed in pants. One can choose to dress to hide disliked body parts or dress to enhance valued physical assets. I find that women with disabilities often do the former. This can lead to a useful treatment technique, namely, having clients literally and figuratively try on different personas. For example, I asked a client with postpolio to wear a dress to the next session. She turned red and said she couldn't possibly, that she never wore dresses. That moment in therapy had the stuff of which therapists dream—core content coupled with powerful and manifest affect. The wearing of pants or dresses became a leit motif in the treatment, and a barometer of her "acceptance" of her disability. It was 8 months before she wore a dress, and then she brought it to therapy, changed into it in the bathroom, and out of it after the session. It was a turning point in treatment wherein the client recognized that she held certain beliefs from the moral and medical models of disability, and that these beliefs controlled much of her behavior and feelings related to the disability.

Goal 2: Empowerment

One of our jobs as therapists is to make ourselves unnecessary, to "empower" clients. This is no less or more true for clients with disabilities. But such clients have a different relationship to issues such as power, choice, independence and interdependence, assistance, and control. As discussed in earlier chapters, persons with disabilities spend more time interacting in settings in which they are in the subservient role. These include hospitals, rehabilitation settings, outpatient care, assistive device fittings, assessments, physical therapy, and so on. Further, there is a quite pronounced and prevalent assumptions by these delivery agencies (and by charities) that "persons with a disability, if left to themselves at best don't know how to take care of themselves and at worst will actually harm themselves" (Gwin, 1995, p. 7). The role of being a passive recipient opposes the goal of self-advocacy. Empowerment involves taking the lead in one's own disability. This includes health care, prevention, social management, control of information, and disclosure of disability.

Persons with disabilities rarely get to set standards, hire, fire, or train persons who assist them. In almost all instances prior expert approval is needed. For example, if a person needed a modified car, the state department of rehabilitation (DOR) is likely to require the following: an assessment by DOR to verify need, a referral from the DOR, an evaluation by a DOR-designated agency of the specific nature of the modifications needed, and written specifications by the DOR-designated agency which puts out the request for bids and selects the vendor. Then, after this process in which the driver-to-be is in a forced passive role, he or she receives the modified vehicle. If there are problems it goes back through the evaluating agency. Thus the end user is disconnected from the process of evaluation, specification, negotiation, and selection. The link between choice and consequences is broken and any corrective feedback loop is bypassed. This "requirement for prior expert approval first permits, and then encourages, passive acceptance or voracious consumption of whatever services the expert approves. Service recipients eventually lose control over events in their lives and can become apathetic or hostile, even if the expert's plan generally meets a recipient's narrowly defined disability-related needs." In contrast, "when service providers are hired directly by the people they are supposed to serve, they avoid the divided loyalties and tensions that inevitably arise from being hired and managed by program staff who are independent from users" (Center for Economic Policy Analysis, cited in Gwin, 1995, p. 7). The issue underlying these situations is that of self-determination. When people with disabilities are denied control over many aspects of their own lives, and prevented from setting their own priorities, the resulting disempowerment can lead to depression, rage, anxiety, passivity, and hopelessness. A key goal of treatment is to help people who encounter situations in which they have little control to gain control of that which is important to them. On a broader scale, in the long run this goal involves ensuring that the end users (i.e., the people with the disabilities) gain control of public funds and decision-making processes that determine funding priorities.

Empowerment does not mean doing everything ourselves. This is an important point, related to the confusion between independence and solitariness. Some people with disabilities try to assert their independence by doing everything by themselves, from opening doors to carrying packages to recovering from surgery. A common theme in the disability community is the need to achieve balance between independent living and being a "supercrip" (see Chapter 2, in the section on language). The history of multiple medical traumas experienced by so many people with disabilities instills a motivation never to be that powerless again. But power and self-determination can become confused with individualism. The disability community has been trying to embrace the concept of interdependence (as opposed to independence), but this is still a tricky distinction for many clients (not to mention therapists).

Goal 3: Values

Four value changes have been hypothesized to be important in the "acceptance of disability" (what I would prefer to call living with the disability):

1. *Enlargement of the scope of values,* such that there is a shift within the hierarchy of the value system. In this shifting, those values that are negatively affected by the disability (e.g., athleti-

cism) take a lower position, and those that remain intact (e.g., creativity) shift to higher positions.

2. *The subordination of physique relative to other values.* This is really a more specific example of the first change in that physique and physical abilities, which are usually affected by disability, shift lower in the hierarchy relative to other values.
3. *The containment of disability effects.* This involves ensuring that values that are unaffected by the disability are not demoted in the hierarchy (by self or others) because of inaccurate association with the effects of the disability.
4. *A change in the process by which one assigns a value to a place on the hierarchy,* such that comparative value (how prized a value is in relation to other values) is replaced by asset value (the intrinsic worth of a value). For example, walking and wheelchair riding are equally valued (asset value) because each allows mobility. Consideration of the value of walking versus wheeling (a comparative value) is eliminated.

Employment campaigns for persons with disabilities state, "It's the ability, not the disability." Cuteness aside, there is a serious message here. The slogan is really about the shifting of values to place those things associated with ability higher on the hierarchy and to demote values affected by impairment to lower on the hierarchy such that they merit less prominence and attention. This is one goal with clients—a refocusing of attention from what has been lost to what remains. This cannot be a superficial Pollyanna-ish switch, or just a "think positive" message. Rather, it must involve development of a genuine appreciation for remaining abilities and values. The position of values related to physique (e.g., beauty, physical strength, and athleticism), inasmuch as they are directly affected by the disability, become subordinate to other values (e.g., friendship, loyalty, creativity, motivation, and work).

A second change is to view values according to their inherent assets as opposed to their status in comparison to other values. Asset values have intrinsic worth, usefulness, and beauty, regardless of their value relative to an external standard. For example, a scooter allows mobility, enables travel to places otherwise too large or taxing to be managed on foot, has a place to store purchases, provides seating, and goes faster than walking. Thus its asset (i.e., intrinsic) value is high. It is only in comparative status to walking that it is judged inferior because walking is more highly valued than using a mobility aid.

Maria, a divorced woman in her 50s, had knee surgery about 8 months ago. Since then she has walked using one crutch. She would do better on two crutches, but in her view one crutch is less stigmatizing than two and doesn't advertise her disability status as much. In this comparison-value model, two crutches has less value than one crutch, which in turn has less value than no crutches. In an asset value, two crutches would be more highly valued because they achieve the goal of walking that is smoother, more pain free, and allows walking for longer distances. Her reliance on the comparison value for determining the use of crutches restricts her mobility more than is necessary. It might be concluded that Maria is having trouble "accepting the disability" (i.e., living with her present level of disability).

A third change involves the ability to find meaning in events, abilities, goals, and life. This is really about the containment of disability effects. The fact of disability cannot be allowed to infiltrate all aspects of life, or to make otherwise positive events negative. Suppose, for example, that a man with SCI is prevented from taking the kind and level of job he held previously because he becomes overly fatigued and then is prone to illness or injury. He then takes a lower-status and -paying job but one that requires fewer hours and allows more flexibility in time management. The health benefits are better, and he gets more sick leave. In this example we can see how this man might have many negative cognitions related to this job change, and hence how his mood would be negatively affected. Conversely, he might relish the simpler lifestyle and the slower pace afforded by the new job and enjoy the extra time he can spend with his family. If he holds this perspective, his mood is likely to be positive and less vulnerable to assault by small setbacks (e.g., a urinary tract infection). Therapists can facilitate this change in perspective by helping clients see the actual and the inevitable. For example, in the previous vignette, it was pointed out to Maria repeatedly how her life was restricted, how there were places where she never went, and how tired she felt most of the time. This may seem mean, but it does not serve Maria well for the therapist to collude in her denial of impairment, any more than it would be wise to ignore the drinking of an alcoholic. It is possible that Maria might say that she has carefully considered all the mobility and lifestyle options, weighing the pros and cons of each, and has chosen to continue the use of one crutch even knowing the restrictions this entails. Should we, as therapists, accept this? In true rabbinical fashion, let me answer with a question: What would you do if an alcoholic client told you she had carefully considered the option of continued drinking and sobriety, had analyzed the pros and cons of each, was well aware of the costs of drinking, but nonetheless had come to the decision to remain an active alcoholic? If you don't think these two situations are analogous because alcohol impairs reasoning while physical disability does not, then you are underestimating the powerful effects of living with a stigmatized condition in a discriminatory world.

Goal 4: Containing Spread Effects

Spread is the power of a single known characteristic to evoke other, unknown, characteristics of a person. One way to contain spread is by viewing the disability as a possession (e.g., "He *has* a physical disability") rather than as a characteristic (e.g., "He *is* physically disabled"). Characteristics (such as friendliness) can be expected to be manifest in a variety of situations and to suggest other characteristics that are likely accompaniments. Possessions, on the other hand, are more delimited. Spread is also contained by defining one's worth as what one *is* (i.e., abilities and inner characteristics) as opposed to how one *appears*. To able-bodied persons this may seem like an artificial division of mind and body, but remember that in disability, anatomy is not destiny.

Spread effects are particularly important in two areas: jobs and dating. In each instance it becomes imperative that the person with the disability be able to convey assets and worth. This must be done even in the face of others' view of disability as a defining characteristic. Families with disabilities may need coaching in how to present the disability to others. It is often the case that families downplay or apologize for the disability. Thus the family may say "He has CP but there's nothing wrong with his brain," or, "She is very minimally mentally retarded but you wouldn't notice it," or, "He has trouble speaking but we all understand him." Families need help understanding the effects of these descriptions and evaluating whether the description has the desired impact. Conversely, the person with the disability may cast an overly positive light, appearing to gloss over the disability, or too negative a light, thereby playing into existing stereotypes. In the following example a new employee achieves a good balance in explaining her MS needs to a supervisor:

> "I wanted to let you know that I have MS, which is a neurological disorder. I have times, usually lasting a few weeks, where it affects me more and other times it affects me very little. The main effects are fatigue and some muscle weakness. Also I have trouble with my memory. However, it should not affect my job performance very much. You'll notice that I take a lot of notes when we talk, and use this Palm Pilot to beep at me for reminders of tasks or meetings. It would be helpful if you think I'm not paying attention if you would say my name and remind me to pay attention. I'm happy to answer any questions you might have about it."

In this example the woman with MS controls the impression of her disability in several ways. First, she takes the lead in bringing up the subject, making it clear that she is comfortable with the topic, and being open to any questions that her boss might have. Second, she focuses only on those aspects her supervisor needs to know. Third, she is concrete about the effects of MS on job-related tasks and specific about how she deals with these. Fourth, she makes it clear that she has taken responsibility for managing her job-related difficulties (memory, notes, reminders). Finally, she asks for a specific accommodation from the supervisor. However, being able to do this is not as simple as it might seem. It requires that the person with the disability feel very comfortable with the disability and is able to take the lead in how the disability is perceived. And even those who are able to do this on the job often find it much more difficult when dating.

Often clients want to discuss when in a relationship (whether dating or business) to let the other person know about the disability. I have found that persons with more visible and/or pronounced disabilities usually want to let the other person know very quickly, say, in a cover letter or over the phone. The rationale seems to be that it pays to weed out quickly those people who are going to have a problem with the disability. And some clients tell me they feel dishonest not disclosing a disability to potential employers. I don't completely buy this; I believe it is a self-protective maneuver. Those of us with disabilities want to avoid that sudden subtle change that comes over others' faces when they first notice the disability, a look that says "something's wrong with you." This is a perfectly understandable goal. But in the effort to avoid that look, the client may be leading with the disability too readily, reinforcing the already-problematic tendency of others to make disability the salient and defining charascteristic. Many clients need help coming up with decision rules on a case-by-case basis, or being good empiricists and trying different methods.

Goal 5: Looking Forward

But have you ever brushed your teeth one evening and suddenly looked in the mirror and thought, "Oh my God, I'm going to have to brush my teeth every morning and every night for the rest of my life, and I don't think I can bear it!" There are aspects of disability that lend themselves to these kinds of thoughts. The endless repetition of impairment-related rituals, the constant saying of "thank-you" as people hold open doors, the familiarity of pain, the recognition of responses to you as a stigmatized person—in the wrong frame of mind it is easy to think wearily, "I've been here so often before." Various strategies are needed to counter the weariness. One is to reframe the task in a different light. For example, saying thank you to people who hold open doors can be an opportunity to practice social skills. For the past 2 years I have reframed nasty things people did or said related to my disability by thinking, "That's a good example for the book!"

Another strategy is to ensure that clients have something to look forward to. *Everyone* needs something to look forward to, not just clients with disabilities, and it is especially important for those clients with negative mood states, such as depression. However, clients with disabilities may need extra help in this area, because the effects of pain, fatigue, and weakness can occupy a large portion of time and erode ability to find pleasure. Clients should have four levels of positive future events: (1) small pleasures that occur at least once a day (e.g., reading in bed and eating two stale marshmallows), (2) slightly larger events that occur at least once a week (listening to Prairie Home Companion), (3) monthly events (e.g., visiting with a good friend and going out for a nice dinner), and (4) larger events that occur maybe once a year (e.g., family vacation and a favorite holiday). Analysis of these four levels of events can help pinpoint where paucity of pleasure occurs and focus treatment on those targeted areas. These distinctions are also important because clients may limit their perspective to noticing only those rarer larger events and need help in finding and enjoying smaller and more frequent events.

Goal 6: Developing a Support Network

Empowerment, hopefulness, meaning, and value cannot survive without support. An essential goal is for clients to develop a support network of people who accept the disability without devaluing the person with the disability. This means the kind of milieu in which one can appear in a bathing suit unselfconsciously; where one can say "my hip hurts" and get sympathy but not pity; where one is free to bring up disability as a part of a discourse without it becoming the primary focus.

Clients with disabilities who have a history of ostracization and stigmatization may come to settle for friendships and relationships that offer too little. Others may have learned early that it is better to have fewer but more accepting friendships but may be having difficulties expanding their network. Sometimes adults with severe congenital disabilities have been kept inside the family as adolescents and young adults and therefore have failed to develop other support networks. Regardless of the history, persons with disabilities need a safe and secure place to be disabled. For some clients therapy is the first place for this to occur. For others this safe haven has been found in friendships but not in a romantic relationship. Clients may need help learning how to discuss disability issues with friends, and in understanding how people feel by observing the ways in which they act.

The relationship of the person with a disability and his or her family can be quite complex. Ideally the family is a part of the support network, but not the sole support. It is here that one should learn what unconditional positive regard truly means. But there is also the possibility that the family, far from being a support, contributes to the difficulties in esteem and valuation of the person with the disability. As is the case for gays and lesbians, the family can be a source of conflict, rejection, and unacceptance. Also, the family is most likely to operate under the medical model of disability. After all, the job of parents usually involved getting a diagnosis of the child, finding doctors, making decisions about surgery and other medical treatments, providing physical therapy, monitoring development, and so on. In addition, parents interact with teachers and the school to ensure appropriate education. Thus parents' role in the disability often is focused on obtaining information and services. This role is particularly intense in the early years of life and schooling, and many families never redefine the role as the child grows older. The child, on the other hand, may come to affiliate with others with disabilities, develop an identity as a person with a disability, espouse the minority model of disability, and reject the models held by the family. In a sense, the child, now adult, outgrows the family. This is not unlike the gay man who is comfortably out in job and community but whose parents secretly hope he'll "outgrow it" if he just meets the right woman. These discrepancies in viewpoints limit the intimacy one can have within the family, as each side feels left out and distanced by the other. Thus therapy with adult clients with disabilities often involves resolving disability issues with the family. As part of this process, the "story" of the disability (see Chapter 6) needs to be turned over to the growing child. That is, the story of how the disability was discovered, what everyone thought and felt, what needed to be done, is usually the parents' story. The child's story is different, and he or she needs room to develop and own his or her own story.

Samuel is a man in his late 20s with muscular dystrophy. He uses an electric wheelchair and for part of the day a respirator. A college graduate in engineering, he's unemployed, and the DOR has been of limited assistance in helping him seek employment. One friend from college lives nearby, but he has lost contact with other college friends and doesn't meet many people in his current state of joblessness. His mother, a widow, lives in town, and he goes there for lunch or dinner twice a week and talks to her almost daily. She remarried 5 years ago and wants more time with her husband.

Although she never states this, she feels Samuel is too dependent on her and doesn't want as much contact as they now have. But she feels guilty about it and unable to take any action unless she knows Samuel has other people close to him. Samuel also would like to expand his social network but is frustrated in doing so. He feels very comfortable with his mother, and others don't measure up in terms of their initial responses to his disability. Thus the cycle of Samuel's overreliance on his mother is continued by both of them.

People with disabilities often are in a position of being helped by others, whether in minor acts such as holding open a door or more major ways such as assistance with daily grooming. The disability rights movement has made a careful distinction between these kinds of assistance and independence—the control over decision making and direction in one's life. But the notions of dependence, independence, and interdependence that are so pertinent to the disabled community can make for complicated psychosocial issues. I find that many of my clients with disabilities have extreme difficulty asking for help from friends. Doing so seems to represent an admission of weakness, even though they know that people without disabilities might ask for the same kind of help. Rosalie packs up to move into a new apartment by herself. Greg only picks up his mail at work once a day rather than ask someone else to collect it for him. Bob stands during a party rather than request that someone give up the one seat he'd be comfortable in. Jessica always declines her neighbor's offer to pick something up for Jessica when she's at the grocery store. Juan pushes the elevator buttons with his chin rather than wait for someone to assist him. In each instance refusing offers or not asking for help is seen as emblematic of independence. In these circumstances people need help seeing and valuing the kind of interdependence that friends, coworkers, and neighbors can develop and in reframing the meaning of "help."

CLINICAL EXAMPLE AND DISCUSSION[2]

This section helps readers translate the many ideas, assumptions, treatment considerations, and goals that have been presented in this chapter into practical application. Readers can see how these are applied more concretely to a case. Further, therapy in two time periods, during two different phases of the disability (diagnosis and 5 years later), are discussed.

---

[2]For a case presentation and discussion of a teenager with a disability, see Olkin (1995).

Jeff, a 30-year-old able-bodied married man with two small children, came to therapy because of uncertainty in his career. He was a
computer programmer, well paid and respected, but he felt he was
unlike most other computer types he met and he was not feeling a
sense of accomplishment or satisfaction in his work. He came for
two sessions, then postponed his third appointment twice to take
his wife to doctor appointments. In the third session he described
some odd symptoms his wife had been experiencing over the past 4
months, such as tingling in her legs and fingers, a feeling of eye
strain, and fatigue. They were having difficulty getting their HMO
(health maintenance organization) to take these symptoms seriously,
and one doctor had prescribed Xanax, which did not ameliorate
symptoms.

In my earlier days, I might have been too quick to think of anxiety
as a possible diagnosis, displaying a therapist's bias for the psychological
over the biological. Now I was fairly certain it was MS. However, I did
not say this to Jeff for several reasons. First, I am not a physician and
should not be making such diagnoses. Second, I could be wrong. Third,
going through the diagnostic process is important; even though it can be
frightening and often frustrating, it cannot be bypassed. Jeff and his wife
were starting to realize the diagnosis possibly was serious and potentially
long term. These realizations involve an emotional development that
takes some time to incorporate. For example, if a client whose mother
died when the client was young thinks now that the mother was "perfect," a clinician can't simply say, "Of course your mother was not perfect," and expect the client to bypass the process of coming to this real-
ization.

Jeff recontacted me about 3 months later. This time he wanted to
discuss his wife's probable diagnosis of MS. I agreed to see him
alone but was shifting my case formulation from individual and
intrapsychic work to a systemic model comprising the whole family,
including the needs of the two children (3 and 7) in this time of family turmoil. It seemed reasonable to see Jeff alone for another session, as I suspected he needed a place separate from his wife to talk
about his responses to the diagnosis, perhaps in ways that were premature for her to have to handle. This was indeed the case, only this
was more apparent to me than to Jeff. He was—on the surface—
being the quintessential supportive spouse, but just below that he
wasn't sure he could love a woman with MS, was worried he might
come to resent her for changing the course of her career and their
marriage (they had been trying to have third child, which they now
put on hold), was worried about her ability to be a mother as her
own needs increased, and was afraid he would have to take care of

her more and more over time (activating his own issues of being the son of an alcoholic mother). These are, frankly, painful things for any newly diagnosed spouse to hear, though common thoughts for the other partner.

I was hoping to encourage Jeff to express these ideas to me, so that we could understand them together, and allow him to maintain the emotional energy he needed to help his wife (Mary) and kids at this time. However, he kept evading these issues. After about the third time that he changed the topic to computers I decided to force the issue a little. I said, "excuse me a second," and went out to the waiting room where I keep my scooter and rode it back into the office. Staying seated on the scooter instead of my usual therapy chair, I said, "Now talk to me." This had the desired effect of immediately bringing the affect to the surface. (My scooter is like some enormous three-dimensional Rorschach inkblot; people see many things in it.) Jeff felt initially guilty, then enormous relief at being able to express these (to him) unacceptable thoughts. The time in individual therapy to say these things without worrying about the effect on his wife increased Jeff's readiness for coming for conjoint therapy. I gave Jeff and Mary the option of starting with another therapist, as I had seen Jeff individually, but they chose to continue with me. Mary worked in a TV newsroom, with occasional air time that she was hoping to increase. She was terrified about the effects of her disorder on her overall energy in a demanding job and her perceived desirability as an on-air reporter. She knew little about MS other than what the doctors had told her. This included their scary admonition that they had to wait 5 years to see what the course of her disorder would be. She knew there were three types of MS.[3] I asked if she knew anyone with MS. She could think of Richard Pryor and Annette Funicello, but no one she knew personally. Her immediate thoughts about these two celebrities is that they disappeared from public view once they had the disorder; this thought buttressed her fears about her own career.

This stage of therapy was focused on two aspects of disability. The first was the diagnostic process itself, entailing many doctor visits, tests of varying degrees of invasiveness (e.g., MRI and spinal tap), feeling captive to a medical system, the scare of alternate and more serious diagnoses which had to be ruled out, and living with uncertainty. A positive sign was that they were clearly going through this process as a team, both as partners and as parents. The second was on figuring out the

---

[3]The literature on MS refers to three types: relapsing and remitting, slowly progressive, and rapidly progressive. In fact there is a newly identified fourth type called secondary progressive, which is a combination of the relapsing and remitting and slowly progressive types.

meaning of the diagnosis: What is MS? In undertaking to learn about this large and emotionally laden topic, the couple closed ranks—they joined forces in keeping others out. This is not uncommon. For example, women with breast cancer often do not seek support groups or other women with breast cancer until they have made the decision about which course of treatment to follow and have begun that process. The initial stage seems to be one of drawing inward, with the second phase of active treatment more one of seeking supports to endure the process. Similarly, until one knows one's own status, it is difficult to comprehend the range of possibilities or to hear information from others, even those with MS. Compounding this is the fact that the course of MS is highly idiosyncratic, treatment options are limited, and some of the most visible media images extremely negative (e.g., about 25% of the cases of Kervorkian-assisted suicides are persons—mostly women—with MS).

These initial tasks and responses are very common—drawing inward, initial coping, processing of diagnosis. However, the next phase is more culture specific. The degree to which people seek information, read on their own, are prone to utilize support groups, talk with their immediate and extended family, tell others, and alter their role in family, work, and social circles is variable, depending not only on culture but on SES, immigration status, cultural views toward the medical profession, resources available, logistical problems (e.g., transportation and childcare), and the meaning of disability in the person's culture.

For Jeff and his wife, the next phase was to increase information. Some people at this point become voracious readers; others titrate the flow of input carefully. I did not at this stage tell them that my spouse has MS and that we'd gone through this process of diagnosis and investigation during our marriage. Although it may have increased my credibility, it seemed a cheap hat trick to pull out the rabbit of similarity. Furthermore, every process is different, and there had to be room for theirs without comparison to mine. Finally, I wanted to counter their increasing belief that no one could understand what they were going through; if they felt understood by me but only because I had been in the same boat it might reinforce this idea. It took a while before they noticed that I had a great number of books on MS on my shelves, and before they asked me directly why this was. I stated only that my husband has MS. I offered no more information than that, waiting to take my lead from them. They did not ask more for quite some time.

An area in which I took the lead concerned their children. I felt strongly that the parents needed to give the children an explanation for increased tension in the house. Jeff and Mary thought the children were too young, wouldn't understand, would have increased and perhaps unmanageable anxiety, that they should wait until they, the parents, knew more information and were more resolved about the issue. I thought their not telling the kids was indicative of their more general difficulty of telling others about the diagnosis— an issue I thought could wait, except in this particular instance. I also thought they had an unrealistic view of what children perceive and what information children can handle. My view prevailed through unfortunate circumstances: Both kids had increased symptoms (nightmares, new separation anxiety, bed wetting in the elder, regression in the younger), and Jeff and Mary became convinced that their children knew something serious was amiss. We discussed and role-played how to tell the children, which elicited a tangible degree of sadness and fear in the therapy room. The parents felt overwhelmed by the emotions aroused and afraid they would become so overpowered by these emotions that they couldn't help their children. However, with some assistance they were able to draw on their experience of one child's ear surgery; they were able to recognize that despite their terror in that situation, they had "been there" for the child.

Models

It is never too early to begin discussion of models of disability. Before any model becomes the family's modus operandi it can be helpful to start linking clients' automatic thoughts with their implications. In this case the moral model was evidenced by the couple's belief that they had done something to deserve the MS. Jeff in particular felt he hadn't done a good enough job with his mother and now was getting a second chance to take care of a woman in his life. They both had thoughts about the MS ruining their kids' lives, that the family was stigmatized, and that this would lead to trouble for the kids with teachers and friends. The medical model also was very much in evidence, particularly in the belief that science would bring hope by discovering a cure for MS. The couple was aware of newer research that showed promise of new treatments. These new treatments had been tried only on mice, and the couple vastly underestimated the time and process from mice to FDA approval. While maintaining hope in science and technology, they also felt that doctors don't know enough. They were angry at doctors who had given an incorrect diagnosis, at the length of time it took to get a more clear diagnosis, and the lack of information about prognosis. The minority model was also in evidence. The couple believed that only other couples with MS could understand what they were going through. They turned to the National MS Society for information and resources. Though they weren't yet ready to become a part of any group, they acknowledged that a support group might be useful in the future. Mary had the thought, "I will lose my job *because of my MS*," but she was shocked to hear me reflect this back as her losing her job *because of discrimination.*

Notice that each model can be used as a source of discomfort or of solace. These models are not progressive, as if one moves from the moral to the medical and finally to the minority model. Usually elements of all three coexist, and the usefulness and costs of each must be carefully examined. It would be highly unusual for a family with a new diagnosis to espouse the minority model unless they were already a part of the disability community. Although I espouse the minority model and believe it to be more useful for people with disabilities, this does not mean that therapists should try to convert clients to this model without judging the client's readiness and the model's appropriateness for the client's stage of development and treatment. In the earlier phases of disability onset and diagnosis, people often resist the idea of changing identities from "us" to "them." Being "them" implies living with the disability forever, at a phase during which people are still hoping for a miracle.

Empowerment

As do most people encountering a new and serious diagnosis, this couple initially felt overwhelmed with information and emotions. But as they got a diagnosis they were able to take more power over the process. For example, they quit one doctor because they disliked how he had handled the diagnostic process, and they found a new doctor to oversee the coordination of medical diagnosis and treatment. They found information for themselves and became more informed consumers. They insisted on a consultation with a specialist on MS. And they kept control over the decision of when and how to tell others. The couple decided to tell family and close friends but not coworkers or supervisors.

Values

As often happens with serious crisis in a family, the value of close family and friends becomes immediately apparent. Painfully, some friends drop out of the picture, but the ones who remain become highly valued. Again, as commonly happens, this couple decided not to continue postponing events. They planned a family vacation for that summer and remodeled their kitchen. I confess I thought this last was a bad idea, in violation of my rule of not tackling too much at once. However, they thought there was no need to wait for something that they would enjoy now. Mary even joked that she didn't want her dream kitchen when she was too ill to use it. I questioned why they were acting as if Mary's disorder were fatal. They responded by asserting that if MS could happen to them, something else could too, so why wait. They started to see small moments with their children and with family as important, not to be taken for granted. On the downside, they felt more impatient with others, particularly when they felt someone was wasting their time. They wished others held their new perspective (roughly summarized as "you never know what can happen so enjoy it now") and sometimes felt isolated when this perspective wasn't shared.

Spread

One way to contain the spread of disability was by controlling when to tell people, particularly at work. Their first impulse was not to tell anyone until they knew what they were dealing with. Their next impulse was to tell everyone because otherwise it felt as if they had a secret life that isolated them from others. They found a happy medium in deciding on a case-by-case basis. For example, they told their son's first-grade teacher because the son was having more difficulty with acting out in class. They did not tell Mary's 90-year-old grandmother.

Jeff needed assistance in understanding what qualities of Mary would and would not be affected by the MS. He visualized Mary in a wheelchair and could not reconcile this image with that of Mary as a competent mother. Mary was having difficulty thinking about career possibilities if she let go of her goal of being on the air, and she needed help with analyzing aspects of her job and how they might be affected by her disability. Each of them was struggling to see the disability as only one aspect of their lives without letting it define them. It was hard to recognize that the vast hugeness of the issue during the diagnostic process would abate.

Looking Forward

As stated earlier, the couple talked about not postponing fun until some undefined future and planned more trips and vacations. On a smaller scale, they bought more premade dinners, something they would have described as needlessly extravagant before. They reserved a weekly time for them as a couple. Thus they were very good at the three larger levels of positive events (weekly, monthly, yearly), but on a daily basis they still felt overwhelmed, suddenly inundated with emotions, and somewhat depressed. It may be that a more fundamental change in values must ensue before more prosaic forms of positive events become available.

Support Network

This couple was lucky in having immediate supports available. Their families, especially Mary's sister, made themselves both physically and emotionally available. Mary had two close women friends in whom she confided and got closer to one mother of her daughter's friend when she told the mother about her MS and the mother confided about her own hidden disability (Crohn's disease). Jeff had more difficulty telling anyone outside his family. Neither wanted to join a support group but could see that they might in the future. The therapy may have served some of the needs a support group would have, and those it couldn't supply were ones the couple didn't yet know they needed.

The Second Phase of Therapy

Five years later Mary and Jeff returned to therapy. There were three presenting problems. The first was that some of Mary's behaviors were having an impact on the relationship. Notably, Jeff wondered if her lability, depression, and memory loss were due to the MS. In addition, during Mary's periods of extreme fatigue she withdrew from family activities and ceased some of her family roles. The second issue was Mary's concern about telling people at work her diagnosis and asking for changes in work duties and load. She knew that she could not continue at her current pace and that she was going to have to "come out" on the job as a person with a disability. Third, they wondered about the impact of the MS on their children, now 8 and 12.

The first issue was helping the couple become more knowledgeable about the range of symptoms possible with MS, and the idiosyncratic nature of symptom patterns. At this point they noticed the books on my shelf, and I reminded them that my husband had MS. They quizzed me about his symptoms, and I disclosed his memory difficulties, among other things. (This level of self-disclosure may seem usual to clinicians ascribing to feminist therapy and more alien to others.) I also shared with them some readings about memory and mood changes in MS. (All the symptoms Jeff mentioned were possibly due to the MS itself.) Regarding Mary's work, she felt pressure to make changes but terrified of the impact of disclosing her MS. She had not disclosed her MS and had moved her career further in the direction of more on-air work. But her hours were grueling and the pace intense. It was in discussing work that the minority model became important. Mary had to make the transition in self-identity. She saw herself as a person with a medical condition for whom allowances had to be made, as if she were out with the flu and everyone had to cover her work for her. This view didn't serve her in the long haul because she always felt beholden to others, and as if she were on probation. However, a therapist cannot simply give someone a new model of disability. Instead, I persuaded Jeff and Mary to join a support group to have contact with other families with disabilities. Because of the similarity in professions I had Mary read Moving Violations (by John Hockenberry, a journalist who uses a wheelchair). I used language reflecting civil rights (e.g., "What kind of reasonable accommodations would help you do your job?" or, "What are your rights in the workplace if you disclose your disability?") and gave them a small amount of reading on the ADA. We role-played telling people about the MS and responding to various reactions. I particularly wanted to teach Mary how to take the lead in helping her coworkers and supervisors feel comfortable in discussing her disability, as this has been demonstrated to be a key factor in successful job interviews for people with disabilities.

Regarding the children, we discussed what the kids needed to know. Jeff and Mary did not need to role-play talking with their children, as they both felt capable of this. The issue was more that they had talked about the MS around the time of diagnosis but had not updated the kids as the MS progressed and, more importantly, as the developmental level of the children changed and their capacity for understanding grew. They did ask in many ways for reassurance from me that the MS would not have any deleterious effects on their children, something I could never give them. But I was able to talk about some positive possible results of growing up in a family with a parent with a disability. They continued to want more, and I continued to be unable to give it to them. Termination began when they finally stopped needing this; this change implied that there were many internal changes in identity, for Mary individually, as a mother, and as a professional, and for them as a couple. They had begun a process of living with the disability rather than viewing it as an alien force that had insinuated itself into the family.

EIGHT

Etiquette with Clients with Disabilities

I've stressed throughout this book that specific clinical behaviors should result from the therapist's understanding of disability experience. If we think of the triad necessary for effective therapy—behavior (skills), attitudes (affect), and knowledge (cognitions)—I have focused on attitudes and knowledge, awareness, and conceptualization. But changes in behavior can effect changes in the other two areas. And a key area of behavior has to do with the small, but important, interaction between therapist and new client with a disability: the etiquette of interchange. Frank discussion of etiquette with persons with disabilities is scarce. Therefore I focus in this chapter on giving guidelines for such interactions. Although many of these may seem self-evident, they merit emphasis and elaboration here. Furthermore, all rules have exceptions, and these bear discussion.

TEN GENERAL RULES

1. Don't stare. Okay, this one is obvious. But in practice it's harder to do. Disabilities often contain oddities, assistive devices, unusual mannerisms—things and actions that draw our attention.

Anna, a college woman with a physical disability and a severe speech dysfluency due to stuttering, arrived to her fourth session at the campus psychological services center wearing thin headphones attached to a small box clipped at her waist. The therapist said, "I see you have a new machine." Anna replied, "Yes, it's to help my

190

stuttering," but immediately went on to discuss other things on her mind—she had failed an important exam and her roommate was pregnant.

While some people might think that Anna's cursory attention to her assistive device with the counselor was "denial," let's reframe it: Anna was trying to do what any other student client would do— bring up problems and concerns that were on her mind. In so doing, she didn't want to have to stop and "be a disabled person." In fact, it was the therapist's interest in the device that made it salient, not the client's behavior. Therefore the therapist, recognizing this, ended the session on time, scheduled the next appointment with Anna, then, clearly on her, not the client's, time, asked, "Do you have a moment to show me your new device?" At that point Anna willingly gave a demonstration of an audio-delay feedback (ADF) machine.[1]

2. Don't tell clients with disabilities about all the other persons with disabilities you know. This is the "some of my best friends have disabilities" routine, and persons with disabilities hear it a lot. There is such a drive to share the fact that this is not the first person with a disability with whom you've come into contact that many people blurt this fact out ("Oh, I sat next to someone on a plane who was disabled!"). Even if the person with a disability is your mother, refrain from sharing it. After all, you don't share other personal information immediately with a client, do you? However, if the person with a disability whom you know really is your mother, this information may be conveyed at a later time, if appropriate. Such a revelation signals the client with a disability that you have some close and intimate experience with disability and may increase your credibility related to disability issues. From your experience with, say, your mother, you may have some notions of how someone with a disability may feel and behave, but these notions may not be applicable to the current client; he or she must be free to feel or behave differently from your expectations.

3. Don't assume the person needs your help, and don't begin to help without asking. Use your judgment here; ask yourself, "What would I normally do in this situation?" or, "What would I do if this were an elderly person?" The elderly-person guide is a useful one; with elderly people we are respectful, not oversolicitous, yet mindful of occasional needs for physical assistance.

If you start rearranging your office ("We'll just move this filing cabi-

---

[1]An ADF machine plays back the wearer's voice with millisecond-delayed timing. Paradoxically, it reduces stuttering in those who usually stutter but creates stuttering in those who usually have good speech fluency.

net over here"), chattering away ("I had no idea that elephant in the doorway was such a problem"), or otherwise behaving in ways that are not your norm, your stance and grace as a therapist will be affected. It's often fairly obvious when people start behaving uncharacteristically, and the client well may become aware of it. This is not a good way to start the therapy. (Usually when we as therapists behave uncharacteristically we've learned to examine that countertransference and often think it is alerting us to something important about the client. However, in this case the more parsimonious explanation is that the you are uncomfortable around the client with the disability and trying to hide it, and more self-conscious about your own behaviors.)

4. Be clear about who is the client. If the client with a disability has a personal assistant, interpreter, or family member who accompanies him or her to the therapy, be clear, direct, and explicit about that person's role in the treatment process. If he or she is there to facilitate communication (e.g., interpreting), nonetheless look at and speak directly to the client. Avoid unnecessary discussion with the interpreter or aide; this is disrespectful to the client.

> Chris, a man with severe CP in his late 20s, came to treatment for help with personal relationships. He used a wheelchair into which he was strapped for stability. His right arm had the most functioning, with partial hand function, and with it he could tether and untether his left arm. His hand moved sporadically, and his mouth manifested uncontrolled movements. His speech was laborious, and about 60% of his words were unintelligible to new listeners. Because of this situation Chris was accompanied by one of his personal assistants, an engaging, attractive, articulate, and sprightly young woman. She knew her job well and would not "translate" Chris automatically but would first verify whether the therapist understood what was said. If not, she repeated Chris's message, using as close to his words as possible. The therapist began the session very mindful of the necessity of addressing Chris, but slowly, by almost imperceptible degrees, started turning her attention away from Chris and toward his assistant. By the end of the session she no longer said "you" (meaning Chris) but "he" (asking assistant about Chris). Chris did not show up for his second appointment.

5. Don't be afraid to say you don't understand either the words themselves or their meaning. We all like to think of ourselves as cross-culturally aware, and we are hesitant to ask persons to repeat words we think we should have understood, or to ask what is meant by them. We worry this will show our ignorance. (I am reminded of a time when I didn't ask an African American client what "fet" was because I thought

it would show how very unhip I am. It turned out to be "phet" as in methamphetamine, which put an entirely different spin on the session. I also discovered that this word use was idiosyncratic to the client. I lost a lot of therapeutic ground by pretending to understand.)

> Deborah, a working woman in her 30s, whose CP was not physically as severe as Chris's, also had difficulties with speech. However, she spoke much more rapidly than did Chris and was in fact a fairly voluble woman. She attended therapy alone and had never used personal assistance for communication. The therapist felt embarrassed to admit he didn't understand Deborah's words; he assumed that if Deborah didn't use an assistant in her career, then most other people must not be having as much difficulty understanding her as he did. He was able to pull off the first session—seemingly doing a lot of listening and asking usual questions. But the second session required more tailored responses, and Deborah confronted the therapist with words along these lines: "It is a lot of work for me to talk. I don't do it just to hear myself. I want to communicate, and if I'm not, if you don't understand me, I want to know. It is rude for people to pretend to understand me." The therapist apologized, and agreed to ask for clarification in the future. He then upped his requests for repetition threefold. However, although he did ask more often for repetition, it was still less than needed for him to really understand Deborah. By the eighth session both therapist and client agreed that treatment wasn't "working," and Deborah quit. She did not want to start again with the new person who this therapist recommended; at this stage, she felt misunderstood, abandoned, angry, and $800 poorer.

6. You don't need to worry about word choices that seem counter to the disability. Examples might be, "Do you see what I mean?" to a person with a visual impairment, or suggesting that a person in a wheelchair take a "walk" as part of a plan to increase activities to counter depression. If you'd normally use these words or phrases there is no reason not to continue them.

However, some words carry great emotive power to persons with disabilities in ways that they don't to able-bodied persons, particularly the word "crippled." An example might be, "You are emotionally crippled by this guilt." It justifiably may be hard for the client not to think that the therapist's choice of words reflects some unconscious hyperawareness of the client's disability status.

7. Don't touch someone's assistive device (wheelchair, voice computer, prosthetic, crutches, etc.) without permission. Suppose you lay your spectacles down on the table, and the person you were talking to

put her hand over one earpiece or traced a finger across the lens; what would you be likely to feel? Now imagine the person did this while the glasses were still on your face. Your space has been violated, yes? Assistive devices are extensions of one's body. Touching the device is like touching the person, even if the person has no physical contact with the device at the moment. Wheelchairs are like one's legs, and I can only presume you don't rub a client's legs. In restaurants I usually lean my crutches against a nearby wall. If a waiter grabs them and says, "Let me just move them over here where they will be more out of the way," I feel as if he had suddenly grabbed my shoulder.

8. Nonverbal cues are often altered by disability. For example, facial grimaces have different meaning in someone with no disabilities than in someone like Chris (the young man with CP in the previous example). Persons who communicate with ASL use their faces and bodies to change meaning of hand signs (e.g., "guilt" is changed to "paranoia" by eye motions back and forth). You will have to learn to understand the interaction among specific disabilities, their severity, the physical manifestations and body movements; above all, be careful in how you interpret body language.

9. Think about the temperature in your office. Many persons with disabilities are very sensitive to heat (e.g., MS) or cold (e.g., arthritis). In my office I cannot control the temperature, and many clients find it very chilly (I love it; my foot swells in heat). Therefore I keep a warm blanket and extra sweaters on hand for clients.

10. Don't take these rules too seriously. They are guidelines, not absolutes. For every person with disabilities who appreciates your sticking to these guidelines, there may be another who resents those very actions. As Radio Shack says, "You have questions, we have answers." Unfortunately, the answers don't always match the questions.

WHEELCHAIRS AND SCOOTERS

For long interactions with a person who is seated, whether on a couch, in a wheelchair, or on a scooter, it is polite to be at his or her physical level. To accomplish this feat most readily you can simply sit down. Another way is to lean back against a desk or table. Finally, you could crouch, although this is not recommended for all; I find some people can get away with crouching and make it look natural, and the same behavior in others tends to come across as patronizing.

Make your office physically accessible to persons on wheels. This may not seem like an etiquette point, but recall the discussion about the experience of a room full of people jumping up to rearrange themselves for you. It is better if you've done this in advance (see also discussion in Chapter 6, in this volume, about accessibility laws for therapists). But of course it often may be that you have a chair, end table, pile of books, and other paraphernalia in the path of someone entering your office. Go move them and begin the session much as you would any other. It is not necessary to fall all over yourself apologizing. A simple statement is fine (e.g., "Let me take a moment to move these," or, "I guess my office is less accessible than I thought").

You can't assume the person will stay in the wheelchair or scooter, so don't automatically move the regular chair to one side until you know where the client would like to sit. Many people who use such devices can walk or transfer to another chair. Another chair may be more comfortable, the person may benefit from movement and change of position, or he or she just may prefer to sit where most clients do. A reasonable question is, "Would you like to stay in your wheelchair or transfer to another chair?"

Be aware of the general accessibility of your area and any places to which you refer the client. Take the time to find out the accessibility of a site before sending the client. For example, don't send the client in a wheelchair for neuropsychological testing to a building that is not accessible. Consider, too, whether the client uses public transportation and whether the referral location is near a stop.

Be aware of what "accessible" means for wheelchairs and scooters. Know the relevant information about grab bars, layout of bathrooms, slope of ramps, curb cuts, doorway width—you don't have to become an expert on building codes, but you should have some sense of general parameters. Do not assume that because there are laws mandating access, most places will be in compliance. In addition there are many exceptions to the laws, and issues as yet untested in the courts. The result is that a good portion of the United States quite simply is not accessible to those on wheels.

Marika, a married woman in her early 40s, set up an initial appointment with a therapist and specifically asked about accessibility of the building, parking, and immediate surrounding area of the therapist's office. She was told that it was accessible. As usual Marika arrived a bit early to allow for unforeseen barriers, but it was more difficult than she expected: The handicapped parking was nowhere in sight, and there was no curb cut. She spent over 20 minutes searching, finally finding the parking spaces and ramps around the side of the building next door, from which locale she had a lengthy trip on the sidewalk to her therapist's building. The front door lacked an automatic opener and was too heavy for her to manage; she had to wait for someone to be going her way to open the door for her. The therapist began the session by interpreting her tardiness. Marika responded with anger and blamed him for his ignorance in how he responded to her request for information on accessibility. He judged her as poorly adjusted to her disability and externalizing of problems. The therapy never got off the ground.

Never push someone's wheelchair unless requested to do so or the wheelchair is in imminent danger of tipping. Electric wheelchairs, especially those with more reclined backs, are much more prone to tipping because the weight of the batteries can create an imbalance. If the grade is too steep there is danger of tipping whether going up or down. For electric wheelchairs, a 1-inch step can make an area inaccessible, whereas manual wheelchair users can usually manage this, and some can even jump up or down a curb (though not two contiguous steps). Manual chairs are not like those in hospitals, which are designed to be pushed; they are made to be operated by the seated person and often lack push handles. Carrying or lifting the person, with or without the wheelchair, is unacceptable. First, there is the danger of injury to the person with the disability (and you need this on your insurance?) and to the carrier. Second, it is an affront to the person's dignity and encroaches on that person's self-determination. It alters roles from collaborative to helper/helpee. And there is no excuse for the necessity to carry people in wheelchairs in an affluent country with the resources ours has.

Outside my building there are two ramps. One, crafted when the building was built, is steeper than regulation grade (which is a 1-foot rise for every 12 feet). The newer ramp is between two handicapped parking spaces. I warn new clients about the steepness of the older ramp. If the newer ramp is blocked by delivery trucks (as if often the case) I might offer to "spot" them (as one spots a gymnast) on the steeper ramp.

SPEECH AND COMMUNICATION DIFFICULTIES

Match listening to speech—if speech is slow, listen more slowly. Don't complete sentences for the client or supply words the client is having difficulty producing. If several attempts at understanding a word or phrase prove unfruitful, have the person write it down (provided hand functioning is sufficient), spell it, substitute another word, or rest for a moment before repeating the phrase.

Communication disorders are varied. Some speech difficulties (e.g., stuttering) are relatively isolated (i.e., do not imply organic deficits). Others (e.g., word finding) imply temporary or permanent brain impairment. For those who cannot produce intelligible speech there are alternate methods of communication, such as sign language, speech boards, and speech synthesizers. Many of these methods slow the pace of conversations; remember, you are on "crip time"!

VISUAL IMPAIRMENTS

Tell the client what materials you have available for clients, and whenever possible offer them in alternate format. For example, if you have brochures in your office on depression and on anxiety, or the brochure "Professional therapy never includes sex" (mandated in California), you might say to the client something like, "I have several brochures in my office that are routinely available to my clients. Would you like me to read you their titles?" Alternate formats means Braille (there are brailling services), cassette, or large print (preferably altered in three ways: print size is around 17 point, bolder, and with more white space around words; some people prefer high-contrast black on white, others have trouble with the glare and prefer black on buff or beige). It also may mean that you read the brochure to the client or send it home with him or her for someone else to read it out loud. Disk versions allow for many accommodations through someone's own computer (e.g., having text read aloud, enlarging print, changing contrast).

When audiotaping materials it is important that the reader have clear enunciation, but not obviously so (e.g., trying saying out loud the word "enunciation" while enunciating each syllable and you will hear an example of what you should not do). In addition to proficient reading skills, readers should be familiar with the terms and phraseology of the material they are reading, or else they tend to stumble over words (examples might be the names of medications, or diagnostic labels).

Convey information about your building, and offer a guided tour. Guide a person with visual impairments by offering your arm and leading; do not take the person's arm and push from behind. Key features such as drinking fountains, entrances and exits, and bathrooms should be located, either in the tour or by description. (People with visual impairments vary tremendously in their navigational skills.)

People with significant visual impairments rely on walking, rides, public transportation, or paratransit. Factors that may be trivial to others can have enhanced importance (distance from transit stops, time of day, number of transfers on buses). Most people with visual impairments, even those "legally" blind, have some residual sight, so daylight appointments may be preferable. Good office lighting may help a person utilize his or her vision. A screen enlarger for the computer and enlarged and bold printouts may help with written information.

DEAFNESS OR HEARING IMPAIRMENTS

This group is diverse. It can be broadly divided into three subgroups: (1) those who are prelingually deaf and whose primary language is ASL; (2) those who are postlingually but early deafened who learned sign and identify with the Deaf community; they are likely to have better reading skills than the first group because English is more familiar to them, and to be more fluid in moving between deaf and hearing worlds; and (3) the later deafened, who are adjusting to the loss of a function they relied on but who will remain in the hearing community. Languages used by these groups include ASL, S.E.E. sign (Signing Exact English), total communication (signing combined with lip reading and speech), lip reading, and English.

You cannot assume any lip-reading skills. Typically lip readers can understand less than half of what is said. Second, those who become deaf prior to language acquisition will not be facile in English. Third, those who are late deafened may not have much experience in lip reading. Thus lip reading works best for those who are hard of hearing and who use lip reading to augment their residual hearing. When talking with someone who does use lip reading be sure to face the person, don't have food in your mouth, and don't obscure your mouth with your hands. Inquire if it helps to increase voice volume; in either case, avoid the tendency to shout. Have good lighting, without shadows, and avoid distracting hand and body movements.

The lighting used in the office can facilitate sign language interpretation. Many therapists prefer soft, filtered lighting in the therapy room, but this can make it more difficult for the client to see the interpreter's signs and for the therapist to see the deaf client's facial expressions, which are so fundamental to getting a feel for the client (especially as his or her "words" are coming from the interpreter's mouth). Also, angle the lighting so that it's not in anyone's eyes as the person looks from client to interpreter to therapist. Although therapists usually give clients a choice of seating, there is a particular arrangement that tends to work best when using a sign language interpreter. This is an isosceles triangle, with the distance between therapist and interpreter the short side of the triangle, and both sitting opposite the client. Thus the client talks (signs) across to both the therapist and interpreter, and the interpreter signs across to the client and speaks next to the therapist. This arrangement also helps remind the therapist to look at the client and not the interpreter, because to do so is to turn away from the client. When using sign interpreters it is imperative that only one person at a time speaks. Desire to interrupt must be signaled through a hand motion rather than by beginning to speak. Interpreters cannot interpret two people at once. If the client stops to write something, communication temporarily stops because the client can neither sign nor look at another person signing, so the therapist should remain silent until the client is finished writing.

The Deaf community relies on and prefers face-to-face interactions. Because so much of signing is in the body language, the words themselves don't convey the full meanings. Thus deaf clients are more likely than others to prefer to discuss everything with you in person, even things that might usually be handled by phone (e.g., changing appointments and questions about insurance forms). This should not be interpreted as neediness, low ego development, enmeshment, acting out, or any other form of pathology; it is normative in the Deaf community. When expecting a deaf client, leave your door open; a deaf person can't hear you say "come in." Also, closed doors carry a different meaning in the Deaf community, of separateness and closing off communication.

Communication between sessions can be facilitated by having available a TTY phone or using a TTY card on computer (available with a fax/modem card), or going through a relay service (by law there is a relay service for every state; it is listed in the phone book, or available by asking information for the State Relay Service number). Another good method is to use electronic mail; this allows you to more directly "hear the voice" of the client. Further, don't be surprised if the client writes you for something you'd expect another client to call about. Finally, remember that for early deafened persons English is the second language, and one they've only seen, never heard.[2] The average reading level for prelingually deaf adults is below fourth grade; this in no way implies subnormal IQ. (Unfortunately, reading scores have slightly declined since Public Law 94-142—"mainstreaming"; this is one population that is better served in special schools for the deaf.) Don't misinterpret your deaf client as ignorant or uneducated based on poor English writing skills.

Pay close attention to body language. Users of sign language use their face and body in pronounced ways, with lots of expression and movement. For example, for deaf people to get someone's attention the usual mode is to wave the hand up and down in someone's line of vision, which hearing people might consider rude. Be careful not to interpret the wide gestures and large fluid motions as histrionic.

Think about how (hearing) clients convey emotions. A depressed client may exhibit lassitude, have few and small gestures, be still and indrawn; the voice might be monotone, soft, with little speech produc-

---

[2] I am reminded of when I ignorantly asked a Deaf woman how her name was pronounced. She laughed and said it didn't matter; Deaf people sometimes choose names by how the letters look together written on a page.

tion. The same could be true for a depressed deaf client; signs would be small, there would be less of them, and body language would be suppressed. Anger, on the other hand, looks different in hearing and deaf clients. "Yelling" in sign language means greater forcefulness in signing, accompanied by more exaggerated facial expressions.

Sign language is a blunt language. People say what they mean without the usual hemming and hawing, disclaimers, and hmmmms. Deaf people tend to see hearing people as too evasive and roundabout in their speech. It is possible for the hearing therapist to view the deaf client as offputting due to bluntness. The majority white culture in the United States is one of small gestures, few facial expressions, minimal body movements, and greater physical distance from our interlocutors. In other words, it is in many ways the opposite of Deaf culture. The therapist must guard against misinterpreting what is culturally normative for clients in the Deaf community. And even with excellent interpretation, there are frequent and considerable misunderstandings in communication due to the tremendous cultural differences between the hearing and Deaf communities. Frequent paraphrasing, feedback, and verification are necessary to avoid larger misunderstandings.

LEARNING DISABILITIES

Discuss with the client (or client and parents, if a child) his or her best learning and retention modes. Some persons with learning disabilities (LD) benefit from more visual presentations; therapy, on the other hand, is a verbal endeavor. It can be useful to make lists, (e.g., to organize how and when between-session tasks will be accomplished) or have clients write down a summary of the main points from the session. Use of colored pens can help: Between-session tasks can be in one color, questions in another, things to think about in a third, and so on. Conversely, written materials also may need to be presented verbally; you might offer to read aloud any written materials you give the client or have available in the office (e.g., informational brochures).

Adults with LD often develop various strategies for maximizing attention and retention. One such strategy, reflected in the previous suggestions, is to have stimuli available in more than one modality. Therefore, some clients want to tape sessions. But it is not always advisable to send clients home with tapes of sessions for them to listen to on their own. For example, a client with an anxiety disorder might get more anxious listening to a discussion of anxiety symptoms or anxiety-provoking stimuli. Clearly there can be no generalizations here; each case must be decided using your best clinical judgment.

NINE

Interviews, Assessment, Evaluation, and Diagnosis

This chapter presents clinicians with guidelines for interviewing, assessing, and diagnosing clients with disabilities. Of course, assessment is fundamental in considering intervention options, and decisions here reverberate through all subsequent treatment decisions. Thus the discussion walks the reader through three main areas necessary for development of a treatment plan: (1) interviewing and the mental status exam (MSE); (2) diagnosis, including the problems of overshadowing and the restricting of diagnostic categories; and (3) testing (e.g., choice of tests, modifications and interpretation of tests). Even if you don't do testing yourself, this chapter should help you read testing reports.

INTERVIEWING AND THE MENTAL STATUS EXAM

A major method we use to understand clients is the clinical interview. This method is such a backbone of clinical work that even small problems can become significant difficulties in later stages. The initial phases of therapy are an opportunity to form a positive relationship and to begin treatment on a hopeful note. How might disability influence this process? This section limits itself to consideration of three particular ways in which the process of interviewing may be shaped by the disability status of the client. These include (1) how presumptions about disability can distort the process of asking questions and interpreting answers, (2) the effects of physical appearance on the MSE and our judgment about clients, and (3) the clinician's response to aspects of clients that are unfamiliar and anxiety provoking. An example sets the stage:

> Nigel is being interviewed to attend a small private college. He has a stiff back due to a neck injury, and one shoulder is higher than the other. His knees touch when he walks and his lower legs splay outward, and he has a bilateral limp. During the interview he sits on the front edge of the chair because it would hurt to lean against the hard back. In conducting the interview the admissions committee has a standard protocol. However, they omit questions about whether he would be interested in living in one of the theme dorms because they assume he would need special housing, and they do not ask about leisure activities because they assume he is not interested in sports, and they don't ask him what electives he would take because they assume he will need a reduced workload. At the end of the interview they conclude that Nigel is "not well rounded."

Interviewing

Interviews are a series of microdecisions on the part of the interviewer, who continually decides what questions to ask, how to ask them, how to interpret the answers, what question to ask next, and so on. If there are small distortions throughout the interview based on bias toward disability, the additive effects of these errors, each perhaps minor on its own, can lead to a significant misunderstanding of clients. It may be through this exact process that clients with disabilities come to feel devalued. It is not sufficient to call for more authentic voices of people with disabilities to be heard, because "what the client says is inseparable from what he or she is asked, so the call should really be for the examination not of the client's voice as such but rather of how the voice is modulated by the encounter with the assessor" (Antaki & Rapley, 1996, p. 435).

Interviews are easily subject to distortion and bias, such that preconceived notions about people with disabilities are seemingly confirmed with "data" from the clinical interview. The stigma and prejudice associated with disability may lead an interviewer to omit questions deemed irrelevant to someone with a disability, to rephrase questions, or to restrict answer choices (Antaki & Rapley, 1996). For example, suppose you ask all your clients, "Are there any problems of substance abuse in your family?" but you ask a client with a disability, "Are there any issues of substance abuse related to your disability?" The second version of the question invites a more restricted range of answers than the first, and valuable contextual information is lost. In addition, the question itself implies that the interviewer is viewing the client primarily in terms of the disability, and this may hamper the initial relationship.

Another type of distortion involves asking prequestion questions. These are questions that introduce topics or lead up to the real questions. For example, a clinician might want to know whether a client who is depressed has contact with other people daily and thus begins by asking, "Do you go out of the apartment most days?" The client might respond by discussing the problems with the automatic door opener in the apartment, but the clinician, hearing that the client does indeed go out several times per week, then focuses on the client's conversations with shopkeepers, and misses the client's feelings of impotence and helplessness engendered by the broken door opener. Had the client not had a disability, the prequestion would not have been asked, nor would the answer to the prequestion have been so vital.

A third type of distortion involves rewording clients. Clinicians tend to think in diagnostic terms. If the client uses nonstandard vocabulary (e.g., "discouraged") the interviewer, who believes that people with disabilities are likely to be depressed, may translate this into a standard word (e.g., "depressed") without verifying the meaning with the client. Thus the clinician's biases about disability erroneously lead to a misunderstanding of the client.

The Effects of Appearance on the MSE

A MSE, whether conducted formally or informally, is a method of collecting and tabulating disparate observations about clients into a cohesive picture. One aspect of the MSE includes the client's appearance. Therefore clinical reports routinely include such phrases as "patient was a well-groomed woman," "patient appeared younger than his stated age," or "patient was disheveled." Appearance is one of the first aspects of the MSE that becomes manifest, and as such is the lens through which we begin to shape our views of new clients. The effects of disability on appearance can influence the MSE, and hence clinical judgments about the client.

In a fascinating article about the role of appearance in impression formation, Nakdimen (1984) argues that although the theory of physiognomy (which holds that physical features are a true representation of one's character) is discredited, we do in fact respond to others as if there were some truth to this theory. A common example is the phrase "he has an honest face." The process by which we notice and respond to another person's appearance is intuitive and unconscious, full of imagery, which can be difficult to translate into a process that is conscious and verbal. Yet this judgment is a standard task of the MSE. Are we, in fact, arguing that someone's physiognomy reveals psychological character? Yes and no. When we describe someone as "haggard," "youthful," or "restless" we are referring to the physiological effects of some psychological states (such as depression) or to a behavior of the body in motion (e.g., foot tapping), and suggesting that these do impart clues about the person's psychological status. I am more concerned here with those more static aspects of appearance to which we respond less consciously. For example, if placement and shape of eyebrows denote emotions (Nakdimen, 1984), what is the effect of a twitch that moves the eyebrows? If body proportions, such as distance from crotch to waist, suggest changes in status, what is the effect of a disability that alters these features? When people with disabilities say, "We are not our bodies," this means in part that others should suspend judgment of character based on unconscious responses to physiognomy. As clinicians write about appearance as part of the MSE, they should try to examine their conscious and unconscious responses to the client's anatomy and consider where their impressions stem from, how they are formed, and whether they are supported by other aspects of the client.

> Clarissa, a petite woman in her early 50s, had a stroke about 2 years ago, leaving her with some residual difficulties with fine motor coordination, word finding, concentration, and speech. Because of the difficulty with her hands she dresses in clothes with simple velcro closures. These come in limited fashions, often meant for juniors. Thus her clothing has the appearance of being for someone much younger. Due to her speech problems she often substitutes a smaller and simpler word at the last minute. And because of her difficulties with concentration, she limits external stimuli by keeping her eyes focused in one spot as she listens, so that she gives the impression of staring blankly when in fact she is listening intently. The overall effect of these disability sequelae is such that the clinician believes Clarissa is "slow" and a poor candidate for insight-oriented psychotherapy.

Clinician Responses

Of interest here is whether clinicians truncate the evaluation process and thereby affect the array of treatment options available to the client. Pollard (1994) documented that this is exactly what happens with deaf clients. In an examination of more than 84,000 mental health records of clients in Rochester, New York (which has the highest per capita population in the world of persons who are deaf: 5.5%), he noted the types of mental health services obtained by each client. He found that deaf and hard-of-hearing clients of community mental health centers received fewer of all types of mental health services, and none of the deaf clients were referred to an innovative new treatment program. Pollard believes that these inequities stem in part from barriers in the interviewing process. A clinician who becomes overwhelmed by the communicative tasks involved in interviewing deaf or hard-of-hearing clients is less likely to be thorough, to look beyond the primary diagnosis or presenting problem to secondary issues or diagnoses, and to feel sure about the absence of Axis II diagnoses. This cycle has been referred to as "fear–shock–paralysis–withdrawal" (Schlesinger & Meadow, as cited in Heller & Harris, 1987, p. 60), in which "otherwise talented professionals fail to use their abilities to the fullest because of the fear or powerlessness they feel when confronted with persons who are deaf" (p. 158). This cycle can occur with any clients with whom communication is altered. If a clinician is distracted by communication tasks, physical tasks (e.g., seating, lighting, access), and countertransference responses to the client, these distractions cannot help but reduce the amount of attention, energy, and focus the clinician retains for the other tasks of the interview. And if the therapist feels incompetent, out of his or her depth, and overwhelmed with affect, he or she becomes "deskilled" (Heller & Harris, 1987, p. 60).

Conclusions about Interviewing

Three different mechanisms by which disability influences interviews have been discussed: distortions in interviewing, the effects of client appearance on the clinician, and clinicians' responses to clients with disabilities. There is nothing about the three that is inherently contradictory, and all three or some combination can operate simultaneously. Furthermore, there are many other routes by which disability might affect the interview process. The result is that the net impact of the disability on the interview itself, and hence on the clinician's judgment, diagnosis, case formulation, and treatment recommendations, can be profound. Nonetheless, problems are not inevitable if the clinician takes the time to examine carefully ways in which he or she is interacting with and understanding the client with a disability.

DIAGNOSIS

There are several key issues in deriving diagnoses of clients with disabilities. The first is the need to ensure that what is being assessed is not merely manifestations of the disability itself. The second issue is stereotyping by therapists, and the effects of these stereotypes on data collection and interpretation, diagnosis, case formulation, and treatment plans.

Stereotyping and Overshadowing

As discussed, the stereotypes clinicians hold about people with disabilities guide the interviewing process itself, influencing what questions clinicians ask, what information they follow up on, and how they conceptualize clients' responses. Stereotypes likewise influence what diagnoses clinicians consider and which they reject, how they formulate the case, their prognosis for improvement and willingness to work with the client, the treatment options that are seen as viable, ways in which treatment is implemented, and how the effects of intervention are assessed. In other words, there is hardly a single facet of treatment that is immune to the effects of stereotyping.

Therapists can misdiagnose clients with disabilities when they harbor mistaken beliefs about what and how strongly people with disabilities should and shouldn't feel. For example, if we expect a client with a recent onset of disability to be "mourning" the loss of more robust physical functioning, we might easily overlook a treatable depression. Anger at oppression or injustice might be misdiagnosed as a personality disorder. Strong self-advocacy might be misinterpreted as entitlement, grandiosity, or narcissism. Persons with newly acquired or exacerbated disabilities are more likely to endorse items on tests related to somatic complaints and obsessive–compulsive disorder (Heinrich & Tate, 1996), but this does not mean they warrant those diagnoses. The increased vulnerability and mortality one feels in these circumstances should not be pathologized. The reality factors associated with disability, "anxiety and worry which can lead to temporary difficulties with decision making, interpersonal concerns and hypersensitivity about dependency and self-image, and finally, feelings of anger and depression" (Heinrich & Tate, 1996, p. 144), must all be considered as part of the diagnostic picture. If the clinician is not familiar with the client's type of disability or with disability issues in general, "gross psychodiagnostic errors" (Belcastro, 1987, p. 97) can occur in how the clinician diagnoses and formulates the case.

Therapists should guard against restricting the range of diagnoses considered for clients with disabilities. Pollard (1994) demonstrated that relative to their hearing counterparts, deaf or hard-of-hearing clients received fewer different diagnoses on Axis I of DSM-III-R, were more likely to receive Axis I deferred or no diagnosis, or to have the diagnosis missing from the record. Substance abuse in particular was significantly less frequently diagnosed (2.9% of deaf or hard-of-hearing clients received this diagnosis, compared with 11.5% of hearing clients). Disorders of childhood were also less likely (4.1% vs. 8.5%). However, on Axis II they were more likely to receive a diagnosis of mental retardation and less likely to receive "no diagnosis." Because the literature does not support the notion that persons who are deaf or hard of hearing have a restricted range of mental health problems, or less substance abuse, Pollard concludes that these differences "reflect problems in service accessibility and clinician expertise rather than valid clinical distinctions" in the deaf and hard-of-hearing population (p. 147). Similarly, another study supports the idea that we should not expect a restricted range of mental disorders among persons with mental retardation (Szymanski, 1988). Indeed, one study demonstrated that children with mental retardation respond to the same types of parental stressors as do other children, and the children with both mental retardation and depression showed a "similar pattern of symptoms and associated characteristics to those found in normal [sic] children with diagnoses of depression" (Kobe & Hammer, 1994, p. 209).

The range of considered diagnoses can be restricted through the phenomenon of overshadowing—the failure to seek or find secondary diagnoses because the disability overshadows other features. The word "overshadowing" in the context of diagnosis comes from an article by Reiss, Levitan, and Szyszko (1982). They describe how the diagnoses of major depression and dysthymia are overlooked in clients with mental retardation because of the "overshadowing" effects of the primary diagnosis of mental retardation.

Let's look at a common clinical example: Think about a client who comes to you in the midst of a severe major depression. This, say, 42-year-old woman sits hunched over, responds to questions in short, barely audible answers, weeps quietly, and wrings her hands. It is hard to imagine that this client might have periods of mania. But training and empirical data tell us that we must ask questions about euphoria, sleeplessness, increased energy, inflated self-esteem, and grandiosity. Although it would be easy for the current diagnosis of depression to overshadow the overall diagnosis of bipolar disorder by making us oblivious to periods of mania, we overcome this tendency by using empirical data to guide the interview, and by explicit questioning.

Now add to the portrait of this women certain features associated with her disability. She sits in a wheelchair, her feet resting on the small metal platforms, and her legs are at odd angles. When she wrings her hands the motion is jerky, and her upper body seems to experience spasms. If the clinician has the "expectation of mourning" (see Chapter 4, in this volume), the disability will be expected to produce depression, the depression may not be diagnosed as a separate disorder, and hence a treatable condition will be overlooked. By elevating disability to the position of defining characteristic, we presume it causes other characteristics, such as the behaviors associated with depression, and other explanations are disregarded. Thus, because of the salience of the disability, we ignore clinical knowledge about depression and mania.

Let's consider another example:

> A young Caucasian man in his mid-20s comes for a first appointment. His head is slightly too large for his body, and he doesn't make any eye contact. His handshake is weak. He reports having been sent (by whom is not clear) for treatment because that person "was worried about me"; he is unable to be more specific. His answers are short and concrete, and he rarely talks spontaneously. His mood in the session is subdued and relatively unvaried.

We have several options to consider here: (1) the man has mental retardation, (2) he has had a head trauma, (3) he has Down syndrome, (4) he is depressed, (5) he is anxious about coming for treatment, and (6) he is guarded and wary due to paranoia. Mental retardation could explain poor social skills (as seen in the lack of eye contact, weak handshake, and minimal conversational input), but so could depression. The problem comes in seeking an answer and then stopping. If both mental retardation *and* depression were true for this gentleman, then a clinician might light on only one of them and fail to entertain the other. Because mental retardation is likely to become apparent with longer contact, through deficits exhibited in session, examination of records, and/or consultation with pertinent others, the danger is that this diagnosis is used as an explanation for all the clinical phenomena and other possibilities are dropped. The client then goes from having a treatable disorder (depression) to a static one (mental retardation).

The Problem of Depression

The diagnosis of depression merits special attention here for several reasons, though it must be noted that "depression . . . is not an inevitable reaction to the onset of acquired physical disability" (Elliott & Umlauf, 1991, p. 326). There are several issues in diagnosing depression in persons with disabilities. Some sizable minority of persons who acquire a disability become depressed after the injury: Estimates vary but are roughly 30% plus or minus 5% (Frank, Elliott, Corcoran, & Wonderlich, 1987; Heinrich & Tate, 1996; Lichtenberg, 1997; Turner & McLean, 1989; Weissman & Myers, 1978). In two studies that tested for depression among geriatric rehabilitation inpatients, the rate of depression was unrelated to gender or ethnicity (Lichtenberg, 1997). Estimates of depression are higher for some types of disorders which may cause depression directly through physiology or brain damage. For example, estimates of depression after stroke range from 23% (Robinson, 1993) to 64% (Stein, Gordon, Hibbard, & Sliwinski, 1992). The depression poststroke is unrelated to gender, ethnicity, SES, or marital status (Robinson, 1993).

Another reason to examine depression in particular is that depression has been shown to complicate the recovery and rehabilitation process, increase length of hospital stay, and reduce independence on ADL. Thus depression should be seen as a primary medical condition, and its diagnosis and treatment a high priority (Lichtenberg, 1997). Third, there is a correlation between degree of insight and depression, at least in persons with TBI (Campodoni & McGlynn, 1995). They found a positive correlation between depression and awareness of TBI deficits. This can be explained in both directions: Those with greater awareness of deficits became more depressed, and those with more depression focused more on their deficits. This supports the idea that depression per se is an important aspect of the rehabilitative process and must not be overlooked. Fourth, the symptoms essential to the diagnosis of depression may be produced by the medical condition itself. For example, appetite change, insomnia, fatigue, attention to somatic complaints, constipation, loss of libido can all be associated with various disorders. Thus it becomes important to understand how to diagnosis depression through analysis of symptoms above and beyond those usually experienced by persons with that type of disability.

Not only should depression be evaluated, but distinctions among the depressions (major depression, dysthymia, adjustment disorder with depressed mood, depression as part of a bipolar disorder, and depression due to a general medical condition) must be assessed. Yet the detection of depression in the context of a major medical condition is difficult and often overlooked. Lichtenberg (1997) studied 150 consecutive rehabilitation admissions who were age 60 or older. He found that of the women who were depressed, only 50% were correctly identified as depressed by the attending physician. The correct identification rate for men was considerably lower (10%), though comparable to previous studies (there are no previous studies on women).

A critical question is whether symptoms of depression in the context of a major medical condition are the same as those in persons without such conditions. A review of studies with patients with stroke or with Parkinson disease (Robinson, 1993) suggests that symptoms of depressive disorder were not widespread in these patients, and conversely that the diseases did not interfere with the typical symptoms of depression. Robinson suggests that insomnia, loss of libido, anxiety with palpitations or lightheadedness, and loss of appetite were unique to those patients with depression, compared to patients with the same medical conditions who were not depressed. However, it is necessary to duplicate this research with other populations of persons with specific disabilities.

Conclusions about Diagnosis

We have seen that stereotyping of clients with disabilities can affect the range and types of diagnoses that clinicians investigate. The diagnosis of depression is particularly problematic. This is because the diagnosis is overlooked when the disability is used to "explain" the mood state, and also because it is tricky to differentiate symptoms of depression from those caused by the disability itself. (Chapter 11 considers the problem of substance abuse separately.)

TESTING

A critical area of concern is the impact of disabling conditions on the reliability and validity of tests. Disability can affect testing in a variety of ways: if tests contain items that measure disability instead of the intended construct, if the process of taking a test is appreciably altered, and if the interpretation of results misapplies able-bodied norms to the client with a disability. A hallmark of testing is standardization, and the essence of disability is individualization. It is the resolution of these two dialectics that is the challenge for the clinician.

Experts have argued both for and against the value of testing versus more informal assessment procedures. Some believe that formal testing is too restricted in scope and type of information collected (Lintula & Miezitis, 1977). Opposing this are those who believe that the use of standardized assessment instruments increases the rate of detection of disorders that might otherwise be overlooked (La Rue & Watson, 1998; Robinson, 1993). Both arguments have merit. Testing guards against overlooking areas of clinical significance and helps ensure attention to multiple issues. But testing should augment, not replace, good clinical interviewing, observation, information from collaterals, and sound judgment.

Much of the literature discusses specific disabilities and specific tests. Some examples are cited here, along with references for further information. But I would caution readers to examine the literature with a critical eye. Authors may know testing well, but some of them are ignorant about disability and alarmingly pathologizing. For example, although the following quote was taken from one article, many echoed the sentiment. It demonstrates the translation of difference into deficit and the overpathologizing of disability:

Although children whose visual deficit falls close to the legal definition *suffer* from a serious disability, they are able to perceive, in some measure, the presence of objects and people in their immediate surroundings, and consequently are far less vulnerable *to the most serious developmental arrests than is the child born lacking any useful vision.* (Freedman, Feinstein, & Berger, 1988, p. 864; emphasis added)

Furthermore, readers should pay close attention to the description of subjects in the studies, as authors may generalize inappropriately in one of three ways. The first is to generalize from a subgroup of persons with a specific disorder to the general population of persons with that disorder. This is exemplified in a study on adolescents with CP (Dorman, Hurley, & Laatsch, 1984). Although the subjects in that study had a mean IQ of 86, were not in mainstream classrooms, and were mostly living in a residential school with other children with disabilities, the authors generalize to all persons with CP. A second type of inappropriate generalization is from one specific type of disability to all persons with disabilities. For examples, titles might use the word "mental handicap" when they mean mental retardation (e.g., Jancar & Gunaratne, 1994), or "disability" when discussing one specific disability. The third type of generalization error is to generalize across ethnicities, usually from studies on Caucasians to those of other ethnicities. The interface of disability and ethnicity has been neglected as a variable in research; "condition-specific issues have been studied in isolated research projects that have yet to be synthesized in any meaningful fashion for rehabilitation psychology" (Uswatte & Elliott, 1997, p. 62).

One concern when testing with persons with disabilities is the lack of appropriate norms for comparison. Most tests are normed on populations that explicitly exclude persons with disabilities, and there is scant research on the impact of the disability on the meaning of test items or on the process of taking the test. Not surprisingly, then, when persons with disabilities are given such tests they tend to incur over- or underinflated scores, which then is interpreted as indicative of pathology. For example:

A teenage male with a visible physical disability received a standard neuropsychological battery which included the Rorschach (Exner system) and TAT. These tests apparently indicated some tangentiality, loosening of associations, cognitive slippage, and macabre themes. The evaluator speculated that this indicated distortions in reality perception or perhaps an early sign of a predisposition toward psychopathology or even psychosis.

I see it differently, due to the effects of this child's disability: He spends extraordinary amounts of time alone, as he is quite ostracized by peers, so he has learned to generate a rich fantasy life. In school he spends a good portion of each day in a resource room with other kids who have been identified as disabled or at risk, which is a social group he shuns. He gets little direct feedback about his behavior from peers, due to his isolation and lack of intimacy, and from adults, due to their benign tolerance of him as a child already "burdened" by disability. His history of invasive and often traumatic medical procedures led to development of the coping technique of distraction, which he now practices in other settings, sometimes inappropriately. His body evokes in others pronounced affective responses such as pity, revulsion, curiosity, and sadness, and he has learned to divide his body into its "good/healthy" and "bad/disabled" parts. This, plus his history of medical procedures, may give rise to the macabre themes he generates. His disability status has had a profound effect on his socialization and psychological and emotional life and can account better for the testing data than can a strict adherence to interpretations based on normative data.

There are three types of testing to be discussed. The first is ability testing, which tries to predict performance. Here a potential problem is the underprediction of future potential of persons with disabilities. The second type is diagnostic testing, and the concern is that persons with disabilities will be overdiagnosed with mental disorders, or conversely that treatable disorders will be overlooked. The third type is neuro-psychological testing, which assesses specific cognitive strengths and weaknesses and how a person functions cognitively as a whole. Finally, I review types of reasonable accommodations made to tests and testing procedures.

Ability Testing

Much of the work here has been conducted by the government (usually for civil service jobs) over the past 40 years, with the focus on employment testing. A second more recent addition is the work by the Educational Testing Service (ETS), which has been concerned with both the reliability of tests of aptitude for persons with various types of disabilities and the validity of the results. ETS examined 5 years' worth of data on its Scholastic Aptitude Test (SAT) and Graduate Record Exam (GRE) for four types of disability groups: learning disabilities, physical impairments, visual impairments, or hearing impairments (for complete results see Willingham et al., 1988). They looked at eight predictors of comparability and found that with the exception of test timing (how long someone is given to complete the test), nonstandard versions were generally comparable to the standard test. However, another study (Ragosta, 1980), also by ETS on the same four disability groups, indicates that the hearing-impaired group scored significantly lower than did the non-disabled group, and lowest of the four disability groups, on all tests. This echoes earlier work by ETS on the SAT in which they concluded that the SAT was not valid for the Deaf. In fact, limitations of utilizing standardized tests with the Deaf is a common refrain, and the clinician is generally safer in assuming that a test will be invalid with this population. In a review of testing of the Deaf, Levine (1974) found that lack of normative deaf samples was a critical problem, as were problems of communication between hearing testers and deaf clients. Interested readers are directed to the following resources: For information on intelligence testing of persons who are prelingually deaf, see Braden and Pacquin (1985) and Phelps and Ensor (1986). See Morgan and Vernon (1994) for discussion of testing deaf children and adults for learning disabilities. Good discussions on testing the Deaf can be found in Belcastro (1987), Briccetti (1994), Gordon, Stump, and Glaser (1996), Heller and Harris (1987), and Zieziula (1988).

Diagnostic and Neuropsychological Testing

Much of the test- and disability-specific literature is organized around disability; that is, the work discusses the process of testing, types of tests, and interpretations of tests for a particular type of disability.[1] But three tests have received more attention across disabilities. These are the Minnesota Multiphasic Personality Inventory (MMPI), the Draw-A-Person test (DAP), and the Brief Symptom Inventory (BSI). Regarding the *MMPI,* several researchers have suggested that interpretation of the MMPI may be unreliable and inaccurate for persons with closed head injury (Gass, 1991), SCI (Kendall, Edinger, & Eberle, 1988; Rodevich & Wanlass, 1995; Taylor, 1970), MS (Meyerink, Reitan, & Selz, 1988; Mueller & Girace, 1988), or deafness (Brauer, 1992, 1993; McGhee, 1995; Rosen, 1967). Among other problems, this is because the MMPI contains symptom profiles that diagnose unusual physical symptoms as

---

[1]Discussion of testing persons with visual impairments is to be found in Davidson and Dolins (1993), Kolk (1987), and Sisson and Van Hasselt (1987). Testing of the Deaf is discussed earlier. Hurley (1993) provides a good discussion of testing on persons who have spina bifida. For a review of general issues related to testing persons with physical disabilities and effects of such disabilities on specific tests, see Elliott and Umlauf (1991) and Wilson (1987); for testing with children with disabilities see Fewell (1991); and for discussion of the use of computers when administering tests to offset physical limitations in the client with a disability, see Wilson (1990). For discussion of testing persons with disabilities for depression, see Campodoni and McGlynn (1995), Dosen and Menolascino (1990), Heinrich and Tate (1996), Jancar and Gunaratne (1994), Kobe and Hammer (1994), and Lichtenberg (1997).

somatization, psychosis, or "fakery." The validity of the *DAP* has been questioned for detection of emotional problems in children who are deaf (Briccetti, 1994) or who have mental retardation (Dykens, 1995), and the interpretation has been questioned for persons with polio (Johnson & Greenberg, 1978). In discussing use of the *BSI* with persons with SCI. Heinrich and Tate (1996) concluded that the new subscales derived from their research were preferable "for clinical usage because standard subscale interpretations of [BSI] scores tend to distort and overpathologize the experience of persons with spinal cord injury" (p. 131). This echoes an earlier study by Elliott and Umlauf (1991) in which they stated that many items on the BSI seem to reflect somatic symptoms common to persons with SCIs.

Not all testing relies on normative data; sometimes testing is done with the person tested serving as his or her own point of comparison. This can be especially useful in tracking changes over time. For example, such testing might be done to assess changes in functioning in a person poststroke. Some studies have examined deficits associated with specific disabilities as documented through neuropsychological testing. (For example, see Beatty's [1996] review of neuropsychological testing results with persons with MS.) Such testing is more resistant to the problems inherent in norm-based comparisons. An assumption is that the results are due to the impairment per se (e.g., word-finding difficulties in someone who had a stroke) and not artifacts resulting from physical sequelae of the disability (e.g., limited English in someone prelingually deaf; block placement in someone with limited hand use).

A head nurse was experiencing pronounced difficulties at work over the past year and had been given two reprimands in her personnel file. This was highly unusual as her previous work record had been exemplary. She had been diagnosed with MS about 5 years prior and currently was experiencing parathesia in her legs, gait and balance problems, and memory difficulties. She wanted to be reassigned within the hospital but was unsure of her capabilities. Testing showed her IQ to be in the high normal range, compared with previous results which would place her in the superior range. Most other tests showed a similar pattern of being within the normal range but much decreased over previous testing. In addition, she showed specific but mild deficits in visual processing, memory, word finding, and, as consistent with a diagnosis of MS, motor function and speed. If her test results were compared to those of other nurses her scores were adequate, though probably not on a par with other head nurses with her level of experience and responsibility. It was only in comparison to her previous levels of functioning that current testing showed the probable effects of the MS. This indicated that although her abilities were not below the norm, she would still need to discover strategies to maximize her work abilities and to adapt and modify her current methods for learning, performing, memorizing, and concentrating.

Reasonable Accommodations on Testing

There are many factors involved in the selection of which tests to use, and how to modify them, when testing persons with disabilities. The first factor is laws. Section 504 of the Rehabilitation Act of 1973 (nondiscrimination on the basis of handicap in employment) stipulated that "appropriate adjustment or modification of examinations" was required. This requirement spread to the private sector with the ADA, and is reflected in the regulations from the EEOC to implement Title I (employment) of the ADA. These laws prescribe "reasonable accommodations" in testing persons with disabilities and proscribe testing in formats that require the use of the impaired skill unless it is job related and essential to the functions of the job (e.g., speech for a dispatch operator). Furthermore, testing procedures that inadvertently screen out persons with disabilities cannot be used unless they are demonstrated to be job related and there are no alternative testing procedures.

In some circumstances the purpose of testing is to maximize learning, but at other times it is to maintain standards of a profession (Keiser, 1998). These two purposes carry with them a change in perspective that has implications for how accommodations are made. It is mandatory in either case to ensure that what is being tested is relevant content and not disability. But the degree to which a test can deviate from standardization is likely to be different in the two scenarios.

Students are covered under the IDEA through age 21 or college but under the Rehabilitation Act and the ADA in graduate programs. These laws critically shift perspective on the role of testing. Under IDEA, the focus is on the right to an appropriate education. For example, a second-grade student has the right to an education that is appropriate to carry him or her through to a third-grade level, so a wide range of testing accommodations would be appropriate. In contrast, a graduate student does not have a right to a degree; that degree is awarded only on merit. The graduate student is covered by the Rehabilitation Act and the ADA but not IDEA. What the ADA guarantees, in this context, is the right to the opportunity to learn, given that the student is an "otherwise qualified individual." The student carries a greater burden for demonstrating a disability, initiating the request for accommodations, and choosing appropriate accommodations. The purpose of the test is to demonstrate competence, which is more narrowly defined than "readiness." In this case testing accommodations would be more narrow. These two examples may seem to denote a change that is inconsequential in focus but is in fact profound.

Much of the research on test accommodations has been in the areas of education, vocational placement, or rehabilitation settings in which the persons with disabilities are not in competition with persons without disabilities. Primary interest in testing accommodations has been demonstrated by the federal government and by large testing organizations, notably ETS. An important impetus for research was the report issued by the National Academy of Sciences' Panel on Testing Handicapped People, in which the authors concluded that "contemporary practices in testing people with disabilities for employment and postsecondary school admission did not comply fully with federal antidiscrimination regulations" (Sherman & Anderson, cited in Nestor, 1993, p. 78). But it was the landmark *Standards for Educational and Psychological Testing* (jointly sponsored by the APA, the American Educational Research Association, and the National Council on Measurement in Education; [1985]) that included a section, for the first time, on "Testing People Who Have Handicapping Conditions." This report raised the notion that modified tests possibly were not valid and hence their interpretation was likewise invalid. A bedrock of testing is standardized procedures. We simply do not know how much we can deviate from any standardized procedures without jeopardizing reliability and validity.

A further issue must be addressed in making testing accommodations: whether the accommodations should be reported along with the results. If a test (e.g., the GRE) is taken in a nonstandardized format, should that score be flagged to indicate nonstandard testing? Doing so alerts recipients that caution in interpretation is necessary, but also identifies which examinees have disabilities. Clients should be informed of their options and may need assistance in thinking through the choices.

Methods of Testing Accommodations

Nestor (1993) considers three types of test modifications: changes in the testing medium (e.g., from written English to Braille and using a reader or audiotape in place of written material), changes to the time limits for taking the test, and changes to the test content. These three types are all specifically noted as appropriate accommodations in the EEOC guidelines for the ADA. The goal of accommodations is to retain validity of testing by altering tests or the process by which they are administered in such a way that the results are relatively unaffected by disability. To take a simple example, suppose we wanted to test "speed": how fast a person could move from point *A* to point *B*. If we made a rule that all contestants had to run, then those in wheelchairs would be excluded from testing. But "speed" does not inherently imply using legs. By modifying the testing process to include other forms of mobility, a wheelchair user could be assessed for speed as well.

But making changes to the process of testing is not always straightforward. There are at least two problems with changes in the testing medium. The first occurs when the test contains lengthy reading passages. Such passages can be more difficult to understand orally, and there is no direct aural equivalent to visual scanning. Also, doing some tasks orally (e.g., finding a pattern) requires the examinees to perform a task of memorization in addition to performing the required task, whereas the written version requires only the pattern-finding task. A second problem is how the test modifier should present tables and figures, which generally have no direct Braille or oral equivalent. Not only is a picture worth a thousand words, it may take that many words to explain the picture and it is still inadequate. Another area to consider is the best way to use readers. These readers must be articulate, clear-spoken, familiar with the vocabulary, and practiced in doing this work. They also must be trained in how to avoid giving answer clues as they read.

Although many people might believe that changing a test from written English to sign language is a change in medium, it is actually a change in language. Thus the total impact of the changes can be enormous. In fact, for the prelingually deaf person, verbal tests are not good measures of anything but verbal ability, and there is almost no correlation between verbal and nonverbal test scores (Brauer, 1993; Gordon et al., 1996; Nestor, 1993). Standardized testing generally should not be used with the Deaf, and alternate means of assessment must be explored.

Another accommodation is to change test limits. In "power tests," time is not a factor, and what is being tested is how many questions are answered correctly. In "speed tests," what is being assessed is how many questions can be answered in a given time frame. However, many supposed power tests also have an element of speed tests, because some examinees (e.g., those taking the psychology licensing exam) do not have time to answer every question. Thus the critical question is how much extra time on tests should be allotted to examinees with disabilities so that they are neither advantaged nor disadvantaged. One answer is to make unlimited time standard. This works for some kinds (e.g., preliminary exams given in graduate school) but not for other kinds of tests (e.g., those more commonly used in neuropsychological testing batteries). Furthermore, ETS found that unlimited time on tests overpredicted future school grades of examinees with learning disabilities. This means that test makers would have to calibrate the necessary but only just sufficient extra time needed for each type of disability. Further, this optimal time would vary with the type of test (e.g., a French comprehension test vs. a calculus test). On speed tests the focus of interest is on speed, and when speed is impaired by disability, extra time is a nonsensical modification. Thus speed tests should not be used unless speed is the essential component of interest. (I am reminded of my junior high physical education class, in which we, a group of students with various disabilities in "Special PE," still were required to take standardized timed tests on such things as how fast we could run around the football field. As I recall, it took me about 45 minutes.)

Changes to test content are another form of accommodation but are more problematic and less common. Changes to content can be accomplished in three ways. First is making changes to specific questions. For example, one might reword a double-negative question (e.g., asking respondents to find the one false answer, when the correct selection is "Hypomania is not a mood disorder"). This is fairly easily accomplished, and for the most part doesn't dramatically impact the validity of a test (and in fact may improve it). The second type of change is to alter the question type (e.g., from a multiple-choice to a short-answer format). This requires that another version of the question be available, and that scores on the new and old version are comparable. If respondents are to be rank-ordered, it is particularly imperative that scores from all versions are comparable.

The third type of change is less straightforward. It is to alter or even delete an area being measured (i.e., a specific area of knowledge, skill, or ability). There are two assumptions when making this type of change, which echo the EEOC testing guidelines. The first assumption is that the content area is not an essential function of the job. The second is that no alternative method of evaluating the content area is possible. An example illustrates:

> All doctoral students in art history at a particular university are required to reach proficiency in translating a foreign language. The rationale for the requirement is that many important writings on art history are available only in their original language. A prelingually deaf student is likely to have great difficulties with learning a second oral language. Should the program waive the foreign language requirement?

The first issue to be addressed is whether there is an alternative method of evaluating the foreign-language content area (probably not). The second issue is whether the essential functions of a doctoral-level trained art historian includes the ability to translate materials from another language. The department might correctly conclude that in this case what is essential is access to the foreign material but not that the historian perform the translation him- or herself. The student might be tested, for example, on his or her ability to develop original material and generate new ideas, given translations done by someone else. Thus one essential function of an art historian is maintained (making original contributions), but the means to achieving that function (reading materials in another language) is substantially altered.

However, I think we can see how merely asking questions about alternative formats and essential functions is a complex and critical task. It can make us uncomfortable by forcing a reexamination of our cherished beliefs and assumptions about what is truly essential in our professions. One fear, of course, is that if we designate something as being a nonessential function of the job description, we open the door for others to challenge the validity of the requirement. However, there is nothing in the ADA, its regulations, or its interpretation in the courts that suggests that altering or deleting a requirement for a person with a disability means that the same requirement should or must be waived for persons without disabilities.

The Assessment Relationship

Assessment, like therapy, requires a working relationship with the client. A critical factor is respect for the client. Respect includes not wasting the client's time or administering unnecessary tests. All evaluators know the importance of the referral question; testing should not be a fishing expedition. An evaluation for eligibility for services would differ from one assessing strengths and weaknesses, or from one measuring outcomes of a treatment program (Fewell, 1991).

The nature of the disability can affect the evaluation relationship. For example, use of an interpreter may mean more time is needed to establish a working rapport. Testing is threatening and anxiety provoking for many clients but may be especially so for clients with disabilities. Questions of malingering, insurance fraud, work abilities, and other types of referral questions can cloud the relationship. Studies, such as one investigating distinctions on scores on the Wechsler Adult Intelligence Scale–Revised of nonlitigating patients with TBI and matched controls instructed to malinger head trauma symptoms (Mittenberg, Theroux-Fichera, Zielinski, & Heilbronner, 1995), can contribute to a distrust and suspiciousness between patient and evaluator. Thus the tester may need to take extra time to create a collaborative stance.

Were I the patient, I would want to ask many questions about who the evaluator worked for, the purpose of the evaluation, confidentiality, and how the results might be used. Recall the discussion in Chapter 4 about how disability affects one's world view and note here a repeat of this theme. Persons with acquired disabilities know that they are suspect, especially if they are involved in litigation or insurance negotiations related to the disability or its exacerbation. The client's perceptions of the tester will shape the degree to which persons will participate in the rehabilitation process. This may be especially so for persons with disabilities who are also ethnic minorities (Asbury, Walker, Belgrave, Maholmes, & Green, 1994).

> Daniella, who had spina bifida and uses crutches, began treatment for "stress" about 6 months after a recent car accident. The accident, in which she was rear-ended at high speed, exacerbated many symptoms and made her back problems considerably worse and potentially serious. She was being evaluated by several doctors, undergoing tests, and possibly facing surgery. She sought me out as a therapist with a disability because she felt her issues and stresses related directly to her disability status, her memories of early hospitalization traumas, and her identity as a woman with a disability. Yet we eyed each other with mutual suspicion for a few sessions. I wanted to know if I was going to be subpoenaed in a suit against an insurance company and asked to attest to the psychological sequelae related to her accident. She wondered if I was asking questions to verify the accident and its severity. For example, when I asked her to describe the accident she said, "Why do you want to know that?" Both of us had to overcome the aura of suspicion that hangs around certain types of disabilities and related events before getting down to the business of therapy.

The relationship is paramount when testing all children, and especially children with disabilities. The nature of the relationship between such children and their parents can affect the testing process. For example, all parents try to spare their children from unnecessary medical incursions, and they have an investment in protecting the child from intrusion. Such protection may be more pronounced in parents of children with disabilities. The parents are used to checking things out and getting as much information as possible before the child is brought into a situation. Thus they may want more information about a test, question whether more testing is even necessary, or try to stay in the room during testing. This should not be thought of as enmeshed or overcontrolling. Similarly, the children may have more difficulty separating from the parents, as similar situations may have been invasive or traumatic. Rapport might be established more slowly, and testing may need to accommodate the extra time needed to establish a working relationship.

Parents of children with disabilities often believe they know the child better than does any professional, and they probably do. Feedback therefore should not come as a surprise or imply that the evaluator has inside knowledge that the parent does not. If parents are more fully integrated into the assessment and interpretation process, "the interpretive conference may serve as a summing up, rather than a presentation of new information that may surprise parents or not fit their perceptions of the child, and thus be unacceptable" (Davidson & Dolins, 1993, p. 259).

Conclusions about Testing

Problems in assessment include inappropriate adherence to standardization of administration such that persons with disabilities are disadvantaged. Furthermore, some tests measure disability and not the construct for which the test was intended. Psychological test items that reflect the disability experience, and have altered meanings compared with someone who does not have a disability, can inflate scores and lead to misperception. Lack of appropriate normative groups and use of inappropriate norms plague the area of testing, leading to erroneous interpretations. However, we must not look only to modifications of tests to rescue us from misdiagnosis of persons with disabilities. Testing is only one way we try to piece together the puzzle of clients. "Psychometric calibrations do not nullify the negative effects of prevailing uninformed professional views of persons with physical disabilities" (Elliott & Umlauf, 1991, p. 326). If a clinician carefully considers, from an informed perspective, the impact of disability on test selection, administration, and interpretation, tests can remain a useful adjunct to diagnosis and treatment planning.

CONCLUSIONS

This chapter has considered the impact of a disability on various aspects of the therapeutic relationship, including interviewing, using the MSE, diagnosis, and testing. All these are components that can help a clinician formulate a case, decide on a therapeutic stance, develop and implement a treatment plan, and evaluate progress. Competent cross-cultural counseling relies on the ability to generate multiple hypotheses that include the role of culture to varying degrees, and to open-mindedly evaluate the evidence for and against each hypothesis. The role of disability in evaluation and treatment can range from incidental to profound, and the clinician cannot prejudge its role. The question, "How might the disability be affecting my [testing, interpretations, assessment, interview, formulation] of this client?" must be a frequent query, and one that is addressed knowledgeably. All clinicians want to provide good therapy, and knowledge of problems that can arise in assessment of clients with disabilities might lead one to self-doubts. Therapists struggle with the incomplete state of our current knowledge and the practical needs of current clients. This chapter reflects that struggle but ultimately places trust in the clinician to make ethical and informed choices despite the lacunae in current knowledge.

TEN

Dating, Romance, Sexuality, Pregnancy, Birthing, and Genetic Testing

DATING AND ROMANCE

For people with disabilities, dating is Mount Everest. Disability discrimination is most felt in the romantic realm. Studies of attitudes toward disability repeatedly show that people's attitudes become more negative as the relationship with the person with the disability gets closer: Those who indicate that they would be fine with the idea of neighbor with a disability draw the line at their children dating a person with a disability, and most people indicate that they would not marry a person with a disability (Olkin & Howson, 1994). Women with disabilities are less likely to marry than are men with disabilities, and both are less likely to marry than are persons without disabilities (Crandell & Streeter, 1977). The stigma and discrimination endemic to disability is a very real and palpable problem in dating and romance: "Once the other person perceives the disability, the switch on the sexual circuit breaker often pops off—the connection is broken. 'Chemistry' is over. I have a lifetime of such experiences, and so does every other disabled woman I know" (King, cited in Resources for Rehabilitation, 1997b, pp. 15–16).

The partner of a person with a disability will experience discrimination by propinquity, or stigma by association (Goffman, 1963; Knight, 1989). The able-bodied partner has to face some of the same questions as does the person with the disability: "Will this place we are going to be accessible?" "Should I tell others in advance about the disability?" "Should I explain the nature of the disability and how much should I say about it?" Such partners will have to contend with others questioning their choice of partner, disparaging the relationship, making assumptions that are not only false but insulting, and commenting publicly about their choice. And if both partners have a disability, the assumption often is that the disability alone was a sufficiently powerful link to create a romantic couple. For example, in a study of students who were and were not blind, the authors concluded, astonishingly, that "the commonality of the blindness between two individuals brings security and a large number of common interests" (Crandell & Streeter, 1977, p. 2). Many people have assumed I chose my husband because his MS gave us a powerful "commonality" (in fact, he was diagnosed after our marriage).

Some problems are particular to persons with early-acquired disabilities, namely, the effects of being a child with a disability. Kids (the little darlings) can be brutal, and early negative experiences paired with high affect can shape durable schemas that carry over to adult life. Thus the person with the disability may have a fear of rejection based on real experiences with negative responses to the disability in childhood, particularly in adolescence. Therefore such persons may have fears and emotions based on old learning. Furthermore, experiences of rejection may have curtailed opportunities for practice in friendships and romantic relationships. Thus such persons may demonstrate skill deficits related to how to present the disability to others, what to look for in potential partners, and how to develop a spectrum of relationships from acquaintance to friends to romantic partners. Two mistakes are common (Knight, 1989). The first is wanting to spend time indiscriminantly with anyone of the right gender and age who is willing to spend time with the person with the disability, in the hope that it will develop into a relationship. This keeps the person with the disability in the position of always being the one chosen and never the one to choose. A second mistake is asking persons out on dates that are too long. This may be as a result of overeagerness when someone is willing to go on a date or trying to maximize use of time given the difficulties of transportation and accessibility (e.g., "it was so hard to get here, let's stay for two days").

People with disabilities need a skill that most people don't need: how to *contain* the disability—that is, how to get people to see them as persons, not as disabilities, and how to help people understand that the disability affects only a small portion of what a person can do. They need to know how to present the disability to others, to decrease others' anxiety, to come across as someone with a positive self-image, to answer questions about the disability, and to fit the depth of the explanation to the situation and level of intimacy. Behavioral rehearsal with a therapist can be helpful in trying out different approaches and developing these skills. The person's comfort level with the disability will set the tone much more than does the extent of the disability. Some persons with disabilities expend considerable energy in trying to minimize their disabilities, whereas others concentrate on the disability presentation. This is a subtle but important distinction. The perpetual need to minimize the disability is degrading, a denial of an essential part of oneself, requiring a great deal of energy, and impeding social interactions because it preoccupies the person with the disability. The management of disability presentation, while also requiring the person's attention, is more ego enhancing and integrative of the disability.

No matter how good the person is at the presentation of the disability, a harsh truth remains: Many people are not interested in a romantic relationship with someone with a visible disability (DeLoach, 1994; Olkin & Howson, 1994). As a therapist you already know what the response to that must be: For a client's well-being he or she simply cannot be in a close relationship with someone who cannot accept the disability. Most people know this already, but some need reminding. Furthermore, the person with a disability can choose a partner with or without a disability. Either choice can represent self-acceptance and esteem or self-loathing. Neither is inherently right or wrong or better or worse; it is the meaning of the choice for the client with the disability that is essential to understand. For example, a person with a disability might think about an able-bodied partner: "Why should I limit my choices only to people with disabilities?" "I mix in a number of circles with both disabled and able-bodied people, and this person was right for me because of our shared values and religion, sense of humor, goals." These thoughts stem from self-esteem. Contrast them with the following ideas: "I would never be with a disabled person." "It's hard enough to be one person with a disability; if we both had disabilities everyone would really stare."

When I met my husband on a blind date (sorry), we spoke by phone to arrange a meeting. I did not disclose my disability on the phone; I felt that to do so at that time gave it too much salience. I also made sure to arrive first for the date and be seated when we met (thus hiding the disability). Only after a good conversational hour when we were deciding to get ice cream did I refer to my disability. Some might think this duplicitous, leaving the other person little choice, but it has been my experience that people feel perfectly free to get up and leave at that juncture. I should also stress that this was the way I chose to

handle the issue; it was right for me, but others may make very different choices. The point is that therapists should not underplay the real
role that disability will play in the romantic arena and should be prepared to help clients develop their own strategies. (For discussion of
disability that occurs after marriage, see Chapter 6.) Knight (1989)
lists some important do's and don'ts for persons with disabilities: (1)
never talk someone into a relationships with you; (2) don't wait for
long, hoping the other person will become more attracted to you; (3)
do look elsewhere for a more satisfying relationship; (4) do not settle
for just anyone's attention; and (5) do not submerge your own desires
and wants to others'. Therapists should know that helplessness and
anger are common reactions of persons with disabilities to the pervasive rejection and discrimination in dating situations and be accepting
and empathic. The therapist should not say, "No one is acceptable to
everyone." This underplays the prejudice that occurs in the romantic
arena for persons with disabilities. It might be analogous to telling an
African American, "Everyone encounters things that aren't fair,"
thereby discounting the pervasiveness and power of racism.

SEXUALITY

Sexuality has been called the "forgotten activity of daily living" (Breske,
1996). Both sex and disability are taboo subjects. But for those clinicians
who believe that part of the therapeutic process is to discuss that which
is taboo, this section provides some parameters to consider about the
confluence of these two subjects. It will not teach you how to do sex
therapy, nor can it give detailed information about the specifics of differing disabilities and their effects on sexuality. Rather, it raises the common issues and gives some insight into this neglected topic.
    A key issue is the absence of discussion about sex and disability
(Boyle, 1993; Sipski & Alexander, 1997). Texts on sexuality barely
acknowledge disability. For example, a review of 25 texts (Calderwood
& Calderwood, cited in Barret, 1990) found that only one had a thorough discussion of sexuality and disability. Conversely, it is startling how
many books on disability do not discuss sexuality, or do so only cursorily. Much is still unknown about the interaction of disability and sexuality. Most of the literature addresses professionals more than consumers, and the focus usually is on adults with acquired disabilities.
However, ignoring persons with congenital disabilities reinforces the prevailing myth that such persons are asexual, as if early onset of a disability prevents healthy psychosexual development. Furthermore, information for two partners with disabilities is virtually nonexistent and quite

scant for gay or lesbian relationships with disabilities[1] (two exceptions are chapters in Nagler, 1993, and Sipski & Alexander, 1997).

For a variety of sociopolitical and economic reasons, the 1970s were a time of burgeoning interest in sex and disability, and much of the literature stems from that period. The journal *Sexuality and Disability* is still the primary source for professional articles. However, a sizable proportion of the literature is about the mechanics of sex (positions, erections, colostomy bags, etc.), to the neglect of psychosocial and interpersonal factors (Boyle, 1993; DeLoach, 1994). Knowledge of mechanics should be thought of as a necessary but insufficient tool for sexuality and disability.

Sexuality comprises sex drive and desire; self-concept and body image; sexual functioning, acts, and behaviors; and interpersonal relationships. These distinctions among components of sexuality are important because disability has differential effects on each of these factors. The therapist who does sex therapy with persons with disabilities must first be a competent sex therapist well versed in all of these aspects of sexuality, as well as able to understand the complex interrelationship of a specific disability with each of these components.

Myths

There are several myths attached to disability and sexuality. The first and most pervasive is that persons with disabilities are asexual, that is, that they lack the basic biological sex drive. This is different from saying that people with disabilities are raised *as if they were* asexual, which is in fact often the case (DeLoach, 1994; Edmonson, 1988; Knight, 1989; Rousso, 1982; Shepperdson, 1988) and probably results from the widespread belief that it is unacceptable for people with disabilities to be sexual beings (Sipski & Alexander, 1997) and that they have "more important" things to think about (Boyle, 1993). (In fact, sterilization of persons with disabilities is more accepted and prevalent than one might think; Brantlinger, 1992; Miller & Morgan, 1980; Shepperdson, 1988.) The second myth is that people with disabilities are incapable of functioning sexually. For example, a friend reported that a new acquaintance, upon hearing that my friend's husband uses a wheelchair, blurted out, "Can you have sex?" That spontaneous (albeit impolitic) question

---

[1]It is estimated that the percentage of gay, lesbian, or bisexual (g/l/b) persons among those with disabilities is the same as among those without disabilities. The percentage of persons with disabilities among the g/l/b population is estimated at 11%, excluding persons with HIV or AIDS (Saad, 1997).

comes up frequently. One of the problems is equating "sex" with "intercourse" and then assuming that the lack of the latter implies absence of the former. The third myth is that persons with disabilities lack the requisite social skills and sound judgment needed to behave in a sexually responsible manner. This myth results from the spread effect (see Chapter 4) (i.e., the physical disability is assumed to affect behavioral and cognitive capacities, impairing interpersonal capabilities). A fourth myth is that no able-bodied people will find persons with disabilities desirable as romantic and sexual partners, or if they do it implies something is wrong with them, or that they are "settling" (stigma by contagion). A fifth myth is that women with disabilities are less affected sexually than are men with disabilities, because of their presumed more passive sexual role. This myth is perpetuated by an astonishing lack of research on sexuality in women with disabilities (Sipski & Alexander, 1997), as if this isn't an important topic. It is also presumed that men's roles, self-concepts, and egos will be more assaulted by disability than will women's. (In fact, men with disabilities are more likely to get married than are women with disabilities, and "fewer socially sanctioned roles are viewed as appropriate for women with disabilities than are viewed as appropriate for men with disabilities" [DeLoach, 1994, p. 19].)

Unfortunately, these myths, singly or cumulatively, can become internalized until the person with the disability believes them as well.[2] It is important that the clinician not believe them also. Furthermore, it is likely that it will be the therapist who must raise and pursue discussion of sexuality, thus developing comfort with these topics is essential. I would warn the clinician that even articulate and educated clients often know much less about sexuality than we give them credit for. Clients with disabilities may know even less, because they may have less exposure to the usual routes of information: touch, vision, hearing and overhearing, experimenting with others, self-exploration, peeping, reading, watching, or discussing. In addition, attitudinal barriers may exclude them from resources and information. Thus their dependence on the family for information is increased, and families, unfortunately, often don't discuss sex, much less sexuality and disability. In the words of one author, this "parental failure to foster sexuality is a form of abuse . . ., albeit an unwitting form, for sexuality is not a minor facet of human life" (Rousso, 1982, p. 83).

---

[2]There is no language for the concept of disability prejudice turned toward the self. Along the lines of "internalized homophobia," I might call it *internalized ableism*. In fact, persons with disabilities may hold prejudices against other people with disabilities, including those with the same disabilities as their own.

Effects of Disability on Physical and Psychosocial Aspects of Sexuality

The effects of disability on sexuality can take numerous routes, including physiology (e.g., sensation, mobility, energy, and pain), psychology (self-concept, body image), and sociology (the relationship, culture). The particulars of the specific disability also must be considered. Other factors include level of knowledge about sexuality and about the effects of one's own disability on sexual functioning, level of comfort or embarrassment in discussing sexual matters, the role of personal attendants in assisting in sexual activities, and fears about sex contributing to or exacerbating disabilities such as stroke or heart conditions. (Generally this is unfounded. Sexual activity and orgasm has been likened to climbing 15 stairs or walking four to five blocks; Badeau, 1995.)

There are many factors to consider just about physiology alone. These include sensation (of erogenous and nonerogenous areas); blood flow; functioning of the central nervous system; muscle tone and mobility, flexibility, and spasticity; arousal; ability to experience erection or lubrication; capability of achieving orgasm, ejaculation, and conception; bladder and bowel control; medications; fatigue; and pain. It is important to list these factors because a disability might affect some of these greatly, others a bit, and some not at all. Thus in discussing sexuality with clients with disabilities it is vital to be quite specific.

It may help to know some general findings related to the physiology of disability and sexuality. Many people in wheelchairs have genital sensation and functioning (Knight, 1989). Kreuter, Sullivan, and Siosteen (1994a, 1994b, 1996) studied men and women with SCI and their partners (in Sweden). The proportion of persons with SCI (80% of whom were male) who were married was 51%, compared with 59% of age- and sex-matched controls. Half the couples engaged in sex at least once a week, and 38% usually had intercourse as one of their sexual activities. Of the sexually active couples, 66% of the partners and 34% of the person with SCI experienced orgasm on most occasions of sexual activity. Partners in relationships that began pre- or postinjury were equally likely to be satisfied with their current sex life (around 87% felt this way). Factors considered important by both partners included use of a varied repertoire of sexual behaviors and the perception that the partner enjoyed and was satisfied with the sexual part of the relationship. The authors concluded that "psychosocial rather than physical factors were important for a satisfying sexual life and relationship" (Kreuter et al., 1996, p. 541). Another study of persons with SCI (Romeo, Wanlass, & Arenas, 1993) found that men with paraplegia or quadriplegia did not differ from each other on any of the scales of the Derogatis Sexual Functioning Inventory. However, when compared with normative samples, men with SCI not surprisingly had below-normal scores on body image, gender role definition, and extent of sexual experience (i.e., in response to specific items such as "intercourse, side by side"). But they did not differ from the normative sample on intensity of sex drive, level of sexual knowledge, breadth of sexual fantasies, and degree of sexual satisfaction. SCI can affect ejaculation (or cause retrograde ejaculation) and, thus, procreation. Procreation can sometimes be achieved through collection of sperm through electroejaculation and artificial insemination (which is costly and about as fun as it sounds).

A study of sexuality in couples where one partner had rheumatic disease (Majerovitz & Revenson, 1994) used a comparison group of couples without disabilities. (For 73% of the couples it was the wife who had rheumatic disease; 94% of the couples were Caucasian.) Results indicated that there was no difference between groups in sexual satisfaction (though women in both groups reported lower satisfaction than did men). Another study of women with disabilities (Nosek et al., 1995) found no differences on sexual desire between women with and without disabilities. However, sexual activity, response and satisfaction were lower for the women with disabilities. The severity of disability was not correlated with sexual activity, and the strongest predictor of sexual activity was living with a significant other.

Disability can affect the psychology of sexuality in several ways. One factor is how one sees oneself. Self-concept and body image affect sexuality; if these are negatively affected by disability, sexuality will be too. If the disability onset was relatively late (postadolescence), there was a prior history of sexuality. This can be problematic in that the person already has been inculcated with prejudice against disability and may apply this prejudice to him- or herself as a disabled person ("internalized ableism"). For those with congenital or early-onset disability the sense of sexual self-identity and development included the disability, though it still might not be fully and realistically integrated into the self-concept and body image. Because many persons with disabilities are raised as if they were asexual, it is a good idea to inquire how the particular client was raised to see him- or herself, if he or she was encouraged or allowed to see the self as a sexual person. Furthermore, this person may have had a lack of opportunities for sexual exploration. Being a teenager with a disability may have inhibited social interactions and reduced dating, romantic, or intimate connections. If early attempts at acquiring information and experience are unsuccessful, this learning, usually in the presence of the high affect associated with adolescence, may lay down a negative blueprint that fails to be challenged for some time. Thus persons with early-onset disabilities may be "late bloomers."[3] Doctors often treat disability as an affected body part—a leg, for example, that only incidentally happens to be attached to a person. Thus sometimes people with disabilities think of themselves this way; many talk about the "good" parts (e.g., the good leg) and bad parts (e.g., the bad leg), thinking of themselves as split into two. Which part contains the sexual self?

There are many effects of disability on the sociology of sexuality. "Research indicates that generally persons without disability are not accepting of intimate relationships with persons with any type of disability. Persons without disabilities are more willing to accept persons with disabilities as fellow employees or casual friends and less willing to accept them as dating or marriage partners" (DeLoach, 1994, p. 19). Because persons with disabilities are often ostracized as children and adolescents, they have less opportunities for social interactions, less practice in social skills, and less feedback on their social functioning. Role models for persons with disabilities, who are active in all spheres of life, including sexuality, are sorely lacking. Persons with disabilities need to learn how to make friends before they can learn how to become lovers and how to make choices in selecting partners and not merely wait to be chosen by someone "willing" to be with them, and not have what Knight (1989) calls "pity sex" (p. 188). It should be noted, however, that early onset of a disability does not mean that the person has more problems or is less "adjusted." In fact, a national survey of parents with disabilities suggests that those with earlier onset had integrated the disability more into their self-concepts (Toms Barker & Maralani, 1997).

Obviously a key factor is the relationship with a partner. Partner issues can include whether the partner also has a disability and the partner's attitudes toward disability and toward sexuality. Partners in general tend to be seen as peripheral for much of rehabilitation, and this is especially so for gay and lesbian partners. Clinicians should assess the relationship and the partner's attitudes and avoid assuming that disability is a problem for the partner or the couple. The amount of caregiving the able-bodied partner does is also an important factor. It may be that sexual feelings and caregiving are somewhat reciprocally inhibitive. Furthermore, as the partner with the disability decreases his or her share of household tasks, the able-bodied partner may need to pick up the slack. This can lead to conflict, blame, guilt, resentment, dependence, and so

---

[3]The literature on development of persons with disabilities is mixed, some saying that this is the case (Resources for Rehabilitation, 1997a; Rousso, 1982) and at least one study failing to support this notion (Silvers, 1996).

on, all of which may be anathema to a sexual relationship. (See also Chapter 6 for more on partners.)

The preceding comments on the effects of disability on sexuality come with a caution: It must not be assumed that current sexual concerns originate in the disability or are entirely explained by it. Other issues (e.g., history of sexual abuse and nature of current relationship) and possible etiologies (e.g., depression) must be kept in mind. Any chronic pain or discomfort should be checked out by a medical professional. Changes in desire or functioning should also be investigated. These may be due to increased fatigue or pain related to the disability, but other causes must be ruled out. For example, for more than 6 months I attributed my considerably lessened energy level to worsening of postpolio syndrome (PPS) symptoms, when it turned out I had a thyroid problem! Furthermore, practitioners must exercise caution in thinking dichotomously in terms of physiological versus psychogenic; impairments and their consequences span both in a fluid bidirectional manner.

Special Issues

Two special issues must be addressed regarding disability and sexuality. The first is sexual abuse. Clearly, this is an area with tremendous implications for sexuality. Although the findings are not consistent, many studies report higher rates of abuse for children with disabilities (for recent reviews, see Kewman, Warschausky, Engel, & Warzak, 1997; Nosek & Howland, 1997; Sobsey & Doe, 1991; Sobsey, Gray, Wells, Pyper, & Reimer-Heck, 1991). Most reports place the risk of sexual abuse for people with disabilities as higher than for those without disabilities (Finkelhor, 1984; Gordon, 1971; Krents et al., 1987; Morgan, 1987; Nosek, 1995; Nosek, Young, et al., 1995; O'Day, cited in Tharinger, Horton, & Millea, 1994; Sobsey & Doe, 1991; Sobsey, Wells, Lucardie, & Mansell, 1995; Zirpoli, 1986). The barriers to information and experience discussed earlier also make children with disabilities vulnerable:

> Children are more likely to be victimized by rejection and abuse when they are ignorant about sex and their own sexuality. They are more likely to misread social cues, ignore danger signals, and to give misleading cues themselves; they are more likely to accept abuse because they feel they have no options; and they are less likely to make assertive, active choices. (Rousso, 1982, p. 83)

It is likely that sexual abuse of children with disabilities is even more underreported than for nondisabled children, because people with disabilities face additional barriers that impede reporting (e.g., access to transportation). The pattern of abuse may be different as well. For example, in the general population about 80% of sexual abuse is by someone known to the victim, but for persons with developmental disabilities, about 99% of the abuse cases are by persons in a caregiving or professional capacity (e.g., relatives, residential staff, bus drivers, volunteers, and supervisors) (Cole, cited in DeLoach, 1994).

We can only speculate about the reasons for any increased rate of abuse of children with disabilities: increased physical dependence, reduced independence, more institutionalization, engendering negative feelings in the adults, increased physical vulnerability, and reduced believability when reporting abuse. Incidence of acquaintance or "date rape" also may be increased; lack of social opportunities can make people with disabilities feel beholden to anyone who seems to take a sexual interest in them, or more willing to "settle" for what they can get. Fewer dating opportunities may mean that the person with a disability has less chance to practice skills in self-assertion and protection, or is less able to recognize early signs of potential danger. Any and all of these reasons could account for increased vulnerability to sexual abuse for people with disabilities. Clinicians should not overlook this area of history taking or let their own countertransference impede this line of inquiry.

The second special issue relates to fetishes. There are occasional anecdotal reports about disability as an object of sexual fetishes. A quick search on the Internet supports this, particularly related to amputation. Videos, chat rooms, web sites, and pictures are all readily available, though only one professional article was found (Everaerd, 1983). Whereas amputation seems to be the most common preference, some seek partners with neck or leg braces. Persons (almost exclusively male) who prefer partners with amputations are called "devotees." Their preferences often are quite specific (e.g., "left leg, above knee"). A subset of persons prefer to simulate disabilities (for sexual gratification, as opposed to the taking on of a sick role associated with Munchausen's). These preferences would be considered paraphilia, NOS (DSM-IV: American Psychiatric Association, 1994) *only* if they caused significant impairment or distress.

Skills and Interventions

The basic model of sex therapy applies to clients with disabilities: support, education, permission, behavior change, and short-term focused treatment on specified difficulties (Knight, 1989). Basic knowledge of sexuality is essential: male and female anatomy and physiology, sexual response cycle, menstruation, masturbation and a range of expressions of sexuality, contraception and conception, sexual lifestyles and orientations, and sexually transmitted diseases. On top of this basic knowledge should be an overlay of information about disability effects on all aspects of sexuality and skills in addressing problem areas. General goals of treatment include putting disability into perspective and understanding its role in sexuality, developing a positive body image, understanding sexual functioning in light of the disability, learning skills needed to address problem areas, and exploring options for remediating difficulties.

The only way to ensure that sexuality does not continue to be overlooked in the rehabilitation and therapy with persons with disabilities is to have all front-line therapists receive appropriate training. Such training must not be focused solely on changing attitudes, values, or beliefs about sexuality and disability but should include an assessment of how these affect professionals' interactions with clients with disabilities and, most important, on building skills in assessment and treatment of these clients. When therapists receive factual information about disabilities and sexuality they feel more empowered through increased comfort and confidence in their own skills.

Not all sexual problems require the same depth of treatment (Sanders, 1984). Many practitioners of sex therapy subscribe to Annon's (1974) notion of four levels of hierarchical skills. The amount of specific training and experience required to be proficient in each is cumulative, with higher levels requiring greater skills. This model is PLISSIT (*p*ermission, *l*imited *i*nformation, *s*pecific *s*uggestions, and *i*ntensive *t*reatment). This model is useful in helping clinician's evaluate their own levels of training, experience, and skills.

The first level is the ability to give *permission*, which involves helping clients to feel okay about being sexual, making it a priority, and being able to initiate and respond sexually. One of the most important aspects in alleviating any sexual difficulties is to help the person feel "normal." Most people think their sexual problems are unique, weird, abnormal, and deviant, and persons with disabilities, who get these messages all the time, are even more likely to experience such feelings. Talking with other people with disabilities can be enormously reassuring and informative. Also, persons with disabilities may need to know that romantic and sexual concerns are common and not unique to persons with disabilities. Generally no special training is necessary for a professional to give the kind of assistance needed at this level. However, therapists must be comfortable talking openly and explicitly about sexuality, able to adopt the client's choice of language, able to process any countertransference issues related to sexuality and disability, and genuine in encouraging and supporting the client's exploration of sexuality. They must be prepared to deal with (but not collude with) the profound disgust a client may feel about his or her own disability and with the rejection the person is likely to encounter from others.

The next level of assistance is *limited information*; this also can be provided by most professionals, though some research outside sessions may be necessary (e.g., about male and female anatomy, the effects of a specific medication on sexual functioning, and whether women with SCI can conceive[4]). Work at this level includes dispelling myths, providing factual information, and answering questions.

The third level is *specific suggestions* tailored to the needs of a client, which usually requires more training. In the PLISSIT model, "specific suggestions" refers to training and experience in sex therapy. But to treat sexual problems of clients with disabilities at this level the clinician also needs information about disability. Unfortunately, professionals often have training and experience in sex *or* disability, making holistic treatment difficult to obtain. To work at this level the clinician must know details about the client and the sexual history, about the specific disability, and about the interaction of the two. For example, strength or weakness of limbs may affect choice of positions and a clinician might suggest other positions. Another example would be for a clinician to give advice about what to do with a Foley catheter (see Halstead, 1998). This level also requires attention to partner/relationship issues, communication, collaboration, and solutions to specific problems. It is useful if the clinician asks for a step-by-step description of a recent sexual encounter; in this way disability-specific difficulties can come to light.

A common specific concern is about fatigue. Suggestions might include finding times in the day or week when energy levels are more optimum. Time of day can be important for some people, taking into consideration needs such as warming up muscles, ensuring reasonable levels of energy and avoiding fatigue, or timing in relation to when medications are taken. Sexual innovation can be useful, such as finding positions that promote relaxation and don't tax muscles or widening the array of pleasurable activities. Sexual encounters may become less spontaneous and more planned.

Another common concern is how to initiate first sexual experiences with a given partner. Behaviors that lead to "spontaneous" sexuality may be limited for the person with the disability. For example, on a date an able-bodied couple may begin to kiss, hold each other closer, make more body contact, and touch increasingly intimate areas, all signaling movement toward sex. But if one partner is in a wheelchair, or body movements include uncontrolled jerks and random motions, the signals

---

[4]The answer is generally, yes.

are less clear and the path to sexual intimacy less marked. Furthermore, there may be requirements for how sex happens that the couple must take care of beforehand (e.g., help with getting into supine position) or during sex (e.g., stimulation of particular areas not usually regarded as erogenous). Thus persons with disabilities may need to have explicit discussions with potential sexual partners about whether they will be sexual together, and if so how it will occur. During this discussion, information can be given to the partner, questions invited, and specific suggestions made. The person with the disability needs to learn how to ask for assistance without losing adult or sexual status and how to reject unneeded assistance without being perceived as rejecting (Rousso, 1982).

The final level of assistance in the PLISSIT model involves *intensive treatment* about issues connected to sexuality (e.g., marital therapy and treatment for the aftermath of sexual abuse). Professionals providing this type of care should be well trained and experienced in this type of work. Ideally they should be well versed in both sexuality and disability. This training may not be specifically in the disability of any given client, but the therapist should understand the general issues related to sexuality and disability and know enough to realize that more specific information is needed. The therapist runs the danger of developing intervention too quickly such that it is aimed at the wrong targets. Lefebvre (1990) developed a systematic method of collecting and evaluating a client's history. The therapist designates categories of interest based on a preliminary overview of the client's history (nature of current relationship, history of abuse, coping skills, religion, etc.). Each category is assigned positive, negative, or no points. Those topics with negative points indicate areas of weakness (not just difference) that will impinge upon sexuality skills, and topics with positive scores indicate strengths that can be marshalled to balance and combat deficiencies. Areas with no points require further investigation until they can be designated as positive or negative. This method can easily incorporate disability issues into the categories and overall assessment. However, therapists should be wary of using existing measures of sexual activities without modifying them first, as many are focused on intercourse.

The hierarchy of assistance needs inherent in the PLISSIT model is not meant to imply that clients with more in-depth needs are hopeless, more damaged, or abnormal. Rather, the model is intended as a way to help clinicians understand different types of assistance that are possible and to evaluate their own level of training and experience in light of the skills required. But clinicians still must be flexible and creative in finding solutions and options for resolving sexual difficulties; deviation from the manual is the name of the game for persons with disabilities. And therapists should consider helping the client with disabilities find peers with disabilities.

The skills necessary for intimacy and sexuality require chaining (i.e., a series of interlinked and cumulative skills that build upon each other). If this chain is curtailed at lower levels, the higher level skills are of necessity also impaired. Thus the clinician must evaluate carefully the range of tasks and behaviors that lead to romantic partnerships and assess skills in this chain. Persons with disabilities have higher rates of victimization, are culturally expected to be passive, have less options in where to go and how to meet people, and are given fewer choices of partners. Thus sex therapy with persons with disabilities often needs to incorporate work on self-advocacy, evaluating choices and decision making, assertiveness, social risk taking, and exploration. Of course, all the factors related to sexuality in general also apply to persons with disabilities. These include issues such as AIDS and safer sexual practices, sexual orientation, history of sexual and/or physical abuse, and substance use or abuse. These factors may be complicated by some types of disabilities. For example, birth control options may be limited: Barrier methods require fine motor control; birth control pills or implants cannot be combined with various medications used for some disabilities (e.g., antiepileptics). A recurrent theme in this section on sexuality and disability is that one must *ask* and *be specific*. Disability effects on sexuality can be minimal to profound, and no set guidelines can convey sufficient information a priori. Furthermore, disability cannot be the scapegoat for all problems, and other issues should not be overshadowed by the fact of disability. Persons with disabilities want to be treated as whole people, so clinicians must think of them this way as well.

PREGNANCY AND BIRTHING[5]

Persons with disabilities who are deciding whether to have children must consider some disability issues. Suggesting such deliberation is not meant to dissuade anyone but to ease the transition to parenthood. It should be remembered that often the disability does not affect fertility. For example, in men with SCI, erection, orgasm and ejaculation are separate func-

---

[5]For a bibliography on reproductive rights of women with disabilities, ask for *Meeting the Needs of Women with Disabilities: A Blueprint for Change* from Berkeley Planning Associates, 440 Grand Avenue, Suite 500, Oakland, CA 94610-5085.

tions, and impairment in one does not necessary mean impairment in the others.

Age is one factor in deciding whether and when to get pregnant. All women do better (i.e., recover faster, have fewer complications) having babies in their 20s compared to their 30s. But this is especially important for many women with disabilities. The effects of aging (even in your 30s), disability, and pregnancy can combine to produce more symptoms in pregnancy. (And having babies later translates into having young children later in life. Nonetheless I had two children at ages 34 and 37. Remember that *possible* and *optimum* are not always synonymous.) The question is not so much how the disability affects the pregnancy but, rather, how the pregnancy affects the disability. Women with physical disabilities may experience significantly increased fatigue beyond that expected from pregnancy and continuing through the three trimesters. They may experience increases in muscle weakness and pain. With the additional weight in the third trimester, mobility may be impaired. None of this is meant to discourage pregnancy but to help women plan for it more realistically.

Once pregnant, it is wise to remember that the woman with the disability knows her body best, so she must be actively involved in all decisions. She is the expert on the disability and is the best one to know if the pregnancy is affecting the disability. But she is first and foremost a pregnant woman, not a disabled woman, and should be treated as such. One difficulty is that the obstetrician/gynecologist (ob/gyn) may be unfamiliar with the disability and with the combination of disability and pregnancy, while physicians expert in disability are unlikely to know much about the interaction with pregnancy and birthing. It may be desirable to seek consultation from outside the ob/gyn group. In any case, a team approach is recommended (possible participants besides the woman are the partner/coach, the primary birth/delivery doctor or nurse midwife, the primary physician for disability, and the anesthesiologist).

Labor and delivery can be affected by several aspects of disability, such as weakened stomach muscles, scoliosis, or pelvic deformity. In some instances a preplanned caesarian birth may be preferable. Careful evaluation of the pros and cons of vaginal versus caesarian births should be undertaken. Recovery from caesarian is generally longer than from vaginal deliveries, but labor may overwork muscles and leave the mother with increased pain, weakness, and even temporary paralysis during postdelivery recovery. Pain medication and anesthesia also need careful analysis. Results of one study of pregnancy and childbirth in mothers with disabilities suggests that epidurals can cause temporary paralysis in disability-affected limbs (as it did in my case, and in several of the cases discussed in Rogers & Matsumura, 1991).

Parents with disabilities also have the option to adopt.[6] Adoption agencies should be accessible to persons with disabilities and are not supposed to discriminate on the basis of disability per se, but they may have some latitude in the name of the "best interests of the child." Some parents with disabilities request a child with a disability, perhaps because there are more such children for adoption, and because some parents feel that they are ideal candidates to parent children with disabilities. For a caregiver with a disability and an infant or toddler with a disability, the first 6 years or so are likely to be physically difficult, and parents should plan for how to meet the physical demands of early parenting.

GENETIC TESTING

This is a hot topic in the disability community and the subject of several disability essays and books (e.g., Finger, 1990; Shakespeare, 1998), though it is rarely discussed in the professional rehabilitation literature. A full review of issues is not possible here, so the goal of this section is simply to raise awareness of how loaded a topic this is. At issue are two factors. The first is the rather pervasive assumption that babies with disabilities should be prevented. The medical and genetic literature (e.g., Rhine, 1993), charity drives, and advertising all focus quite matter-of-factly on the prevention of such births. The second issue is the identification many people with disabilities feel with children with disabilities. A common sentiment in the disability community is that preventing the birth of babies with disabilities is preventing *people like us,* and preventing the putative suffering associated with our disabilities. But most of us are not suffering and would not choose to have been aborted over our present lives with a disability.

Sentiment about genetic testing runs deep. Two examples illustrate this sentiment. In the first, two women with disabilities include the following in their list of six empowerment issues in a manifesto for "disabled feminists":

> We want all women to understand that they can refuse to have these [prenatal screening] tests if they don't want them. We want children with disabilities to feel welcome in the world. (Waxman Fiduccia & Saxton, 1997, p. 61)

---

[6]A useful guidebook is *You May Be Able to Adopt!: A Guide to the Adoption Option for Women with Disabilities and Their Partners* by L. Toms Barker, S. Haight-Liotta, M. Kirshbaum, M. Jakobson, and F. Nisen (1997), available for $10 from Through the Looking Glass, 2198 Sixth Street, Suite 100, Berkeley, CA 94710-9863.

And from a recent book on disability studies:

> Most of us would be horrified if a scientist offered to develop a test to diag-
> nose skin color prenatally so as to enable racially mixed people . . . to have
> light-skinned children. And if the scientist explained that because it is diffi-
> cult to grow up black in America, he or she wanted to spare people suffer-
> ing because of the color of their skin, we would counter that it is irresponsi-
> ble to use scientific means to reinforce racial prejudices. Yet we see nothing
> wrong, and indeed hail as progress, tests that enable us to try to avoid hav-
> ing children who have disabilities or are said to have a tendency to acquire
> a specific disease or disability later in life. (Hubbard, 1997, p. 187)

There are people who have no difficulties with the ethical, emotional, and practical issues raised by genetic testing. Some people desire
the testing and welcome the information to aid in decision making. Others eschew testing. And many, like myself, are profoundly ambivalent.
To complicate matters further, partners may feel differently and advocate
different courses of action. All these issues will test the abilities of the clinician to remain neutral and facilitative. What is important here is to
understand the profound depth of psychological meaning and emotion
that are likely to be attached to these topics by persons with disabilities.

ELEVEN

Special Issues
in Therapy with Clients
with Disabilities

This chapter helps increase clinician's competence in cross-cultural therapy by covering several issues likely to arise when treating clients with
disabilities. These issues include living with a progressive disorder, pain,
or fatigue; dealing with discrimination and stigma; aging; substance
abuse; use of support groups and readings; and physician-assisted suicide. Admittedly this is an odd assortment of topics, and there are many
others that could have been covered. The ones selected for inclusion are
those that are more common, those that may be less intuitive for the
able-bodied therapist to understand, and those that are key concerns in
the disability community.

LIVING WITH A PROGRESSIVE DISORDER

Most disabilities progress (i.e., get worse), even if they are not considered "progressive" disorders, just because of the effects of aging and the
accrual of new infirmities. For example, my limp did not get more pronounced, but its impact became more troublesome once I acquired a
back problem. Thus the total effect is that my impairment is worse (i.e.,
more disabling in daily functioning) than before. Other disabilities do
progress in severity, some slowly, some rapidly, some with sudden decre-
ments in functioning, and some with unpredictable and idiosyncratic
courses. This feature of getting more disabled means we have the task of

constantly adjusting, and then when we think we've adjusted, adjusting again. Sometimes the changes are slowly progressive but experienced as sudden because at one point they cross an important line of functioning. Like a rain barrel that's filling with water, all it takes is one drop to make it overflow, but that drop can be a long time coming when the barrel is barely full. Thus a seemingly small change, a single drop of water, suddenly can mean a pronounced change in functioning. From the outside this seems very harsh, a hard part of disability to cope with. In some ways it is; uncertainty—about future, financial and job security, health, relationships, and support structures—is psychologically and emotionally difficult to contend with. But in another way it is not as hard as ABs think. Remember being in, say, fourth grade, and thinking about going to high school? It seemed impossible, uncopable, unimaginable. But of course by the time you got to high school you were more than ready; the transition to first-year high school, although still a jump, was less of a leap than it seemed it would be back in fourth grade. Progressive disability is like sliding into high school; by the time you get there it's only a small increment from the grade before and isn't as psychologically jarring as you might think. It is rather like growing—from the inside it's barely discernable, but if your aunt hasn't seen you in a year she'll exclaim how much you've grown. And yes, you can look back a year and see you have grown, just like you can look back a year or two and see the progression of your disability. But day-to-day experience is not taken up with this knowledge.

I'm making it sound as if one is always ready for the next stage of decline. But one of the paradoxes of disability is that one is always ready and never ready. Every decrement seems to come too soon and before we are prepared. People rarely explore options for electric wheelchairs before they need one or consider the relative merits of scooters versus wheelchairs while they are still ambulatory. We all deny, and sometimes that denial serves us—who wants or needs to dwell on declining abilities? It is only when the denial prevents useful action or planning that it becomes a problem. Otherwise a bit of repression serves the soul.

LIVING WITH PAIN

When thinking about pain I am often reminded of the orthopedist who told me that after surgery (in which they broke several bones, and reshaped and fused my ankle) that I would experience a little "discomfort." To me, that "discomfort" was an 11 on a 10-point scale. This anecdote begins a discussion of pain that includes its many variables—its severity, frequency, description, disruptiveness, and management.

In working with clients with disabilities, pain is likely to be a factor. It can become a treatment issue if variability and unpredictability of pain interfere with keeping appointments (I discussed therapist and treatment flexibility in Chapter 6). Clients may need help living with chronic pain, adjusting to new levels of pain, or facing a period of exacerbated pain (e.g., during or following a medical procedure). Many articles and books deal with the topic of chronic pain, so I limit myself here to those issues I think are most applicable to people with disabilities.

Disability-related pain may stem from a variety of sources. Impairments can lead to tendinitis, bursitis, arthritis, muscle pain (myalgia), and muscle spasms. Sitting, prolonged inactivity, and bed rest can lead to decubitus ulcers ("bed sores") which are not only very painful but potentially life threatening. Back pain is a common concomitant of orthopedic impairments. Pain is a symptom for some persons with MS but not all. Thus pain is an idiosyncratic part of the subjective experience of impairment.

Describing Pain

Often we talk about pain as if it were a bimodal state—I am in pain, I am not in pain. But pain has gradations, from none to severe. The point at which it is labeled "pain" varies from person to person. My orthopedist's "discomfort" was my "intolerable." Clients often need help in understanding and labeling the gradations as a first step to deciding how to respond to or deal with the pain. But because pain is so often a corollary of disability, having more labels for it than simply pain/no pain is necessary to begin to understand and live with it. An analogy that may be familiar to many clinicians is the client with anxiety. On intake the client may complain of "always" feeling anxious and when asked to rate anxiety on a scale of 1 to 100, gives it a 90. But when the client is instructed to self-monitor at different times of day, he or she may come to discover that the anxiety does in fact fluctuate, and even go down to 20 or 30. Only then does it become possible to discuss the link between anxiety levels and behavior (e.g., ratings above 50 lead to avoidance). Just by learning to make finer discriminations in levels of anxiety more options of response become available. The same is true for pain. Thus self-monitoring (e.g., a pain diary) is an important initial step. Care should be taken to sample times of day that will demonstrate variability. For example, if I assessed pain levels three times per day at 8 A.M. (poor circulation upon rising), 4 P.M. (sharp drop in temperature and barometric pressure), and 9 P.M. (fatigue, swelling), I could falsely conclude that I experience a consistently high level of pain. But if I assessed at 10 A.M. (movement and hot shower increase circulation) and 2 P.M. (minimal swelling, not yet fatigued), the levels would be much lower. Thus a client can "rig" the data to fulfill his or her own prophecy.

Pain is subjective; it is difficult to define and measure. There are different meanings of the word "pain." It may denote psychological or emotional pain, spiritual void, physical sensation, or some combination. Various words can be used to describe pain: sharp, stabbing, tingly, burning, pinching, dull, achy, pulling, pressure, throbbing. Some commonality of definition and understanding of the meaning of pain are necessary for client and therapist. Discussion of levels of pain that occur during the therapy hour are useful in developing a common understanding. For example, after discussing something absorbing and not related to the disability, the therapist could ask for a reading of pain level. Or, when a client shifts uncomfortably, another opportunity presents itself to generate words that describe the pain. Again, a key point is the idiosyncratic nature of the experience and meaning of pain, requiring some mutual exploration before therapy can begin to address intervention.

Acute versus Chronic Pain

The most common type of pain is acute, and this is the model of pain most people think about in considering pain. In acute pain the pain is often well localized, described as sharp, intense, or burning. The cause of the pain is usually apparent, and if that cause is treated the pain subsides. The pain signals are carried through the body to the brain by large, myelinated, A-delta nerve fibers, which send messages quickly and efficiently. The pain serves as a signal that the body has been or is being damaged. When pain is a signal (e.g., slow down, stop what you're doing), it pays to listen to the message. For example, I get certain types and severity of ankle and foot pain which indicate that if I don't stop walking, I'll fall because my knee will give out. I therefore don't medicate any pain at or below that level of severity because I need the early-warning system. On the other hand, I recently slipped and twisted my ankle, immediately elevating the pain level above that threshold, alerting me to ice and elevate my ankle.

In contrast to acute pain, chronic pain is usually dull, more poorly localized, and often the cause is indeterminate. The duration is long term (most pain clinics set the entry criterion at 6 months). The pain is not signaling damage; thus it sends false messages, which are carried by small, unmyelinated, C-nerve fibers, a less efficient messaging system. There are several theories of why chronic pain persists. It may be that there are overdeveloped pathways in the central nervous system, or an increased number of pain receptors, or an impaired inhibitory system in the descending nerve pathways (from brain to body).

Chronic pain patients represent medical failures—failure to diagnosis the cause or ameliorate the sensation. They are viewed as having pain of unknown or psychogenic origin, "out of proportion" to the injury. Such persons may be dependent on pain killers, often narcotics, depressed or angry, lacking in sleep and may have sought multiple physicians, had multiple surgeries, and made many visits to emergency rooms without any clinical findings. They are more disabled by the pain than seems medically warranted by the level of impairment. In addition, their rate of depression, somatization, and utilization of medical services is higher. (Chronic pain seems to have the effect of reducing serotonin levels, as does depression, which may be one reason for the high overlap.) All these issues may be part of the reason that such patients have a terrible reputation. Instead of being viewed as a failure on the part of the medical system, such persons are usually seen as being "treatment resistant." The therapist who ascribes to this view of such patients is likely to hold certain beliefs (e.g., the person could feel better if he or she tried harder or the person is making the pain worse) that may impede the treatment. The point is not whether such beliefs are "true" or not but rather whether they are "useful." I would argue that such beliefs undermine chances of a more successful outcome.

The Relationship between Person and Pain

Pain can be viewed as avoidable or unavoidable. Beliefs about the purpose of the pain affect how the pain is experienced. For example, because some of my ankle pain provides useful information I don't think of it as pain but as a *signal*. But the pain in my lower back serves no useful purpose, and I label it needless and painful. However, rather than medicating it on a long-term basis, I try to alter my lifestyle (seating, bending, lifting, carrying) to minimize the pain. This relationship to chronic pain carries over to my experience of acute pain. When I get a headache I often forget to medicate it; without being aware of it, I'm waiting to see if the headache is a signal for something amiss. Persons with disabilities have a relationship to their pain, and it is important for the clinician to understand and respect that relationship.

Chronic pain can occur outside conscious awareness. I am in pain some portion of every day, yet if you ask me, "Do you experience pain?" I have to think very hard about how to answer the question. Much of the time the pain occurs and I respond to it without consciously being aware of it or directing my response. Pain can be like white noise; if you really stop and listen to a white noise machine, the noise is somewhat annoying, but if you tune it out, it is in the background and blocks out other noises. Pain is in the background and blocks out other awareness; it can distract without making itself known.

Treatment

As discussed earlier, it is useful for clinicians working with clients with disabilities to avoid labeling such clients as "chronic pain patients." Persons with disabilities may experience chronic pain, but that does not make them chronic pain patients. Although many chronic pain patients have greatly reduced their activities, persons with disabilities usually have been taught not to "give in" to their disabilities and have an early cognitive template for coping with adversity. They are used to accommodating to the environment, and the pain becomes another environmental handicap to be overcome. Studies on chronic pain patients have generally been in medical settings and excluded people with disabilities, so readers should be cautious in generalizing from this literature to clients with disabilities.

For many people with disabilities pain has a diurnal variation. For some it's worse in the morning when joints are stiff. For others, pain increases as the day wears on. In some cases the weather (heat, cold, drops in barometric pressure) affects pain levels. The temperature of your office may become an issue, and the time of day for appointments may be more restricted. This should not be viewed as acting out, and accommodating these physical needs can be useful in helping a client be more available to the therapeutic process.

Some clients remain on medication on a long-term basis, such as nonsteroidal antiinflammatories, steroids, narcotics, muscle relaxants, antiseizure medication, or small doses of antidepressants (tricyclics, below levels used for treatment of clinical depression, or selective serotonin reuptake inhibitors). Generally, discussion of medication is inevitable when treating chronic pain. Most medically oriented pain treatment programs insist on cessation of analgesics and narcotics prior to beginning other treatments. The process of ceasing such medications usually involves several steps. The first is to demonstrate to the client that the pain is not being regulated by the medication. For example, clients often report a reduction in pain after ingesting a medication but before it has had a chance to effect physiological changes. A pain diary with times of medication and frequent assessment of pain levels can also demonstrate the disconnect between the two. The second step is to induce the belief that the client can cope without the medication, and the hope that other methods not only will be as effective but more so. The third step (under medical supervision) is to reduce the amount of the medication until it is zero. One such method is to administer real and placebo medication, decreasing the former and increasing the latter over time. Clients usually agree to this method only if they are guaranteed that they will not be asked to go "cold turkey."

Pain treatments can include surgery, injections (e.g., cortisone), ultrasound, nerve blocks, and implantable pumps for medication delivery in small doses (some people are able to take small doses chronically without addictive behavior). Unfortunately, these more invasive procedures are often the first rather than the last methods tried, and they have side effects. Noninvasive procedures should be tried earlier. So-called alternative medicine (better called adjunctive medicine) such as acupuncture, massage, and chiropractic methods can be useful. Another noninvasive procedure is *transcutaneous electrical neurostimulation*, commonly referred to as TENS units. Such units are about the size of a pager. They have two wires, each splitting into two, and attaching to four (replaceable) electrodes. These electrodes are placed on the skin surrounding the pain area. For example, I used one for my lower back, placing the electrodes at the four outer quadrants of the area. The TENS unit has two volume switches (one per wire). As the volume is turned up the unit delivers electrical stimulation to the electrodes. The feeling is somewhat like a strong tingling, though too high a volume can be the sharp pain of an electric shock. It can be worn safely for several hours, though usually a shorter period of about half an hour can interrupt a pain cycle and reduce pain for a day. No one knows why TENS units work, and to further complicate matters they work for some people and not others, or sometimes for a while and then not at all. But it is a noninvasive method without side effects. TENS units can be rented at some medical supply stores or borrowed (with prescription) from a physical therapy department.

Changing activity level is another pain reduction technique. It is not always a lessening of activity level, as often persons with chronic pain have reduced their activity levels too drastically and need help to resume more normal activities even in the presence of pain (remembering that chronic pain is a "false" signal). But energy conservation and joint protection are often desirable for persons with disabilities, so any activity program must balance the varying needs. Exercise, conditioning, and stretching muscles are important to reduce spasms and possibility of injuries. Education about chronic pain is an important ingredient of any program. Links between mind and body should be explored, and distraction, coping, and relaxation techniques may need to be taught and practiced. Humor should not be overlooked, and communication skills and family therapy may be beneficial, as chronic pain often has involved changes in family relationships.

"Pain" is not the same as "suffering." This is an important distinction, because persons with chronic pain often do suffer, and in a sense the treatment mostly is to reduce the suffering and less so the pain. When thinking about living with chronic pain over the long term, a client needs to understand that it is not synonymous with long-term suffering. A second important distinction is between cognitions that tend to exacerbate the experience of pain and *causing* or being responsible for one's own pain. When clients are taught ways to ameliorate pain by changing beliefs and behaviors, it is easy for them to hear this as blame for causing or exacerbating their pain. After many doctor visits in which they are told their pain is psychogenic or disproportionate to an injury, such persons become sensitized to intimations of blame. Treatment can inadvertently tap into such feelings by suggesting responsibility for lessening pain. The best way to handle such feelings is directly and openly, with a discussion of the meaning of getting better, and if the client doesn't raise these issues the therapist should.

LIVING WITH FATIGUE

It is fitting to discuss pain and fatigue in the same breath, because pain is fatiguing. Of course, everyone feels fatigue at some time or other. The mistake is in thinking that this experience is what persons with disabilities mean when they say they have problems with fatigue. The difference between quotidian fatigue and that which plagues persons with disabilities is a difference not just of degree but of quality. To illustrate, think of body temperature. The quantitative difference between 98.6 and 101 degrees is slight, only 2.4 degrees. But the clinical difference is profound. At a certain temperature the clinical phenomenon shifts from "well" to "ill." The fatigue that able-bodied persons experience might be akin to a temperature of 99.0. It impinges upon activities, reducing functional capacities. The remedy is usually a good night's sleep. The fatigue—really *over*fatigue—associated with many disabilities is more akin to a temperature of 101 or higher. A good night's sleep is not sufficient to reduce it appreciably. The remedy is often a more prolonged period of significantly reduced activity, body rest (sitting or lying down), and increased sleep. But, of course, the better long-term remedy for such overfatigue is prevention.

When fatigued, body movements can be difficult, including gross motor (e.g., getting out of a chair to go into another room), smaller gestures (e.g., raising an arm), and fine motor behaviors (e.g., opening a can, or writing). The effects of fatigue can be experienced cognitively as well as physically. Concentration, attention, memory, learning, and tracking—all can be impaired. Such an acute episode of overfatigue can last from a few hours to several days or even weeks. During these periods of pronounced fatigue the body is more vulnerable to injury. For example, when I'm fatigued I'm more likely to cut myself with a kitchen knife because my hand slips, to drop something I'm holding, or to trip over the nap in the rug. Thus an episode of overfatigue can lead to injury.

Clearly such states of overfatigue are best avoided. Remember the rehabilitation slogan of our times: Preserve it to conserve it. What does this mean in practice? One thing it means is that every decision to do something (e.g., go out to dinner on Tuesday) means a decision not to do something else (stay at work late on Wednesday). It becomes necessary to make continual choices and to set priorities, to rate one thing over another (e.g., my kid's birthday party this Saturday versus getting this chapter finished this week). These decisions may not even be conscious if the person with a disability is used to operating in this way. For example, if I want to make plans for the weekend I open my calendar and scan the shape of my week; that is, I don't look only at whether I'm free on the weekend but how my Monday to Friday week has been, to see how fatigued I might be. In exercising the constant choices of one thing over another the person with the disability may not explicitly state the reason for the choice to others. Thus from others' perspectives it may look as if the person is uncooperative (e.g., because of not volunteering for a task), antisocial (e.g., not participating in social festivities), aloof (resting alone in the office behind closed doors while others are in the company cafeteria), lazy (asking others to take the mail up to the mail room), uncaring (not participating in the Brownie troop outings), or unconcerned (refusing all the myriad invitations from your child's elementary school to bake, plant, clean, drive, organize, etc.). Yet all these behaviors can be explained as part of a program of managing one's energy levels. The goal is to keep on an even keel, with few significant dips. This goal requires constant management. The easy choices usually get made early on—hiring a gardener to lay the patio bricks, shopping in only one grocery store regardless of bargains across town, curtailing socializing on weekday evenings. Then come the harder choices—living with a messy and perhaps dirty house, unless one has the money to hire a cleaner; deciding that not every work task is worth giving 100%. After that come the really tough changes, the ones that seem to go to the core of one's identity—type of work, hours on the job, having or adopting children and number of children, using a wheelchair or scooter rather than crutches.

Vonda, a single mother in her 30s with two children under 8, works in a small neighborhood library 30 hours per week. She has MS, which has slowly progressed over time though she is still ambulatory, and has periods of more acute exacerbation that usually last about 6 weeks. When she is overfatigued, she feels a profound desire to lie down and has to employ great effort to move. In addition, she has difficulty tracking conversations, translating thoughts into behaviors, anticipating needs, and speaking clearly. She came to treatment at the suggestion of her support group because she seemed depressed. Her initial complaint and presenting problem was that she felt "boxed in." Every change she thought of making seemed unacceptable to her. In treatment she was helped to see the inevitability of having to choose among equally pressing needs. She narrowed her primary focus down to three items: (1) her children, (2) earning a living, and (3) her closest friends. This meant letting go of many activities that also commanded attention. For example, she tried to take the children to visit their grandmother twice a month, in a town about 2 hours away. She reduced this to once a month and took the train instead of driving. Although the train ride took longer, it gave her time to be with the children without any competing tasks to distract the family. Although the choices Vonda made were ones she probably would have been forced to make by the limits imposed on her time and energy by the MS, by talking about them and thinking them through in treatment she was able to be more accepting of the choices and to feel more proactive than reactive in making them.

Clinicians are trained to analyze motives of clients. It is our inclination to be wary of clients, students, or supervisees who make seemingly excessive demands. In the case of persons with disabilities who must regulate their lives to avoid overfatigue, this wariness may be a mistake. It is another way in which we overpathologize people with disabilities out of ignorance of the norms for such persons. One might wonder why the person doesn't just say the reason for the request. For example, a student may apply for practica in only a small geographical area close to home and not tell the director of training the reason. The director may then think that the student is being unreasonable or unrealistic. Why doesn't the student just tell the director the rationale for the choices? There can be many reasons: The disability may be hidden and the student may choose not to disclose it; the student may be having a hard time accepting some of the limitations imposed by the disability, and verbalizing it gives it greater reality; the student may be unaware of the choice, i.e., may so automatically operate to minimize fatigue that he or she is no longer aware of when fatigue is the issue; the student may worry that making an issue of the disability and acknowledging that it could impinge upon practicum will make him or her seem less competent, less able to become an accomplished practitioner, and maybe even jeopardize his or her standing in the program; students with disabilities often don't like to ask for special considerations. As much as administrators worry that students with disabilities will try to "get away with" something, I cannot stress enough how much the opposite is true. For any or all of these reasons the student may not disclose the reason for the request. With these ideas in mind, I overcompensated and mismanaged the following case:

> A man in his early 50s with a neuromuscular disorder called about therapy. He was not actually requesting an appointment but wished to explore his treatment options. He requested a therapist who was (1) cognitive-behavioral in orientation, (2) experienced with disability issues—and his disability in particular, and (3) within a small geographic radius of his home, preferably next to a bus stop (though in a pinch his wife could sometimes drive him). I was able to find several therapists (myself included) who fit some combination of two of the three requirements, but no one who met them all. Because I did not meet requirement (3), he did not want to see me. I gave him several referrals in his area. A year later he called again and we had the same conversation from scratch. It took several more iterations of this scenario over time before I began to see how resistant he was to the idea of therapy. I had overlooked several times that he never actually saw a single therapist despite getting many names of highly respected practitioners, until I finally was forced to recognize that this man was making no movement at all in the direction of treatment beyond calling me once every year or so.

This example illustrates once again a common refrain in this book. In treating clients with disabilities one can err in either direction, by overpathologizing the client through misinterpretation of disability sequelae or by allowing the disability to overshadow other presenting problems.

ADVOCACY AND DISCRIMINATION

Being an adult with a disability means being your own advocate. This includes finding doctors knowledgeable about your disability and gaining access to them in this time of managed care. It means self-monitoring and adjusting activities and lifestyles, renegotiating job descriptions, finding new ways to accomplish tasks, learning about assistive technologies, and acquiring new skills. For those who were children or young adults at the onset of the disability, parents were the advocates. But as adults, persons with disabilities have to take on the role, usually without any specific training, modeling, or guidance on how best to achieve this. It is on-the-job training. For example, I became an expert on scooters and insurance rules for obtaining durable medical equipment. I found jar openers, spring-loaded scissors, grabbers, electronic lamp switches that allow me to turn off the light from bed, and other labor-saving devices. At work I had to get an elevator installed, handicapped parking near my office, a doorway moved to lessen hallway obstruction, and many other accommodations. In every sphere of my life changes were needed, ranging from small (a device to hold bagels while I sliced them) to large (a new van, scooter, and lift that would all work together). Some were necessitated by newer symptoms (e.g., a different keyboard for the computer), others were extensions of older long-term needs (finding shoemakers to correctly alter my shoes), and others were specific to particular life stages (finding someone to attach a child seat to the back of my scooter). In all cases I had to advocate for myself, know my rights, and feel confident in pursuing them. Instead, I felt overwhelmed.

This list of accomplishments represents a full *decade* of work. Often I did nothing. Many times my husband shouldered much of the responsibility of getting something done. Other times I made do. The main lesson is this: Persons with disabilities have to learn to use their time and energy effectively, often by tackling only *one* thing at a time. This rule is essential for those disabilities that siphon off energy. The list of tasks may seem impressive, but everyone's list adds up over time. It's vital to keep perspective on what's essential (mobility), what makes life easier (new curb cut) or reduces pain (better desk chair) or fatigue (closer light switch), and what's nice (bagel holder). No one signs on for the job of advocate; it comes with the territory. However, in the attempts to juggle competing needs, make lives easier, deal with discrimination, and advocate for ourselves and for disability rights, persons with disabilities must be mindful of the overall load, as should therapists. If a person is embarking on a fight with the insurance company over getting an assistive device, it is not the time to tackle getting the city to install a curb cut, not to mention buffing the kitchen floor.

There is a part of having a disability that we cannot control, which is the stigma, prejudice, and discrimination attendant to persons with disabilities. People vary in how aware they will be of these factors, what their responses will be, and how they want to handle them. For example:

Greg, who uses a wheelchair, has been seeing you for therapy for issues related to his recent divorce and some overall dissatisfaction in life. One week he reports to you an incident that is troubling him. He attended a meeting at the Casa Hospitality Hotel. It was the third time he had been to a meeting at this hotel, and each time there was a problem with access to the handicapped parking. The first time an overnight mail truck blocked the ramp, the second time a delivery truck blocked the space, and this time a housekeeping cart was in the parking spot. The previous two times Greg complained to the manager and was assured that the hotel would attend to the problem. This third time Greg got extremely angry and parked on the lawn near the front door, blocking access to the hotel. The manager was called and was upset that guests could not enter or exit by the front door. He and Greg got into a shouting match, each threatening to sue the other. Greg was too riled up to attend his meeting and went home instead. He now has to decide if he will carry through on his threat of a lawsuit.

As we can see from this example, there are many factors to consider. First, what do we, the therapists, think of what happened? To some it may seem that Greg has badly overreacted. To me, as a person with a disability, I can completely empathize with Greg's frustration and anger, especially given that he had tried to address the problem twice already. Yet what course of action serves Greg best? Do we understand that question to mean Greg individually or Greg as a member of a disenfranchised class? We might encourage action that lowers Greg's frustration (e.g., we might do automatic thought records, attend to physiological cues, and practice relaxation techniques) and reduces his likelihood of taking legal action (e.g., we might have him list pros and cons of doing so, noting energy expenditure on each action item), but is this in Greg's best interest? How do we decide? The answer, "We let the client decide," begs the question and promulgates the myth of value free therapy (see Chapter 13). The point here is that the issues of discrimination and advocacy are salient ones for clients with disabilities, and therapists will be forced to take actions or inactions that address these issues.

Just when I think I've figured out my stance on these issues, a client inevitably challenges them. For example, Joshua, a man in his early 30s who has CP, which greatly affects his gait, speech, and gross and fine motor coordination, has been unable to procure a job, never getting past first interviews. When I raise the issue of discrimination he says to me, "I don't want to feel like a victim," and fights my attempts to redefine his problems in terms of civil rights. How do we understand this? Doesn't Joshua have the "right" to his opinion? Is it in his best interest for me to take his perspective and work within it? Is doing so perpetuating the discrimination he incurs? Is insisting on a minority model of disability clinically and tactically an error? Let's change the example a bit, and see how these changes affect our thinking in this case. Suppose Greg had mild mental retardation. How do our responsibilities change in that case, and would we make different decisions? Suppose Greg were a father and the issue was that he wouldn't let his 10-year-old son, the star of the team, play in the baseball games that were in fields inaccessible to the father? How do we then think about Greg's rights in light of the child? Whose best interests are we bound to uphold? These questions have, in a sense, all possible answers and no answer. They are simply unavoidable conundrums in treating families with disabilities.

AGING AND LONG-TERM CARE

Persons who are older and have disabilities fall into two camps: those with disabilities who are aging and those who become older and acquire a disability. The experiences of these two groups are not equivalent. People with disabilities acquired early in life are not entering the later years from a level playing field. They come with some disadvantages: Those with disabilities generally have less education, more unemployment, lower income, and higher levels of poverty. In addition, the disabilities may have increased the need for support from family or service agencies, higher medical costs, and more costs associated with assistive devices and modifying the environment to increase accessibility. Further, relatively minor physical deterioration with aging may be more pronounced for persons with disabilities when combined with previous disability symptoms. Thus persons with disabilities may experience a decrease in functioning earlier than do others. However, people with disabilities also come with some strengths: They have been members of a disadvantaged group of lower status (persons with disabilities) and hence have learned ways of coping prior to entering a second group of lower status (the elderly). They often have developed ways to cope with functional losses. Further, they may have gained wisdom through experience. One lesson is that *everything* has to be prioritized, giving up on some items further down the list of priorities and continually making compromises.

Disability is not an inevitable experience of aging, and most older people do not have disabilities; over 60% report that their health is good or excellent (though some might take their age into consideration in making this evaluation—"I'm in pretty good shape considering my years"). Most (about 80%) can live independently and care for themselves, even with chronic health problems. Nonetheless, aging usually means deterioration of some functions (often hearing and vision), more susceptibility to injury, and quicker onset of fatigue. All this may be more noticeable for people with disabilities, and unlike the gradual onset for able-bodied peers, those with disabilities may experience sudden decreases of functioning. Once again people with disabilities are faced with an unpredictable course of the disability, one requiring continual readjustment.

Getting older combines synergistically with the effects of disability. Although many people slow with age, this process is more rapid or pronounced for persons with disabilities. The effects of aging coupled with disability can be like acquiring a second disability. The meaning of aging for persons with disabilities is different than it is for others because it reawakens old feelings associated with disability onset. It becomes necessary to integrate the increasing disability into a self-concept that is also being assaulted by the aging process.

Most persons with disabilities must be especially mindful of increased physical vulnerability with age. Women with physical disabilities in particular should be taking extra calcium to offset osteoporosis. It is a good idea to install aids before they are needed (or worse, you injure yourself), such as grab bars around a shower/tub, handles around the toilet, ramps to the front step, and an extra handrail on stairs. These seemingly small changes can ease the physical load. For example, just putting a phone book, pen, and notepad next to each phone in the house avoids walking to get supplies.

The changes in our disabilities affect not only us but our families as well. Parents of adult children with disabilities may feel a reawakening of some of their earlier feelings associated with the disability onset. Our spouses and partners may have to readjust their thinking and participate in altering lifestyles to accommodate new losses. For those with children still in the home, the combined demands of childrearing and disability have to be managed.

One hallmark of older age is retirement. Retirement is often the result of poor health. Persons with disabilities may retire at earlier ages than those without disabilities or take advantage of a job change to leave the work force. Before retiring, employees with disabilities should take advantage of any group insurance plans offered, because such persons may be denied long-term care insurance if they try to buy it individually. Retirement at earlier ages puts retirees out of synch with peers, who may continue working for at least another decade. But retirement also can free up time and energy and allow a more evenly paced lifestyle without overfatigue. However, with retirement comes a change in roles in the family; a fluid definition of roles and functions within the family eases the transition.

Many people, with and without disabilities, find that discussing long-term care, wills and durable medical powers of attorney, and children's guardianship after parents' death are all anxiety-producing topics. For the person with the disability, with the heightened sense of vulnerability, the anxiety can be even greater. Unfortunately, it may also be more difficult as the person must meet many financial, health, and insurance demands. The type of lawyer who is best able to assist in these matters is someone who specializes in "elder care" (even if you are not elderly). Some locations may have assistance in finding an expert and providing consultation.[1]

Another frequent occurrence with age is widowhood. This is the single most disruptive and deleterious event affecting older persons. It is associated with increased illness and death in the surviving spouse. For those with disabilities it brings additional stresses. Any negative changes to income may be more pronounced for persons with disabilities due to increased need for aid (e.g., shopping), accessibility (e.g., installing grab bars), or convenience (e.g., buying prepared meals). The loss of daily practical, physical, and emotional support makes persons with disabilities more vulnerable to institutionalization. Because losing a spouse is so emotionally overwhelming, it is difficult to cope with the loss and make new practical plans simultaneously. For example, the spouse may have provided tangible support (e.g., aiding a spouse with a disability in and out of the bathtub, driving, preparing meals, and helping with shopping and laundry) which has to be found elsewhere. It is wise to set up backup plans, a support system, and alternate means of aid before they are needed; even if these plans are not used, just knowing the options can alleviate anxiety and be immediately useful at a time of loss. Other losses also are more common in older age, such as losing other significant persons to illness and death. Family members (parents, siblings, spouses, children) are also aging and may become less able to provide support. Hospitalization of loved ones or of oneself can reevoke earlier traumas connected with disability onset or surgeries. Thus aging for people with disabilities carries some increased liabilities and multiple losses: of support at a time of increased physical need, of people, of previous levels of functioning, and of independence.

Although there are many potential negatives associated with aging, there are also many positives. One is that having a disability becomes more "normal" among peers. As people age, some begin to acquire disabilities, so having a disability is no longer unusual; people with disabilities become one of the gang. Furthermore, older age can be a time for evaluation and reflection, increased wisdom and maturity, freedom from caring so much about what others think, and new interests and fewer demands. To enjoy these, it is important that people with disabilities maintain good health practices, continue to get exercise, and be active. Too often the view of older age as a time of inevitably declining health leads people (including professionals) to minimize the benefits of reha-

[1]For example, in the San Francisco Bay Area, the Family Caregiver Alliance assists families of persons with some types of disabilities in finding legal assistance and pays for a 1-hour consultation.

bilitation. Because rehabilitation usually means restoring function and increasing independence, these goals may not been seen as realistic for older persons. Further, our health care system is more oriented toward treatment of acute, short-term problems and less proficient in providing ongoing care, while persons with disabilities have chronic conditions. These views of older persons with disabilities unnecessarily limit their options; they must resist giving in too readily to these notions and strive to remain active and involved.

As people with disabilities age, money helps enormously. People generally need either time (to do the task) or money (to hire someone else to do the task); having neither is no good. Money does wonders. But even without lots of it little things can make a difference. Sometimes the problem is in not knowing how valuable a change, addition, or assistive device will be until one tries it. For example, we raised our living room so it was no longer sunken by one step. Only then did I realize how much I had previously avoided the living room. That one step made all the difference. People with disabilities have to look for the steps in life, real and metaphorical, and ramp them. Aging is just another step.

SUBSTANCE ABUSE AND MEDICATIONS

Disability is correlated with several risk factors: high school dropout, injury, physical and sexual abuse, reduced options for dealing with family violence. Another such risk is substance abuse. The unhappy link between disability and substance abuse is entrenched in several ways. First, the alcohol industry is a leading and public contributor to disability charities. For example, the Muscular Dystrophy Association received $50 million from Anheuser-Busch over a 13-year period, United Cerebral Palsy Associations took in more than $8 million from the Miller Brewing Company over a 10-year period, and alcohol ads often link increased consumption with charitable donations (e.g., for every case of beer purchased $1 goes to a charity) (Marin Institute, 1993). Second, use of substances can lead to disability, especially when combined with driving, guns, boating, skiing, swimming, diving, or other sports.[2] Third, the ages and gender of persons with certain types of impairments, such as SCI, are those associated with increased substance abuse. The higher rate of substance abuse predisability carries over to a high rate postinjury

---

[2] A study of patients with spinal cord injuries in Chicago found that causes were motor vehicle crashes (including bikes and motorcycles) (38%), gunshot wounds (22%), swimming and diving injuries (17%), falls (17%), and other (6%).

(Greer, Roberts, & Jenkins, 1990). And the use of drugs and alcohol can greatly complicate and lengthen the recovery process (Sparadeo & Gill, 1989). Further, the effects of substances may be more pronounced and problematic when combined with a physical, sensory, or cognitive disability.

Most studies of rates of substance abuse in persons with disabilities have found rates that are substantially higher than those in the general population. The exception seems to be persons with mental retardation; two studies (DiNitto & Krischef, 1984; Edgerton, 1986) found a reduced rate of alcohol and drug abuse (less than 7% and less than comparison friends, relatives, and spouses), but another study (Rivinus, 1988) found that alcohol abuse in persons with MR was a "serious problem" (data not supplied to support this contention).

Many authors have posited reasons for the increased risk of substance abuse among persons with disabilities (Freeman, Ferreyra, & Calabrese, 1997; Greer, 1986; Greer et al., 1990). These include the stress and frustration of facing daily discrimination and stigma; increased social isolation[3]; reduced rates of employment with its attendant increase in unstructured time and isolation; increased history of sexual abuse—a known risk factor for substance abuse; decreased attention by service providers to sexuality and histories of abuse in women with disabilities; overmedication[4]; easier access to medications, many with mood-altering properties, and many with high potential for abuse (e.g., medications used for spasticity, pain, or sleep); enabling on the part of family and service providers due to pity, reluctance to confront the substance abuser, avoidance of hostility, or belief that life with a disability is so hard that drug abuse is necessary to make it tolerable; higher rates of chronic pain; high rates of predisability substance abuse in some categories of persons with disabilities (e.g., those with spinal cord injuries); and use of medications in childhood, which seems to predispose one to later substance abuse (Greer et al., 1990).

There are numerous barriers to substance abuse treatment for persons with disabilities. One is the lack of attention paid to substance abuse problems within rehabilitation. A review of the major rehabilitation journals from 1978–1988 (Benshoff, Janikowski, Taricone, & Brenner, 1990) found that of 1,743 articles, only 20 (1.14%) were drug

---

[3]For example, about 42% of women with disabilities are married, compared with 60% of women without disabilities (Freeman et al., 1997).

[4]For example, one study of clients of a center for independent living found that 41% reported having been prescribed drugs which the recipient did not feel was needed (Hepner, Kirshbaum, & Landes, 1980/1981).

or alcohol abuse related. These authors note that "while these journals may provide helpful information, they typically do not adequately address substance abuse in the context of traditional rehabilitation practices, procedures, and processes, and they do not address the interaction between alcohol, drugs, and the presence of other disabling conditions" (p. 11). Even a section on alcohol rehabilitation in a text on disability rehabilitation (Dell Orto & Marinelli, 1995) fails to integrate alcohol and disability, discussing the former without the context of the latter. Two special issues of the *Journal of Counseling and Development* (vol. 58, 1979 and vol. 68, 1989) on counseling persons with disabilities and their families had no articles on substance abuse. A study of attitudes, beliefs, and policies at 68 physical medicine rehabilitation training programs (Rohe & DePompolo, 1985) indicated that only 25% routinely screened all patients for alcohol or drug use, 45% had written guidelines on substance use, 55% routinely provided access to drug counselors, and 29% provided education to patients and 22% to staff. The lack of education of patients and staff is a serious problem in light of the fact that many persons with disabilities will be on at least one prescribed medication, and that medications interact synergistically with alcohol and illicit drugs.

It seems that disability-centered agencies have been slow in recognizing the need for substance abuse assessment. A study of three counties in northern California found that only 17% of the disability service agencies had conducted any significant assessment of alcohol or drug use, and only 15% offered information on substance abuse to clients (De Miranda & Cherry, 1989). A study of CILs in California found that almost two thirds did not routinely ask about alcohol or drug use (Frieden, 1990). A study of persons with SCI living in the community (Heinemann, 1991) found that of the 16% who believed they needed substance abuse treatment (probably an undercount), less than half had actually received such treatment. One study of rehabilitation counselors found that their attitudes toward alcoholics were quite negative (Allen, Peterson, & Keating, 1982). Texts on psychosocial aspects of disability mostly omit the topic of substance abuse, and those that include it do so only very cursorily. The reason for the delay in tackling substance abuse may be, in part, that persons who abuse substances incur a great deal of stigma, and "physical or mental disabilities have enough social stigmata attached to them without adding the extra stigma of substance abuse or chemical dependence" (Greer, 1986, p. 34). Further, medical and rehabilitation personnel may erroneously ascribe signs of substance abuse to disability (e.g., irresponsibility, lateness, lack of motivation, and poor health) and fail to make an appropriate intervention or referral (Freeman et al., 1997).

Conversely, substance abuse agencies seem to overlook persons with disabilities. One study (De Miranda & Cherry, 1989) found that only an estimated 0.5% of persons with both a disability and substance abuse problem had been in treatment in the previous year. Their data provide a partial explanation: Sign language interpreters were available in only 13% of the substance abuse programs, and 50% of the programs prohibited use of one or more medications required for control of certain types of physical disabilities. In a listing of the 100 best treatment centers in the nation (Sunshine & Wright, 1988), only eight facilities had special programs for persons with disabilities who abused substances. In a directory of Alcoholics Anonymous (AA) meetings in Memphis, only 7 of 95 were listed as wheelchair accessible (Greer et al., 1990).

There are numerous barriers to substance abuse treatment for persons with disabilities. Physical access is a tremendous problem. The agency may be in a two-story building with no elevator, far from transportation with no nearby stop, on a block without curb cuts, or on a street with lots of traffic and little parking, with no handicapped spaces. There may not be a TTY number available, the front door may be too heavy and/or have handles that are difficult to open and no automatic door opener, the bathroom may be inaccessible, the pathways may be less than the required 3-foot width or contain boxes and file cabinets that reduce the passageway. Sign language interpretation and sound amplification may not be offered, written materials may not be available in alternate formats (cassette, Braille, large print, disk). Required meetings may start too early in the morning for someone who takes several hours to complete a bowel program, bathe, dress, and eat, perhaps with assistance. The cost of treatment may be prohibitive, especially given higher underemployment rates, lower overall income, and lower probability of health insurance, for persons with disabilities. Each of these barriers alone may pose problems but when combined make an agency very disability-unfriendly. In addition, there are attitudinal barriers: the belief that substance abuse doesn't exist for people with disabilities or, conversely, that substance abuse is unavoidable due to the trauma and loss associated with disability. Preacceptance intakes may inquire about medical or chronic conditions, outreach efforts may be in inaccessible places or formats, and there are unlikely to be staff members with disabilities. Substance abuse programs often disallow or discourage use of any medications, especially ones such as Valium, which are more commonly used by persons with disabilities. This wall of obstacles is distressing, because there is a critical window of opportunity during which a person abusing substances may seek help, and if the person encounters barriers during this brief phase, the obstacles may foreclose the opportunity for treatment

In keeping with the philosophy of this book, "intervention" must occur at multiple levels. The first level is that of the individual therapist providing treatment to an individual with a disability and his or her family. At this level the clinician should keep in mind several considerations:

1. Substance abuse tends to be overlooked in persons with disabilities. There are several explanations for this, one of which is the overshadowing effect (discussed in Chapter 7). Another is the misattribution of substance abuse behaviors and symptoms to the disability. A third is the myth that people with disabilities are not substance abusers. The bottom line is that all clinicians must do routine screening for alcohol, drugs, and medication misuse.

2. A history of substance abuse prior to disability onset is the best predictor of substance abuse after disability. Glass (1980/1981) distinguishes between Type A substance abuse, which predates the disability, is an entrenched pattern of substance use as a means of coping, and is more recalcitrant to treatment, with Type B, in which disability predates substance abuse and the substance abuse is a response to the multiple stressors of disability. He posits that Type B is best remediated through intervention directly on disability coping, living skills, and independence, and Type A by more traditional substance abuse treatment methods. Certainly for some types of disabilities (e.g., TBI and SCI) disability onset is associated with a high rate of substance abuse that may continue postinjury, complicating and prolonging recovery and rehabilitation. When substance abuse or dependence is present in a client with a disability, the clinician must carefully evaluate whether substance abuse should be the initial and primary focus of treatment or whether amelioration of some of the stressors associated with disability coupled with increased coping and skills will result in cessation of substance abuse.

3. There seem to be some differences in beliefs and affect between persons with disabilities who do and do not abuse substances. For example, Greer and Walls (1997) found that measures of anger and anxiety differentiated "between those for whom substance abuse was always a problem versus never a problem" (p. 7) among clients in vocational rehabilitation. Moore, Greer, and Li (1994) found that persons with disabilities with higher levels of alcohol abuse were significantly more likely to endorse the belief that people with disabilities were entitled to use alcohol and drugs. Thus one way disability interacts with substance abuse is through cognitive mediators that promote or inhibit substance misuse.

4. Predictors of substance abuse in the general population are also risk factors for those with disabilities. These include sexual abuse, early onset of drinking, and history of alcohol or drug abuse in the family. Some persons with disabilities are more exposed to these risk factors, and thus it is not the disability per se that accounts for an increase in

rates of substance abuse but the increase in known risk factors. As is true for any client, a careful collation of relevant history is essential.

5. Persons with disabilities are likely to be on one or more medications, some—but not necessarily all—of which may be medically required. Any substance abuse pattern may be complicated by use of prescribed medication. The person may be unaware of the potential dangers of mixing medications, alcohol, and/or illicit substances. The types of medications frequently used for pain or for spasms or spasticity potentiate the effects of alcohol and other drugs. Thus the complete picture of all substances taken must be considered, and consultation with a primary care physician may be essential.

6. Making referrals to AA or other self-help groups or to treatment facilities requires preinvestigation by the therapist as to the accessibility of meetings and treatment centers. The effects of encountering a physical or attitudinal barrier at the delicate juncture of new recovery may be disastrous, and clinicians have to take some responsibility for ensuring that their clients are referred to settings, agencies, and treatment centers with appropriate accommodations. It is important that the therapist not assume accessibility, even if the meetings are held in a place that should be accessible (e.g., a hospital). It is also helpful if the therapist can paint a clear picture of the physical layout of a place before sending a client there. For example, I might say, "There are two handicapped spots right near the front entrance, but they tend to be taken by late morning. An alternative would be the side entrance, and that section of the parking lot usually has empty spaces." Furthermore, the group's philosophy about medication should be considered.

7. The physiology of some disabilities can increase the risks associated with substance abuse (e.g., decreased tolerance, decreased levels required for toxicity, greater cognitive impairment, more lethargy, and more quickly impaired judgment). Further, intoxication can lead to unsteadiness that carries increased risk of injury.

The second level of intervention relates to the various other roles of clinicians, such as supervisors, instructors, consultants, researchers, and board members. We can ensure that our clinical work and research related to substance abuse includes people with disabilities, and that our consideration of persons with disabilities includes attention to assessment and treatment of substance abuse. We can encourage agencies and coworkers to challenge their assumptions about persons with disabilities and substance abuse. We can ensure that all institutions with which we affiliate have and publicize a TTY number, or at the very least indicate whether the phone line is voice only and note that callers can use the state relay number. We can make all agency and clinical materials available in alternate formats and become familiar with how to hire interpreters and how to use sound amplification systems. We can support staff, coworkers, and administrators in their efforts to improve outreach and treatment to the disabled community and advertise our agencies' accessibility in all ads, announcements, flyers and brochures, letterhead, talks, and informal networking.

The third level of intervention is in the realm of policy and politics. The issue of substance abuse among persons with disabilities must be addressed "not just as problems of individuals seeking access to services, but also as political and sociological phenomena that must be addressed at cultural and societal levels" (Cherry & Tusler, 1991, p. 1). Strategies for dealing with substance abuse for persons with disabilities are similar to those for other members of the underclass in the United States. The social context of the lives of persons with disabilities must be addressed holistically. Rates of employment, and hence income and health insurance, must rise dramatically, as stigmatization, discrimination, and alienation are addressed directly. Funding sources related to disability should include substance abuse identification, assessment, and treatment, and funding for substance abuse treatment should require accessibility for and inclusion of persons with disabilities. Issues of housing, poverty, transportation, and civil rights are fundamental to the problems of persons with disabilities, and attention to these ills could do much to improve the health of the body politic.

One resource for understanding disability combined with substance abuse is a bibliography from the National Clearinghouse for Alcohol and Drug Information (1987).[5] There is a version of AA's 12 steps written for the Deaf (Watson, Boros, & Zrimec, 1979/1980). A paper titled "Identifying Substance Abuse in Persons with Disabilities" has a list of questions and symptoms (Ford & Moore, 1992).

USE OF SUPPORT GROUPS AND READINGS

Most metropolitan areas have support groups for many of the conditions that result in disability. Even rare disorders often have support groups, though they may meet less often (e.g., once a year) and cover a wide range of territory (e.g., all of northern California). There are several ways to find out about such groups.

1. Call the national organization and request information for your locality. Often they have the times and places of local meetings and the first name and phone number of a contact person.

---

[5]P.O. Box 2345, Rockville, MD 20852; (301) 468-2600.

2. Call the nearest CIL.
3. Find a doctor who specializes in that disability.
4. Look up the name of the disability on the Internet.

In making any referral to a support group, or in working with a client who is already in a support group, clinicians should be mindful of the role of such groups, and the potential ways in which they can further or hinder a particular client's process. Of course, there are many types and variations of support groups, so all cannot be painted with the same brush. They vary in amount and type of structure. Most are run by persons in the group rather than by a trained counselor. Some alternate between invited speakers and unstructured meetings.

Some support group problems are common. First, support groups are mixed blessings. They do provide, in a way that individual therapy never can, access to other persons with similar diagnoses, struggles, needs, and responses. But they also raise scenarios that can detract or even be counterproductive to progress, and possibly be at odds with the goals of the therapy. The persons in a support group can carry great weight, and things they say can have tremendous impact on an individual. Thus, any advice or judgment from group members, coming from such authenticity of experience, can outweigh what the therapist says.

Second, support groups can be scary propositions for the newly diagnosed person. Typical fears are that the group will be composed of persons worse off than oneself, who are depressed and whiny about their bleak futures. In actuality, I've rarely heard of groups that meet this fantasy. Often in groups there is a wide range of severity of symptoms and function among members and an almost upbeat, supportive tone. But this doesn't mean the fantasy is completely off base. In meeting with a group of people with the same or similar disorders one will encounter persons with greater quantity and severity of symptoms, and this can be frightening. Hearing about, say, incontinence or colostomies, declining cognitive abilities, or loss of ambulation can create great anxiety in a person more recently diagnosed with MS. Another fear is that the group will force its members to emote publicly. This fantasy is even less true. More often groups collude to avoid difficult topics and to bring strongly emotive material back to a more intellectualized plain. Occasionally some members of a group may have the zeal of converts; having found something that made a big difference for them, they want to cajole others into following suit. But this can actually be useful in treatment, in helping clients articulate their own position.

Monty had been HIV positive for more than 12 years but had not converted to AIDS. He attended a support group once a month.

One of the men in the group, Tim, had found that he had more energy after he'd changed to a macrobiotic diet, and he was encouraging everyone else to do the same. He thought it was especially important for Monty, however, because Tim also had been HIV positive for a long time. Monty, a thoughtful and introspective man, brought the issue into his therapy and wondered about his own openness to the constantly changing field of HIV and AIDS treatments. He had elected not to try any of the drug regimens and now was reluctant to try a change in diet. He asked, "Am I just being passive, accepting my fate? Do I think that what will be will be, and therefore have I given up my own power?" In formulating answers to these questions Monty came to a clearer understanding of the role of HIV in his life and his relationship to his disorder and to the various systems of treatment, both medical and nontraditional. Thus the support group served as a catalyst for fruitful exploration, because of who Monty was and the nature of the therapeutic alliance; another individual might have responded by dropping out of the group, or hopping on yet another bandwagon and being disappointed.

There are certain tasks of living with a disability with which support groups can be particularly helpful. A new diagnosis or exacerbation of an older diagnosis is an extremely stressful time, and some find the stories of others reassuring. When my husband was newly diagnosed with MS an acquaintance called me and disclosed her own MS. We talked for an hour, and now, over 15 years later, I still remember much of what she said. This experience is not uncommon. It is as if there is a semihypnotic state around diagnosis in which attention becomes sharper and more focused on issues related to the diagnosis. Contact with other persons in similar situations can be comforting, can help impart information, and can provide support for the process. However, for others receiving a new diagnosis is a time for consulting medical professionals, seeking information, talking with a few select close people, and making decisions. In such cases it might be only after this initial phase that an individual is ready to hear about and learn from others. For example, women with breast cancer are more likely to join support groups once they begin treatment and not as likely during the initial diagnostic and decision-making period. In any case, just going to a support group, just saying, "Yes, now I need help and support, to be with peers with this disability," connotes a psychological change, irrespective of what happens at the group.

Most people want to read about their disorders. They might ask their therapist for advice about what to read, or go to a bookstore and browse, or search on the Internet. Each of these options has merits and pitfalls. It is helpful if therapists have prescreened reading materials, but even if that is not the case, it is important to discuss with the client some common reactions to readings. First, reading about what can happen can be frightening. For example, a book on MS designed specifically for newly diagnosed persons (Scheinberg, 1983) covers bladder and bowel management—symptoms that may be in the distant future, or even irrelevant for that particular person. It also covers nursing care, which can be a terrifying idea when one is still ambulatory, employed, and active. Second, in seeming contradiction of the first point, some readings are unbearably upbeat and can leave the reader feeling isolated in his or her more demoralized state.

Third, readings tend to cover all possible parameters of a disorder, and readers can get "medical student syndrome" (i.e., they develop symptoms based on reading about them). For example, I stopped subscribing to the *Post-Polio Network News* because each month after reading about breathing difficulties I developed breathing difficulties. Fourth, readings tend to cover the diagnosis and symptoms of a disorder more than treatment, or indicate that there is no known treatment. Thus readers can be left feeling very bleak and hopeless. Fifth, much of the disorder-based readings ignore families or emphasize the "burden" of the disorder on the family. And finally, although there is a seemingly boundless plethora of books on diseases, there may be scant literature about a specific disorder, or a specific symptom, or a particular aspect of a disorder, leaving the reader feeling isolated.[6]

Despite all these caveats, readings—from pamphlets to books—can be a valuable source of information and comfort. They can make a person feel less alone, encourage affiliation with others with a similar diagnosis, address myths, and correct misinformation. Clearly, they can provide such information and comfort for the therapist as well as for the client, and therapists are encouraged to read some of the literature available about the diagnoses of clients they are treating.

"PHYSICIAN-ASSISTED SUICIDE"
AND THE "RIGHT TO DIE"

It may seem odd to have a section devoted to this rather auxiliary issue. However, there are three reasons to include it here. First, familiarity with

---

[6]The National Organization for Rare Disorders (NORD) is a good starting place for locating literature. Their address is 100 Route 37, P.O. Box 8923, New Fairfield, CT 06812-8923; (800) 999-6673.

the social history of persons with disabilities can facilitate a more empathic understanding of the client with a disability. The disability rights movement currently focuses on three major issues: personal attendant services, transportation, and physician-assisted suicide (P-AS). Thus these are the issues that drive the disability rights movement and define the parameters of the disability community. For example, more than a dozen disability rights groups, including the National Council on Independent Living and the National Council on Disability, have officially opposed legislation to legalize P-AS. Second, although therapists are unlikely to get involved in issues related to transportation and attendant services for persons with disabilities, P-AS is an issue that falls well within the psychological domain. This is especially true for aspects related to voluntariness, informed consent, and assessment of confounding psychological factors such as depression. It is important that therapists be informed about the disability community's perspective on P-AS. Third, disability represents a human vulnerability to morbidity and mortality. Disability reminds us that able-bodied status can be undone in a second, that we all have a hidden vulnerability that can be tapped unexpectedly. Thus it is hard to discuss disability at any length without considerations of life and death.

In October 1996, the U.S. Supreme Court agreed to hear two cases on the right to physician-assisted death, coming from the Courts of Appeals for the Second and Ninth Circuits. In their ruling in June 1997, they failed to affirm a "right" to assisted suicide. But several states have passed laws on P-AS. In Oregon, the first such state, the law's implementation was delayed by a court injunction, then cleared for implementation in the spring of 1998. A key problem was the lack of any existing infrastructure to support and implement the law, and lack of clarity on the roles of various health service providers. (For example, should pharmacists be required to dispense lethal combinations or dosages of medication?) Mental health services are an important part of such an infrastructure.

Critical questions related to P-AS arise for therapists: What are my beliefs regarding this issue? Can I opt out of participation if I work in a setting in which P-AS becomes available? If I opt out, can I still take referrals of elderly or seriously ill clients who might choose P-AS? What are the appropriate interventions with families facing loss of a member through P-AS? How should the issue of remaining minor children be handled? How are "voluntariness" and "capacity" best assessed, and by whom? How do we assess for underlying treatable depression when many symptoms of serious or terminal illness overlap with those of depression?

Why is P-AS of particular concern to the disability community? Perhaps one of the foremost reasons is the perennial conflation of disability and illness. As discussed in Chapter 1, disability is not the same as illness—it is possible to have a serious disability and be in otherwise excellent health. Therefore, disability should not be viewed as in any way synonymous with terminal illness. This point may seem obvious, but in fact the two conditions are routinely confused. In three famous court cases involving persons with disabilities and the "right to die" (Elizabeth Bouvier in California, David Rivlin in Michigan, and Larry McAfee in Georgia), advocates for P-AS, judges, and the news media made the two concepts synonymous. In addition, of the first 56 cases of Kervorkian-assisted suicide, over one fifth were persons with MS. None of the media reports of these deaths of which I'm aware pointed out that MS is not a terminal illness.[7]

Trying to define eligibility for P-AS in such a way that it includes the imminently dying but excludes those with disabilities is a huge problem. Often when we think of terminal illness we think of cancer. In fact, cancer is a more clear-cut illness because diagnosis and prognosis are relatively accurate and correlated. In such cases of agreed-on poor prognosis—and increasing pain, diminished well-being, impaired breathing—it seems cruel to disallow persons in such a state the "right" to hasten and control their own death. The problem comes as soon as we move away from the cancers (cancer, leukemia, Hodgkin disease) yet try to apply the same criteria of sure diagnosis and terminality. Take, for example, ALS (better known as Lou Gehrig's disease). The general life expectancy for a patient with ALS is 5 years from diagnosis. But Stephen Hawking, the notable physicist who has made great contributions to his field, has survived ALS for more than 25 years. True, he is an anomaly, but nothing about his case early on suggested he would be; he might well have chosen P-AS and aborted several productive and creative decades of his life.

The definition of eligibility is further complicated by technology. How do we think of someone who is machine dependent? Many persons with disabilities are machine dependent. Take, for example, the case of Ed Roberts, the former head of the California State Department of Rehabilitation. He was ventilator dependent. Without the ventilator he would die within 2 to 4 days; from that perspective he was "incurable" and "terminally ill." In the wrong social circumstances (e.g., absent family or forced to live in a nursing home), personal attributes (e.g., low self-

---

[7]In 1999, after assisting in over 150 suicides, Kervorkian was convicted of murder in a Michigan court.

esteem, hopelessness, and poor coping), and economic straits (e.g., unemployed and on a low fixed income), Ed might have "chosen" to die. Others viewing his situation from the outside might say to themselves that they too would "rather die than be like that." Disability cannot be considered separately from social class.

This brings us to the second problem with P-AS, which is guarding against the right to die becoming a mandate to die. Those with disabilities are a devalued and disadvantaged group. They "require and increasingly demand alternative physical and social arrangements to accommodate them and in some cases need a larger share of societal resources" (Longmore, 1987, p. 141). As medical resources shrink, difficult choices are made about maximizing precious resources. Will we agree to utilize some of those resources on people with disabilities when able-bodied people think they'd rather be dead than to live "like that"?

In the Netherlands, P-AS has been tolerated since approximately the early 1970s for "ill, competent patients." By the 1980s, guidelines for P-AS were established:

> In 1984 the Supreme Court of the Netherlands accepted physician-assisted suicide and euthanasia, not only for terminally ill patients, but also for chronically ill or elderly patients. Most startlingly, in 1990, there were more than 1,000 cases in which Dutch physicians terminated patients' lives *without* their consent. . . . The Netherlands has moved from assisted suicide to euthanasia, from euthanasia for terminally ill people to euthanasia for chronically ill people, from euthanasia for physical illnesses to euthanasia for psychological distress, and from voluntary euthanasia to involuntary euthanasia. (House Judiciary Constitution Subcommittee, 1996, p. 10 [emphasis in original; p. 10])

When I attended an invited conference on P-AS at Stanford University, I found that my perspective, from a disability vantage point, differed in some important ways from that of the majority. (See Young et al., 1997, for a report from the conference.) These include the following:

1. The framework from which we ask questions about P-AS; the question at the conference was about how P-AS should be implemented, whereas I would ask the question, "How can we prevent the acceptance of P-AS?" As one African American participant wrote (as quoted in Young et al., 1997, p. 383): "This is a white question. My people aren't asking to die; we're afraid you're going to kill us." The disability community echoes this sentiment.

2. The definition of "terminal illness" seemed to include too many people with disabilities (e.g., those dependent on iron lungs or ventilators).

3. The question of who should be the second opinion in ascertaining voluntariness, mental status, and consent (majority opinion placed it in the hands of the medical establishment, and I wanted it anywhere but there).

4. The guidelines call for an assessment of mental status but not for an evaluation of socioeconomic or political context.

5. The model is too either/or: Either the medical professionals decide *for* the patient, or the patient decides *by* him- or herself; there is no model for deciding *with*.

6. How do we understand "voluntariness" in light of a family that is anxious to be relieved of the financial and physical care of a suffering patient?

7. The family (and hence the family's culture) is delegated to an ancillary and dispensable role. As the report notes: "The patient should be the primary decision-maker. Families, as defined by patients, should be involved as much as possible, but should not be able to veto the patients' decisions" (p. 385). Thus my husband could be arrested if he flew off to Tahiti without providing for his children, but is able to decide to die and carry through the act without providing for them. I might learn of his wish for P-AS only after the fact.

In each of these questions certain values became clear and were in contrast to those of the disability community. These values have to do with the primacy of individual versus family rights, autonomy, models of paternalistic versus communal decision making, the subservience of community and group to the individual, the perceived compromise of the quality of life imposed by a chronic disability, and the underplaying of the impact of inequality and oppression on the mental status of minority individuals.

A complete discussion of P-AS is not possible here. The main point for therapists to take away with them from this brief introduction is this: Their clients with disabilities often have a markedly different perspective on this issue. An analogy might be differences in opinions between whites and African Americans on the police. The latter group is more likely to report negative interactions with the police, to hold more negative views about police, and to distrust the police to look after their interests. Whites, with generally more positive and less negative interactions with the police, view the African American perspective as "paranoid." The differing experiences lead to shifts in resulting vantage points, each pathologized by the other. In a similar way, the experiences of those with disabilities have provided different lessons, leading to alternative conclusions. One such conclusion has to do with doctors. Being a physician is a profession in high esteem in the United States. Yet those with disabilities often have histories of negative interactions with doctors, encompassing powerlessness, pain, subservience, and denial of psychoemotional needs. These histories promote a more negative view of doctors and the medical profession. Doctors are integral to P-AS. If we can't trust them with our lives will we trust them with our deaths?

A man in his early 50s called a therapist with a disability, whose name he'd gotten from a help line. He'd been diagnosed with MS about 12 years prior, after seeing multiple doctors and not getting answers about why his hands and feet were numb and tingly. Since then he'd gone from unassisted walking to using a cane, then from a manual wheelchair to an electric wheelchair; lost significant vision in both eyes; and experienced chronic fatigue. His driver's license was denied 4 years ago, and he took early retirement. He'd called the help line requesting information on physician- assisted death— he wanted help in killing himself.

Over the next few months, with the support of the therapist, he began going to MS support groups twice a month, subscribed to four disability magazines (cassette versions), and met by phone several people active in the disability community. He began to understand that his wish to die stemmed in large part from his clinical depression and the isolation that had resulted from his disability. As the depression and isolation were alleviated he no longer requested assisted suicide. Many significant problems remained (he couldn't afford a wheelchair-accessible van; his marital relationship had deteriorated; he needed more personal attendant services than could or should be provided by the spouse), but he had better coping and social supports to help him tackle these issues. Most important, he felt hope about how to live with his disability. He felt he had a community of people like himself and had seen that people more disabled than himself had sufficient "quality of life" that they chose to live rather than seeking means to die.

TWELVE

Assistive Technology and Devices

A focus on technology with reference to persons with disabilities is only about a decade old. Two key events in the mid-1980s mark the beginning of this inquiry. First is the landmark legislation, the Technology-Related Assistance of Individuals with Disabilities Act of 1988 (Public Law 100-407; reauthorized in 1994). The second is the appearance beginning in 1986 of dissertations on "technology studies" (Leahy, VanTol, Habeck, & Fabiano, 1990). Rehabilitation engineering is the discipline that trains designers and makers of assistive technology (AT).

Various terms are used to describe AT, including assistive devices and durable medical products. All these terms refer to *things* (e.g., lifts, wheelchairs, and modified utensils) as opposed to *services* performed by or with the aid of another person (e.g., interpreting, dressing, and exercising). The goal of AT is generally to increase the independence of persons with disabilities, replace or reduce the amount or degree of assistance needed by others, minimize disability and maximize functioning. The Technology Act defines AT as follows, a definition that has become standard in all relevant legislation since 1988: "Any item, piece of equipment, or product system, whether acquired commercially off the shelf, modified, or customized, that is used to increase, maintain, or improve functional capabilities of individuals with disabilities" (p. 3).

There are an array of assistive technologies ranging from no-tech (e.g., modified items such as altered handle shapes on utensils) to low-tech (e.g., mechanical items such as grabbers) to what we might call medium-tech (electric items such as scooters, remote controls for lights or TV) to high-tech (electronics and computers, such as computers that respond to eye blinks of the user). Assistive technologies can aid almost any human sensory, communicative, motoric, or other function. Examples include aid in locomotion (scooters, wheelchairs, lifts, canes, orthotics), speaking (voice synthesizers, communication boards, programmed "smart keys" on computers), reading and comprehension (magnifiers, books on tape or disk, Braille signage), hearing or communicating (TTYs, hearing aids, personal FM radio systems, vibrating pagers, visual alarms), and self-care and self-management (electronic memory storage devices, modified kitchenware, buttoners, environmental control systems).

A closely related concept to AT is *adapted equipment.* This concept refers both to equipment available for general use, but which is used by persons with disabilities in a new way or for a purpose other than intended, and equipment for general use that comes with adaptations for persons with disabilities. The first adaptation is probably quite common (Toms Barker & Maralani, 1997; Conley-Jung, 1996), but there is no way to know how often it occurs. The second is so routine we often may not even notice. For example, loudness buttons on pay phones become so ubiquitous that we stop thinking of them as adaptations. Other "adaptations" are built into the original design so post hoc changes are unnecessary. In architecture, this approach is manifested in the idea of universal design. According to this view, designs are intended to work for the greatest number of people and to be easily tailored to the needs of each user. For example, curb cuts are essential for most wheelchair users but also helpful for persons with limited mobility, strollers, bikes, shopping carts, and package delivery services. A curb cut can be thought of as a universal design. A different kind of universal design builds adaptability into a product. A good "secretary's" chair, for example, often allows manipulation of seat and back height and back position, making it fit more users.

Sometimes technology creates inaccessibility as well as providing solutions. An example would be the public toilet kiosks installed by the Decaux company in several cities around the United States. During negotiations for their installation in San Francisco, the kiosks were the subject of much controversy. At issue were how many of the kiosks should be the larger wheelchair-accessible models which are more costly and take up more sidewalk space. Suppose, for technological reasons, that only larger models could be made. Then all kiosks would be wheelchair accessible and no distinction would exist between "normal" and "accessible" models. It is only the company's ability to manufacture smaller and cheaper units that brings the discrepancy to light. Thus, technology creates a separate class of users.

"Durable medical equipment" (DME) is a phrase used by insurance companies to denote certain types of assistive technologies. These technologies include crutches, wheelchairs, walkers, scooters, manual and electric wheelchairs, prostheses (artificial limbs), and orthotics (devices that support and strengthen arm, hand, ankle, and/or foot). Usually insurance limits the frequency it will pay for replacement of DME, and often some DME is excluded from coverage.

The relationship of the person (with a disability) to assistive technology was virtually ignored until quite recently. For example, in reviews of dissertation topics from 1954 through 1993, the topic of "technology studies" appeared only in the years 1986 to 1991. There were only 20 dissertations on the topic in those years, from a total of over 900 dissertations. This is not because AT is new—it isn't. Only high-tech assistive technologies are recent. However, it seems that the phenomenal growth of the computer industry and the advent of electronics into our daily lives has spurred an examination of man and machine not seen since the industrial revolution (D. H. Lawrence would be having a field day). However, we must remember that assistive devices have been around for a long time.

The history of wheelchairs provides an illustrative case of the relationship of equipment to people and vice versa (this brief wheelchair history is adapted from Kamenetz, 1969). Mobility devices for those ill or with disabilities are seen in depictions dating back to 4,000 B.C. At that time people were transported in a recumbent position (in a "litter") and carried by others. This method was primary for thousands of years. However, as this mode of transport was also used by able-bodied wealthier persons, it didn't connote stigma. A child's bed on wheels—the first indoor vehicle—appears in the 6th century B.C. The next advance came from China in the 3rd century A.D. with the advent of the wheelbarrow, but it wasn't until the 12th century that this invention made its way to Europe (via the crusades). In 1595, King Philip II (Spain) had a "gout chair" built for him, with four small wheels, reclining back, and adjustable elevating leg rest—features found on wheelchairs today. By the 1680s there were 20 such chairs in the French king's castle at Versailles. However, they were heavy, had small wheels, and were not designed for self-propulsion. Clearly these were chairs only for the wealthy and high of station, who had servants to move them. Self-propelled chairs were first made in Germany; a German watchmaker with paraplegia built himself what would now be called a wheelchair using cogwheels turned by two cranks (similar to a watch mechanism). Forward movement was achieved by turning the crank (as opposed to directly turning the wheels of the chair). However, despite some advances in design, the carrying chair was still the easiest for short outdoor travel. Thus mobility was limited to those who had people to carry them. One carrier could be replaced by a pair of wheels in a wheelbarrow, and these were much in use in France and England in the 17th and 18th centuries. A wheelchair was developed in Bath, England at the end of the 1700s. The "Bath chair" had two large wheels in the rear, smaller wheels in front, framework and wheels of iron, a canvas hood, open in front, which could be raised or lowered, and hinged flaps to protect legs. It was pushed from the rear while the occupant steered with a handle, or else pulled by the handle. Overall it had a dark, heavy appearance, and its bulk and weight made it unfeasible for indoor use. By 1766 chairs were made with wheels large enough to be turned directly by the user without intervening cranks or chains. Such chairs changed over time (wood vs. wicker, two vs. one front wheel) and are the direct forerunner of modern wheelchairs. They began to be manufactured in the United States by 1871 and included a hand rim for users to turn the large back wheels—the first example of designing wheelchairs specifically for ease of propulsion by the user. The bicycle craze at the end of 1800s led to improvements in wheels—from wood to wire spokes, and then covered with rubber; wheelchair tires were bought from the same manufacturers. Then World War I led to increased need for wheelchairs. Thus by the 1930s the United States was mass producing collapsible, lightweight chairs. Usage continued to increase due to more people surviving illness, injury, and surgery due to improvements in medicine, more wheelchairs made, and improvements to wheelchairs which made their use easier. It was only at this point, when more people using wheelchairs began to move out into the community, that the needs of users began to influence design. This is a modern idea. It comes at the end of a long path of developing notions about the interplay of person and machine. From being carried by servants (or slaves) to being pushed outdoors to indoor use to self-propulsion—these changes reciprocally determine and are determined by social forces. What has changed along with advances in technology is our conceptual framework for assistive technologies. The focus is now more clearly on the increased function and independence of the user than on needs of the care provider. With the introduction of motorized wheelchairs (first in the 1950s, though not more widely available until the 1970s) another perceptual shift has come about; AT is not just about replacement of body parts or functions but about aids to self-determination.

RELATIONSHIP OF USER/OWNER
TO ASSISTIVE TECHNOLOGY

We can understand the relationship of an assistive device to the body and self-image of the user by examining how it feels when someone first gets eyeglasses. Remember how it was a bit jarring every time you caught sight of yourself in the new glasses—"Who *is* that?" How aware you were of them, of their weight, of their feel on your face? How conspicuous you were sure your new glasses were? The fact that they improved your vision was secondary at first. But after a while their utility became the more salient feature, you and others got more used to seeing you with your glasses than without, and you felt naked without them. But suppose that transition happened only within you but not for everyone else in response to you. Suppose each new person you met looked first at your glasses, commented on your glasses, tried hard to look everywhere but at your glasses, and thought of you predominantly as an eyeglass wearer. Suppose people asked to hold or try on your glasses, or reached out and felt them on your face?

This example highlights several points. First, the use of assistive devices alters one's self-image. There is a period of acclimatization during which the assistive device is incorporated into one's body image; the assistive device becomes a part of the body. Second, as a part of the body, it is no more open to touch, stares, personal questions, or lending than are other body parts. Third, although those close to you acclimate to your new "look," strangers often focus initially on the assistive device, to the exclusion of "you."

A fourth point (less exemplified by glasses) is that assistive devices can and often do fail—they break, don't fit, hurt, wear out, run out of batteries, and bend. Some assistive devices require no more attention than, say, your toes, but others demand constant upkeep and attention. I'll use myself to illustrate both extremes. I wear an orthotic on my right ankle and foot, called an AFO (ankle–foot orthosis). It's made of a hard plastic resin of "skin color" (only within the past decade did manufacturers realize that skin color included coffee and chocolate), and sculpted to a plaster mold of my foot and ankle. It's held on by my shoe and two hook-and-loop straps around my lower leg. Once made and fitted, I can basically ignore it—I put it on with my shoes in the morning and take it off with my shoes in the evening. It does its job: strengthening my ankle, forcing my knee back into a locked position, and allowing me to use a $\frac{5}{8}$-inch buildup on my right shoe. It is virtually maintenance free for about 3 years. Then a small stress crack starts at the ankle and grows infinitesimally each day. At that point I begin a prolonged and intensive round of negotiations with my insurance company, which has a policy about the frequency of replacing "durable medical products" (no more than every 5 years) which is out of synch with real-world durability. It is a nerve-wracking race between the length of crack and the obtuseness of my insurance company. Ultimately I am fitted with a new AFO, and I can ignore it happily once again.

I also ride an electric scooter. Scooters are three- (and occasionally four-) wheeled cousins of the golf-cart. They can go up to 4 miles per hour, with a range of up to 20 miles. Power is supplied by one or two 12-volt batteries which are plugged into a converter which in turn plugs into any three-pronged outlet. A full charge is usually achieved in 8 hours, so I plug mine in overnight. I transport the scooter on a lift that puts it in the back of my van. (Scooter manufacturers claim that scooters can be easily taken apart and put in the trunk, but each battery weighs about 30 pounds, so this is not an option for most persons with disabilities.) Scooters cost about $2,000 and up, lift plus installment another $2,000 (lifts are not covered by medical insurance). Batteries need to be replaced every year or more, depending on use. Tires go flat suddenly and with annoying frequency. The electronics fail with some regularity, rain causes it to "short," and the whole scooter easily can be stolen with a phillips-head screwdriver. Upkeep involves constant attention to small and hard-to-find parts. Manufacturers consider the lifetime of a scooter to be 7 years maximum and stop making replacement parts after that time. Insurance companies are unwilling to replace scooters at the same rate as they wear out and do not cover many upkeep costs.

We see in these examples two extremes in terms of maintenance and upkeep. As the end user, several skills are essential to successful assistive device procurement and use. First, active participation in selection and fit is essential. Indeed, research supports the notion that consumer involvement decreases likelihood of AT abandonment (Phillips & Zhao, 1993), and most researchers call for increased consumer choice and involvement (Batavia & Hammer, 1990; Enders, 1991; Grady, Kovach, Lange, & Shannon, 1991). Even in fitting my AFO, which may seem a more passive role than selecting a scooter, it is vital that I evaluate, complain, and demand alteration of any parts that don't feel perfectly comfortable. Any small deviation will turn into a major irritant with daily wear, so early detection and correction are important. A good working relationship with the fitter eases this process. Hard negotiation skills and firm self-advocacy are needed to negotiate with insurance. Savvy consumer shopping skills are key to finding the right product and price. Knowledge of electronics and handiness with a screwdriver will help immeasurably. Time—to make calls, locate equipment or parts, peruse catalogues, fill out insurance forms, get referrals from your primary care physician—is needed each step of the way.

Matching person and/or need with technology is often a difficult process. First, many persons with disabilities don't know what products are available. There are no menus of assistive devices, and consumers simply are not aware of their options. For example, in the largest survey to date of parents with disabilities (Toms Barker & Maralani, 1997),

56% of parents identified at least one type of adaptive equipment that could have helped them with parenting, but they cited costs and not knowing where to go to get information as the major reasons for not obtaining adaptive equipment. Thus even though adaptive equipment for parenting has many benefits for both parent and child, lack of information is a large barrier to adaptive equipment use. In a study on mothers with visual impairments (Conley-Jung, 1996), mothers lamented that they would have used AT if it had been available but also that they couldn't think of any AT they could have used—that is, they can't imagine what to ask for without knowing what exists.

The second problem in matching is that professionals are equally unaware of the array of available products. Specialists (e.g., at a hand clinic) might know about a limited number of assistive devices related to their specialty, but not those in other areas. Occupational therapists are probably the most informed about assistive devices, but this presumes the potential user has access to occupational therapy, which is probably available to only a small percentage of persons with disabilities.

The third problem is knowing where to find assistive technologies. Any one item (scooters, page magnifiers, baby carriers, voice-activated computers) requires intensive research to find what options are available. Medical supply stores are one source. However, these are only in larger cities; limited in variety of items sold; focused more on self-care, hygiene, and grooming items than on the full array of options to increase independence; not sources for electronic devices; and hugely expensive. The minute something is labeled "medical" its price goes up exorbitantly. For example, a small piece of latex for a hand orthotic is less than one tenth the size of exercise or biking shorts made from the same material but more than three times the price. A really good pair of scissors might be $30 at a sewing store but double that price at a medical supply store. Therefore, locating nonmedical sources, if available, is a good idea. Another source is mail-order medical supply companies, but these share the same limitations as medical-supply stores. Further, about half of each catalogue often is devoted to incontinence products, and this view of disability can be jarring or scary to those more newly disabled. Other sources include pharmacies, sports stores, large discount stores, medical professionals, computer bulletin boards, and association newsletters. Computer manufacturers often have (800) numbers for information on computer AT. American car manufacturers also have (800) numbers for inquiries about their rebate programs for vehicle modifications for buyers with disabilities ($750–1,000) and most will send you a free videotape of the most common modifications.

A significant barrier to matching AT and persons with disabilities is the reluctance of many persons with disabilities to think of themselves as such. Thus they refuse to avail themselves of the most accessible, reliable, and comprehensive data source, namely, the disability community and its various service agencies (e.g., CILs). Making the call, visiting the agency, requesting information about disability products and giving out the home address, saying out loud, "I have X disorder/diagnosis/disability"—all are large psychological steps for many people, especially those whose disability is recently acquired or worsened.

Stan's disability had been relatively stable for the first 10 years since diagnosis. However, over time his energy levels decreased and his fatigue increased, with a rapid decrement around the 12th year. He had to make choices about how he expended his energy. Doing action A implied less available energy to do action B; day-to-day tasks were a constant juggling of priorities and trade-offs. One day, faced with walking to the back of the grocery store to pick up some milk, for the first time Stan used the store's electric scooter. It was a transformative moment. Suddenly he was bombarded with new thoughts, awareness, reactions from others, and physical demands. He noticed for the first time that (1) a half gallon of milk is harder to pick up from a sitting than from a standing position; (2) the fruit and vegetable area, with its more circular and less linear traffic patterns, was more crowded and difficult to negotiate; (3) displays that intruded on aisle space made it necessary to take turns with shopping carts for passage; (4) the automated teller machine/credit card machines on most check out lanes were too high; (5) aisle one was designated as reserved for those with less than nine items and those with disabilities, leading him to wonder how those in line would react if he had a full basket; (6) the handicapped logo on aisle one was a person in a wheelchair, and although he could begin to think of himself as a person with a disability, he didn't identify with the wheelchair logo. The store clerks, used to seeing him ambulatory, were giving signs of wanting to—but refraining from—asking him about his change in locomotion. More people than usual seemed to make a point of smiling at him, and he felt self-conscious, no longer able to slip in and out as just-another-man-picking-up-milk-on-his-way-home; now he was the-guy-in-the-scooter. He emerged from the store aware of having expended less physical energy than usual for the task but a great deal of emotional and psychic energy. Was the trade-off worth it?

Other persons with disabilities are an excellent source of information. Magazines geared toward the disability community often carry ads of products. Some metropolitan areas hold "disability expos," usually in a large venue such as a coliseum or warehouse, to display disability-related products. At these expos, persons with disabilities can try out products, sign up for mailing lists, and find sources for products. For example, there are disability expos in Edison, New Jersey, in April; Anaheim, California, in May; Chicago, Illinois, in August; Washington, DC, in September; and San Mateo, California, in November. Going to the San Mateo expo ($5 entry fee; free with coupons from disability magazines) was the only way for me to find a scooter, lift, and van in one place and see which models of each three would work together.

This brings us to the fourth problem with matching person and AT—time. Finding easier-to-use scissors is only one need related to more limited hand use; what about the time to find writing implements, can openers, jar looseners, buttoners, car controls and auto-alteration specialists, automatic curtain openers, door openers, tools, kitchen utensils, and so on? For example, my feet are two different sizes: one an adult size for socks, the other a child size. I spend an extraordinary amount of time finding socks that come in both sizes and match in color and in frills (e.g., bows or absence thereof). Most persons with disabilities are subject to these hidden time stealers.

Fifth, most products cannot be borrowed or rented before making the purchase. However, a critical strategy to reduce product abandonment is to increase prefitting of product to user (McGrath et al., 1985; Phillips & Zhao, 1993). Prefitting would increase consumer use and satisfaction, save money, and prevent valuable assistive technologies from sitting useless in closets. It would also prevent society from losing valuable assets among its population, namely, the contributions of persons with disabilities. And everyone seems to agree that increasing consumer involvement and choice would maximize usage. Unfortunately, this practice does not seem to be the norm. One study found that under 29% of respondents answered affirmatively to the question, "Were you given any choice in equipment?" (McGrath et al., 1985, p. 432). Another study found that "the odds that the device will be retained were significantly greater when users feel their opinions were taken into account in the selection process" (Phillips & Zhao, 1993, p. 41).

ASSISTIVE TECHNOLOGY USE AND ABANDONMENT

Assistive technologies are big business. Since 1982, the medical device industry has grown from 5,900 to 16,900 companies. About $40 billion was spent on medical devices in 1994. According to the 1990 U.S. Census National Health Interview Survey, more than 13.1 million people in the United States—5% of the population—used assistive technologies, and the number is growing, due to greater survival rates of persons with disabilities, the aging of the population, availability of newer technologies, and the Technology Assistance Act of 1988. But the use of an AT is not dictated purely by need and availability; other factors also influence their use.

Device "abandonment," as it is referred to in the literature, is determined by a complex interaction of many variables, including characteristics of the user; utility, appropriateness, and match of the device to need(s); and availability of the AT. Some early studies indicate that usage rates were very low. For example, only 32% to 65% of children wear their hearing aids (Gaeth & Lounsbury, 1966; Karchmer & Kirwin, 1977), and a paltry 16% to 27% of adults prescribed braces actually wore them (Kaplan, Grynbaum, Rusk, Anastasia, & Gassler, 1966). In light of these data, several authors have hypothesized about factors predicting a greater likelihood of use. Some authors (Scherer, 1987; Vash, 1983; Wright, 1983) suggest that some "acceptance" of the disability and a positive approach (i.e., what activity the AT potentiates) are associated with higher likelihood of assistive technology use. Other authors (Brooks, 1990; Zola, 1982a) place more emphasis on the interpersonal and social factors such as the person's conceptualization of independence and the meaning of assistive device use, as opposed to just physical functioning. Scherer (1995) uses the concepts of "technophobe" and "technophile" to explain large differences in response to AT. However, even technophiles may acquire assistive technologies but not use them; the pleasure may be in procuring each new device as it comes along. The technophobe, however, is more apt to resist new technology and assistive devices that require new learning, especially of controls or electronics. Unfortunately, the concepts of technophobes and technophiles are not unrelated to gender. Girls and women, especially those with disabilities, are less exposed to technologies and thus may be intimidated by or avoid them. On the other hand, one small ($n = 10$) study (Scherer, 1988) indicated that women were more likely to emphasize their abilities to do things because of their assistive devices, whereas men were more likely to interpret their assistive devices as poor substitutes for the lost functions they were meant to replace or augment (Scherer, 1988).

The largest U.S. study of abandonment (most studies have been conducted in Europe) showed that just under 30% of all assistive devices were abandoned (Phillips & Zhao, 1993). The rates were highest in the first year, with a smaller peak of abandonment in year 5 (this may be related to insurance company policies on frequency of replacement). Mobility aids were more frequently abandoned, at a rate six times that of any other category of device. The authors posit that because mobility devices are often used in work, social, and community settings, users may use different standards and criteria for evaluation of the devices. It may be also that in these more socially interactive settings, stigma and other negative effects on interpersonal interactions are more pronounced.

Of course, the abandonment of assistive devices is not always a negative thing; among the reasons given for abandonment is "change in needs/priorities" (Phillips & Zhao, 1993, p. 40). Two factors that predicted device abandonment were "device performance" and "personal opinion considered in selection" (this latter has profound policy and procedures implications). But an unexpected finding was that "ease of obtaining device" also was correlated positively with device abandonment. It may be that devices that were easier to obtain were more off-the-rack and less well matched to the user. Such devices may be routinely sent home with patients, or easily located (in stores or catalogs) but not fully explained or illustrated, or useful for inpatients but not at home or at work. For example, when I attended a hand clinic for physical therapy I was given two different hand splints, each billed directly to my insurance company, with no copayment from me. Thus I had no disincentive to try them out—"it couldn't hurt." But within 2 months I used neither, as they didn't alleviate the problem. Being allowed to borrow or rent them could have facilitated my learning this, without an expenditure for useless products.

A large proportion of device abandonment occurs between hospital and home. Several factors influence this abandonment. The user may not have been adequately trained in device use. For example, many patients are handed a pair of crutches with little or no lessons in their fit and use (*always* land in a tripod position; crutches that hit your armpit are too tall). Also, devices that work well in the hospital setting (e.g., walker over a linoleum floor) may not translate well to home use (e.g., walker over plush carpet). The device may be one-size-fits-most but prove not to fit well with extended wear or use. Further, to be useful, the device has to be where the user is. In the hospital, the nurses may have diligently put the device next to the bed after each use, but at home it always seems to be in the other room when needed. Most important, family members may not be prepared to see the family member as an assistive device user, with all that this use implies. Their associations to the assistive device may be negatively conditioned to illness, injury, surgery, trauma, hospitalization, and separation. Their focus may be on the loss of function, not on how the assistive device increases independence and functionality.

As this chapter has repeatedly demonstrated, psychoemotional and interpersonal factors are important determinants of assistive device use and satisfaction. Scherer (1996) conceptualizes this as a pyramid, with needs arranged hierarchically (as in Maslow's motivational needs hierarchy). Lower-level needs (functional need for the AT) must be met before a person considers or is motivated to meet a higher level (usability and performance). If not, "the likely outcome is avoidance, dissatisfaction, or non-use of the technology" (Scherer, 1996, p. 160). Further, a person may be at different need levels for different functional losses. Moreover, the use of assistive devices may be synergistic and increasing the number of assistive devices not simply additive.

Successful matching of person and technology depends on myriad interacting factors. Scherer (1995) organizes these into an MPT model: *m*atching *p*erson and *t*echnology by assessing *m*ilieu, *p*ersonality, and *t*echnology (Scherer, 1993). A person might be an ideal candidate in terms of personality and technology, but the milieu may be physically difficult (in which case the best intervention would be structural or building modifications) or may create psychosocial difficulties (in which case the person may need help in self-assertion, teaching others about the disability, or self-disclosure of needs and limitations, or in-service training at the workplace could be offered). Thus the MPT model not only helps assess where any impediments to AT use may lie but also points toward the area(s) in which intervention may be most effective.

Milieu

Assistive technologies used in the hospital or rehabilitation often fail to make the transition to home use. There may be practical reasons for this occurrence (e.g., the device is difficult to get in and out of the car), but psychosocial factors in the milieu should not be underestimated. The user may have accepted use of the assistive device while in the sick role in the medical facility but not at home, in the community, or at work. An individual may have difficulty in handling others' questions, which may entail an alteration in self-image that the individual has not yet attained. Family members and friends also might be embarrassed by the obvious display of disability involved in using an assistive device. Further, the use of AT may alter familial routines and require more—or less—help from a family member. Employers may be concerned that the device will impede work, break or fail, or create the "wrong image" to customers. Each of these issues can mean the difference between AT use and abandonment. Therefore, it is essential that assistive technologies are tried out in the milieu in which they will be used prior to purchase or commitment, especially for higher-priced assistive technologies. (Of course, this is not always possible, for example, in the case of home dialysis.)

Other factors of the milieu are availability of alternatives (e.g., personal assistance rather than device use), whether tasks can be modified to be performed without assistive device use (e.g., using an enlarged computer screen rather than a typewriter), or environment altered so an assistive device is unnecessary (raising a table so transfer from wheelchair is unnecessary). However, pointing out these factors is not meant to suggest that the use of assistive devices is a less desirable, attractive, or functional solution that should be avoided.

Assistive technologies should rarely if ever be imposed on a person. Such imposition occurs when the use of AT is made a condition of discharge to home. Family members also may insist on the use of such AT. They may be tired of performing various functions and seeking relief from certain helping activities. The person with a disability may hear this as rejection, fatigue, lack of nurturance, or distancing. Thus the device can convey intense symbolism and become the focus of an interpersonal struggle.

> Sam and Phyllis sought therapy at a point of great impasse in their 18-year marriage. Sam had used a manual wheelchair for the past 2 years, after surgery to remove a cancerous tumor from his spine left him paraplegic. He stopped working as a food products developer and went on Supplemental Security Disability Insurance (SSDI). His wife worked for an insurance company. Whenever Sam went out of the house by car he was accompanied by his wife, who removed the wheels and collapsed the wheelchair and put it in the trunk. She was tired of doing this, but felt responsible for ensuring that Sam left the house. Although money was a consideration, Phyllis felt Sam's monetary objections to getting a van and wheelchair lift were spurious. The therapist asked each of them for one good thing and one bad thing that would result from getting a van or wheelchair lift.
>
> For Phyllis, the good thing was that "Sam could go out more." She couldn't think of a bad thing and had to be pressed; finally she offered that she'd have to fill Sam's car with gas for him because most stations were self-service, which Sam couldn't do. For Sam, the good thing was that Phyllis wouldn't have to haul his wheelchair into the trunk anymore. The bad thing was that it would cost a lot of money. Because this issue had already surfaced, the therapist pushed Sam for another answer. He replied that his wife wouldn't want to go places with him anymore.
>
> These answers bring several issues to light. First, Sam's good thing about the AT was a positive for Phyllis, not for himself, raising the question of what was in it for him. Second, Phyllis's frame for thinking about AT was a positive one of increased independence for both herself and Sam; Sam's frame was a negative one of decreased intimacy and togetherness. Third, Sam resented that Phyllis at first couldn't even think of one bad thing; he took a meta-message from this that his views hadn't been heard. Thus the therapy needed to address three issues: (1) the symbolic meaning of the

AT; (2) the communication between the couple that was being played out through the AT; and (3) the dance of distance and intimacy in which they were engaged, and the important distinction between the concepts of independence and intimacy.

Personality

As previously discussed, a critical factor in acceptance of AT is that the devices be perceived as enablers of activities and functions that would otherwise be difficult or impossible. This half-full perspective comes more readily to some than to others. But this reframe is an essential one for clinicians. An important distinction is that loss of function does not equal loss of control—decision making and self-determination as they relate to the function should be retained. Take a common example: In the hospital, patients may have to use a bedpan. But the patient should be able to retain control over timing of urination rather than conforming to the nursing staff's schedule.

People's needs and life circumstances change such that assistive devices may cease to serve their purpose, or new AT becomes necessary. For example, parents with disabilities identify "getting infant or toddler in and out of car seat" as a task for which an assistive device would be useful (Toms Barker & Maralani, 1997). However, once children can accomplish this task for themselves the parent no longer needs an assistive device. Conversely, some decisions about AT choice require allowing for future needs. For example, in selecting my van I had to think about not just present functioning but how my physical abilities might change over the next 5 years.

People change in ways other than physical, and these changes too will affect assistive device use. Someone who is married may worry less about superficial appearance than they did when dating. Someone who has children will place greater emphasis on conserving energy. A person may resist aging and hence become increasingly averse to assistive device use. Many assistive technologies don't have built in flexibility to allow for changing needs of users. This fact, coupled with minimal time allotments between purchases imposed by insurance companies, makes the decision of when and which assistive technologies to invest in more difficult. One feature of personality that affects this process is tolerance of ambiguity, or, conversely, rigidity. Obviously, decision-making abilities also play a strong role. Particular skills discussed earlier, such as self-advocacy, can be key to assistive device procurement.

Janelle is a young woman in her 20s with osteoarthritis, now working in her first full-time job since graduating from college a year ago. She has difficulty with fine motor movements, especially with her hands, and finds using a computer mouse makes her hands freeze up in one position and her arms tired. Although she prefers using the keyboard rather than the mouse, her computer at work would need some reconfiguring to allow keyboard control for some applications. Janelle would like the company's computer support services to make these modifications for her, get her a more ergonomic keyboard, and replace the mouse with a finger touch pad. Costs would be under $300 plus staff time for computer support services.

On the MPT model Janelle would have the following profile: Milieu—mostly unknown psychosocial variables at the workplace. Janelle views her supervisors as intimidating, judgmental and demanding. However, Janelle is shy, young, and relatively inexperienced and new to the work world; hence her fears may be unfounded. Personality—Janelle is neither extreme of technophobe nor -phile but very comfortable with computer use. However, she has little experience in self-advocacy and is shy with strangers and persons in authority. Technology—the required modifications are relatively inexpensive and readily available and achievable.

Technology

Questions we might ask about AT include the following: (1) Does any technology exist that could aid a particular function; (2) are there choices of technologies or, if only one kind of technology, are there different versions of it; (3) does the device adequately enable the function to be accomplished; (4) how readily available is such technology in terms of expense, availability, ease of learning use and ongoing use, portability, and social stigma; (5) is the person with a disability psychologically and emotionally ready to use the technology; (6) is the family able to accept and support the technology; and (7) does everyone who needs to know how to operate the technology. As discussed earlier, it is hard to comparison-shop AT because of the lack of compiled information about it. And altered use of readily available equipment should not be overlooked. For example, when my first child was still too young to sit, I bought the largest basket made for my scooter and installed it on the front handlebars. I then put my son in his carry-all and placed it into the basket. This worked well for several months (though the sun was always in his eyes) until he could sit, at which time we installed a regular bicycle kid's seat on the back of the scooter, in which each of my children happily rode until he or she reached 25 pounds. (One unintentional result of these arrangements is that my children felt for some time that it was their God-given right to ride and would complain about why they "had" to walk.)

It is easy to assume that no assistive device exists for a particular function or purpose because you've never seen or heard of one. I fell into that trap: I helped an adolescent girl with the use of one hand and limited use of the other to learn how to tie her shoes. Although I'm a fairly savvy AT aficionado, I didn't discover until 2 years later, and then only by accident, that there are devices that help people with the use of only one hand tie their shoes. It just didn't occur to me that such a device might exist, so I didn't even look for one. (Also consider those springy, coiled shoelaces that don't need to be tied at all and come in all sorts of cool colors.)

CHILDREN AND ASSISTIVE TECHNOLOGY

Children may use AT to sustain life or for one or more of the many other functions of childhood. AT includes leg or back braces, wheelchairs, communication boards, talking watches, asthma inhalers, and so on. One of the themes of this book is that we have to stop thinking of children with disabilities as tragedies, and this extends to how we view their assistive devices. Although the goal of most AT is to increase independence and functioning, for children the primary goal is to allow users to be children. I am reminded of this by a catalog I received recently of communication aids for children with disabilities. On the front cover is a photo of a girl around 6 years old. She sits in a wheelchair, the position of her hands suggests spasticity, and the wideness of her open-mouthed smile implies some loss of motoric function. In front of her is a talking aid, and she is saying, through this device, "I want to go see *101 Dalmatians*." So profoundly ordinary.

Children develop a relationship to their assistive devices in a way adults don't. For children who acquire such devices early on, or who learn a new skill (e.g., "talking") simultaneously to learning how to use the assistive device (a communication board) may come to see the two as inseparable, normal, and routine. For example, a child who has used a combination stroller/wheelchair for mobility since age 2 will see the two (AT and mobility) as inextricably entwined. Some children are introduced to an assistive device later. The device may be associated with unpleasant events, such as doctor visits, hospitalization, surgery, or pain. The anxieties about the child of the adults in his or her life may communicate negative messages about the device. Teachers may be unfamiliar with devices' functions and usage, and peers may want to play with it or may deride its use. Adults must help prepare the child for assistive device use, and a therapist may have to help prepare the adults.

Perhaps one of the most pervasive but easily avoidable mistakes adults make with children is an act of omission—they fail to explain the purpose, nature, duration, and functions of the assistive device. Clearly explanations have to be provided at an age-appropriate level and updated as the child matures. Parents often tell me "he knows" (about the device) because "he was right there when the doctor explained it." Studies of adults going to doctors indicate that they only remember about 50% of what is said, and of that 50% they get about half wrong. So expecting children to attend to, understand, and retain what the doctor said, especially in an emotionally laden setting, is unrealistic. Further, adults have to respond to the unspoken questions and fears of children. For example, it is possible, perhaps even common, for children to "interpret the orthotic appliance as a punishment for having a deformity" (Fredrick & Fletcher, 1985, p. 230). Children may not understand the temporal aspects of the device—whether it's forever, for a period of correction, for a developmental phase, or for a prespecified or indeterminate amount of time. The child may not be motivated to wear or use the appliance/device because of lack of information about how it can help. Too often parents and teachers use long-term negative reinforcement (avoidance of a negative outcome that is far in the future) to induce usage—do this to avoid that (e.g., "If you don't wear your back brace you'll grow up all crooked."). But having a preponderance of negative reinforcers with a paucity of positive reinforcers leads to depression in adults; it can hardly be expected to have a more positive effect on children. And we certainly know from antismoking campaigns that threats of dire possible long-term outcomes (e.g., lung cancer or emphysema) have little effect on a behavior that is more immediately gratifying. But parents often need help in finding and articulating what's in it for the child. For example, help them switch from "If you don't wear your eyepatch you'll end up cross-eyed forever," to "If you wear your eyepatch for a few months you'll get fewer headaches and be able to get your homework done more quickly because you can focus your eyes more easily."

It is good to bear in mind that it is often easier to be the one doing an unpleasant task than to be the one watching, especially if the one doing is a child and the one watching is that child's parent. Adults may overestimate the degree of discomfort. For example, it might seem intuitive that any devices made of metal, plastic, or leather would be uncomfortable (though this is not necessarily the case). Thus adults may be more concerned about discomfort than is warranted. Conversely, they may ignore complaints because they think there is nothing that can be done. But anything more than minimal discomfort after initial adjustment indicates a problem that should be addressed and rectified. The device or appliance may need adjusting, repairing, refitting; it may be being used incorrectly or outgrown. For orthotics and prostheses, skin rashes are a common complication. On occasion, rashes result from a contact allergy, though often they are due to more prosaic reasons. They are reduced through proper hygiene, adequate ventilation of the area, good fit without rubbing, and regular cleaning of skin and appliance.

Many devices for children, whether prosthetic, orthotic, or assistive, are meant to be worn or used both at home and in school. Thus teachers need some information and instruction. Fredrick and Fletcher (1985) cite five questions that teachers should be able to answer:

1. Is there a specific schedule for use of the device?
2. How will the teacher know if the device is not functioning properly?
3. What are the restrictions, if any, on activities when using or not using the device?
4. What type of assistance should be provided to the child?
5. How is the device to be applied and used?

The Office of Technology Assessment (U.S. Congress, Office of Technology Assessment, 1987) has developed a scheme for categorizing children dependent on some form of life-sustaining medical technology. These four categories have differing degrees of technological complexity and level of skill required of caregiver. All are necessary for life support, imply prolonged dependence, and require some skilled care. Conversely, a premature infant might require a ventilator for some time, but ultimately its lungs will mature and the baby will no longer be dependent on the ventilator. Such use of technology is not part of the classification that follows. A rough estimate of the number of children who fall into one or more of the following categories is 64,000 (Palfrey et al., 1991): (1) dependence on mechanical ventilation; (2) dependence on parenteral (usually intravenous) nutrition or medicine; (3) dependence on other device-based respiratory or nutritional support (e.g., tracheostomy or gastrostomy tubes, suctioning, and oxygen support); (4) dependence on medical technology to compensate or replace compromised or lost body function (e.g., sleep apnea monitors, renal dialysis, urinary catheters, and colostomy bags), which requires daily nursing or other skilled care.

Any of these categories of devices mean that a technology has joined the *family*. The family must respond; the family must learn about the device and its use; the family's routines must be reformed to incorporate the device. In two-parent families, parents initially should go with their strengths—one parent may be better at comforting a child during procedures, giving injections, or suctioning a child. The other may be better at distracting and entertaining the child during periods of waiting (e.g.,

when waiting for medicine to take effect). However, some degree of flexibility of roles is more adaptive in the long run.

Jennifer is 5, and has insulin-dependent diabetes. Her mother gives
her daily injections, but her father has been unable to do so. He is
squeamish about needles and injections, especially so for his little
girl. However, this arrangement restricted the mother's activities to
the point where she gave up her job to be available for the task. She
was extremely fearful that Jennifer would have a severe insulin
depletion and be unable to get help. It wasn't long before mother's
activities became more and more restricted to ones where she was at
or near home. She was angry with her husband for his refusal to
participate in the diabetes control and for his resultant greater freedom of movement.

   At this point the mother sought therapy. She insisted on coming
alone to the first session, and maintained that her husband wasn't
able to leave work during the hours the therapist had available.
However, it soon became clear that the mother wanted time alone
with the therapist to vent her anger and frustration. These emotions
were easier for her to maintain than her fear for her daughter's
safety. Thus she helped maintain a system that kept her angry. The
therapist was able to get the mother to agree to ask the father to
join them for the second session, and they role-played how to
accomplish this. With both parents present the therapist and couple
came to an agreement that it was impractical and potentially dangerous for only one parent to be able to give injections, and that one
goal of treatment was that both parents know how to give injections and have sufficient practice in this task. This required two
simultaneous therapeutic tracks. One was to help the father with his
needle and injection phobia (beginning first with his own ability to
have injections before turning to his daughter's insulin shots). The
second was to elicit the parents' fears about their daughter, and help
them find more ways of coping with them. The father's disclosure of
his terror of losing his daughter decreased the mother's anger
toward him. As they felt increased empathy from each other, they
turned more toward each other. Intimacy increased, and the mother
was able to make some initial steps in letting go of her vigilance as
the father participated more in the daughter's care.

   This couple returned to treatment when Jennifer was about 10.
The presenting problem was again about letting go: The father
agreed with the daughter's wish to give herself her injections, and
the mother felt that the daughter was too young, the task was too
important, and the potential consequences of mistakes too costly.
This time the daughter was included in treatment, which focused on
deriving a family contract about injections—at what age the daughter could begin self-injections, when and where they were to take

place, what the backup system was, and how the parents could be assured that she was behaving responsibly in giving injections, eating, and lifestyle. They finally compromised (after many weeks of stalemate) by agreeing that the daughter could learn to inject herself the summer after fifth grade, when she was 11 and would be entering middle school in the fall.

CONCLUDING REMARKS

None of the discussion in this chapter is meant to imply that AT use is the desired outcome, or that it is in some way "better" for a person to use an assistive device than not to do so. Although increased acceptance of disability may facilitate AT use, use of AT should not be taken to mean better "adjustment" to disability. If Cindy walks slowly with a cane while Sally, with similar level of functioning, zips down the hall in a manual wheelchair, this does not imply that Sally is more accepting of her disability than Cindy. This is a very important distinction because it is easy to infuse assistive technologies with meanings they don't warrant.

Conversely, persons with disabilities are often importuned to use their own limited functions rather than an AT that would make the task easier. Lisa Fay (1993) writes an eloquent account of her ultimate decision to forgo yet more speech therapy and instead to use a speech synthesizer to improve her communicative abilities rather than her own impaired speech. She describes the pervasive bias of speech therapists, the mental health community, and rehabilitation facilities toward her using her own voice, despite years of little therapeutic gains, increased fatigue, and mounting frustration that deleteriously affected her quality of life. This was true despite evidence that communication impairments are among those least amenable to rehabilitative treatment (Baker, 1983; Baker, Stump, Nyberg, & Conti, 1991). In other instances a family might resist the implications of an AT and insist that the family member rely on his or her own limited facilities, despite the drain on personal energy and emotional resources it may entail. Either bias is not helpful to the person with the disability and in fact can be very psychologically wounding. The minority model of disability and the basic tenets of the ILM lead us to conclude, as Gloria Steinem did in another context, that it is the people who have the problem (in this case persons with disabilities) who are the experts; the experts aren't the experts. This discussion has tried to emphasize freedom of choice and self-determination for persons with disabilities. Thus assistive technologies should be adapted to persons with disabilities, not the other way around. AT choice should include the right to choose or to reject AT.

AT is not a luxury. For some it can mean the difference between keeping a job or not, retaining custody of children or losing them, going outside the house or being housebound, needing assistance or doing a task independently. For example, when my children were babies, going up a single stair required the following steps: I put the baby on the floor up the stair. I held onto a piece of furniture and climbed up the step myself. I knelt down and picked up the baby and put him or her on a chair placed there for that purpose. I stood up, keeping one hand on the baby to prevent him or her from rolling off the chair. Then, from a standing position I picked up the baby and we went our merry way. A ramp or lift would have changed my life in early motherhood. Over and over we come to the same theme—AT changes lives, but people with disabilities can't ask for technology they don't know exists and thus can't imagine how it would improve quality of life. In this case, information is power.

SUMMARY OF KEY POINTS

1. The study of the relationship between person and AT is recent and scarce. Few theoretical models (besides Scherer's) have guided inquiry. The notion that machines should fit the user and not the reverse is a modern idea that has not yet fully taken hold. Scherer's MPT model can help assess readiness for AT use and pinpoint where intervention may be most effective.

2. Assistive technologies are imbued with symbolic meanings. On a societal level they may reflect prevailing paradigms of relations between man and machine. On more individual levels the symbolic meanings can increase or inhibit the use of AT. Admitting to the need for an assistive device can be a large psychological step.

3. Having access to AT may mean the difference between two widely discrepant outcomes (living in the community vs. in a nursing home; retaining custody of one's children).

4. Assistive devices can become extensions of the body. As such they need to be incorporated into one's self-image. They must also be respected as part of the user's body and personal space.

5. Assistive technologies communicate messages about the user to others. These messages may be misleading (e.g., the flat tone of a speech synthesizer) or misunderstood. They may also engender a range of reactions, including curiosity or stigma.

6. Finding and procuring appropriate assistive technologies can require time, concerted effort, ingenuity, strong self-advocacy skills, creative financing, and ingenuity. The process is made more complicated by

insurance restrictions and by uncertainty about future health needs and course of disorder. Clients are likely to need help in learning what is available and in locating assistive technologies. This is an area in which connections to the disability community can be invaluable.

7. AT use or abandonment is determined by a complex set of factors, only a few of which concern the device itself. Factors associated with increased likelihood of assistive device use are a greater degree of acceptance of disability, a focus on what the AT enables and association of the AT with positive values (e.g., independence and freedom), comfort with technology, greater consumer control over choice and selection of device, proper training in device use, and performance of device. Because assistive devices affect not only the user but the user's family, the family can play a large role in determining device use or abandonment.

8. Children's AT use may be routine for them if introduced early in life, or if a task has always been accomplished through AT use. For the later addition of AT parents and teachers need information, training, and a chance to ask questions and express concerns, so that they are then in a better position to help the child with transition to the AT.

9. Loss of functions and use of AT should not be equated with loss of control or self-determination. Requiring or deciding to use AT should not imply less self-determination but more; assistive technologies can facilitate the goals of independent living.

THIRTEEN

The Personal, the Professional, and the Political

When the client has a disability, what is the boundary between client and therapist, when and how does therapy incorporate advocacy, and how does therapy fuse personal and political agendas? For some populations of consumers (women and gays and lesbians), these questions are addressed in specific theories (feminist therapy and gay-affirmative therapy). But what about clients with disabilities? How do the personal, professional, and political arenas coexist or collide? What are the responsibilities of therapists treating clients with disabilities? What might constitute *disability-affirmative therapy*? What are the implications for psychologists of this model for training, teaching and research? The purpose of this chapter is to address areas of responsibility for psychologists in their roles as clinicians, teachers, and researchers.

Why should mental health professionals care about disability issues? First, persons with disabilities constitute the largest minority group in the United States. Second, social justice cannot be achieved by advancing the cause of one group while continuing to subjugate another. Third, we can no longer assume that psychology is exempt, that disability issues are "special," as in "special education" and "special Olympics." Disability studies must join the mainstream in psychology, in part because, according to Linton (1998):

> [S]ome basic tenets of psychology run counter to core ideas in disability studies in at least three fundamental ways. First, psychology is responsible for the formulations and research conventions that cement the ideas of

294

"normal," "deviant," "abnormal," and "pathology" in place. . . . Second, psychology's emphasis on empiricism and its repudiation of standpoint theory or positionality as legitimate starting points for research work against the types of . . . analyses necessary to explicate the social construction of disability. . . . Third . . . psychology primarily trains practitioners to intervene on the personal level rather than intervene to alter the environment. (p. 6)

Thus we as individuals and collectively as members of a profession have a responsibility to challenge the assumptions about the place of disability issues in training, curricula, research, and therapy.

It should be clear that embracing a disability-affirmative model is a rejection of competing models, most notably rehabilitation psychology and the medical model, with their focus on impairment and deemphasis on disability. When we reject the medicalization of disability, the study of disability "contests the current academic division of labor in which the study of the phenomenon rests in the specialized applied fields . . . and the rest of the academy is largely exempt from meaningful inquiry into the subject of disability" (Linton, 1998, p. 2).

Therapists incur several responsibilities when providing treatment for clients with disabilities. It was my original intent to present these responsibilities separately in three overlapping areas: the personal, the professional, and the political, but doing so would imply a distinction among the three. Yet it is a basic tenet of this book that disability-affirmative therapy, like its cousins for women and gays and lesbians, rejects the artificial separation of these domains. Therefore what follows are points that span the three domains, moving roughly through the roles of clinician, teacher, and researcher.

The *personal* might be defined as those aspects of psychotherapeutic work which are inside the therapist—interior debates, cognitions, expectations, attributions, values, and beliefs. The *professional* might be defined as those aspects of psychotherapeutic work which comprise the various roles and functions of the psychologist. These may include clinician, teacher, supervisor, consultant, and researcher. Less apparent but no less important are our functions as role models, activists, and advocates. The *political* might be defined as those aspects of work which carry implications and power beyond the individual(s) in treatment or training, and/or which encourage or empower clients or students to influence organizational, social, legal, or political change. The political also incorporates the inverse direction: the effects of politics and oppression on the person.

The literature on culturally competent therapy typically refers to three domains: *awareness*, *skills*, and *knowledge*, to which I would add *relationship*. Skills and knowledge may be more amenable to classroom training, whereas awareness and relationship may be more responsive to experience. How are awareness, skills, knowledge, and relationship affected by disability issues? What areas should clinicians who work with clients with disabilities be aware of? What are the responsibilities of psychologists in their roles as teachers and researchers? This chapter first addresses whether clients with disabilities are best served by clinicians with disabilities and then discusses 15 disability-related areas to consider in our roles as clinicians, teachers, and researchers.

DO YOU HAVE TO HAVE A DISABILITY TO COUNSEL THOSE WHO DO?

A common assumption about therapy is that shared characteristics (e.g., ethnicity, culture, and gender) between client and therapist enhance treatment. With regard to disability, we might add several other assumptions. The first is that those without disabilities can never truly understand what it is like to have a disability; even temporary disabilities fundamentally differ because they are temporary. Peer counseling (i.e., counseling of those with disabilities by those with disabilities) is a fundamental tenet of the ILM. Are these sound assumptions?

In a review of the literature on the effects of counselors' disability status (Strohmer, Leierer, Cochran, & Arokiasamy, 1996), the authors question the assumption of client–counselor similarity. These authors examine the evidence for similarity in disability status between counselor and client having an appreciable impact on treatment. However, there are several major problems with the literature reviewed. First, studies of client–counselor disability status have assessed clients' reactions to counselors but not actual treatment outcomes. Second, the concepts of personal experience (i.e., of having a disability) and expertise (i.e., of having special knowledge, skills, and experience) are treated as if they are the same. Third, disability is treated as a bimodal state (i.e., you either have one or you don't) without regard to type or degree of disability. Fourth, the emphasis has been predominantly on the client, most studies focusing on the perceptions of clients (with and without disabilities) about the counselor (with and without disabilities). The effects of client disability status on the counselor are barely discussed. Thus potential bias, stereotyping, or misperceptions by counselors are not the focus of study. It is as if we threw away all we know about therapy and instead are asking merely whether clients like us. The core question of whether clients with disabilities are better served by clinicians with disabilities remains empirically unanswered.

RESPONSIBILITIES

Disability as Minority

Psychologists should recognize and acknowledge that persons with disabilities constitute a minority group. Therapists generally are aware of their responsibilities for developing cultural competence, but unless we see persons with disabilities as a minority we will fail to apply our methods and process of increasing cultural competence to this group. From this awareness of disability as minority, it follows that persons with disabilities are bicultural, living in both a disability minority world and an "able-ist" majority world. Thus, therapy with clients with disabilities by able-bodied therapists is cross-cultural therapy. The clinician must be open to the culture of disability and flexible in ways of understanding the cross-cultural client. Without this openness and flexibility, the clinician's perspective is narrowed through the lens of his or her own culture, seeking and finding only what is sought (Tseng & Streltzer, 1997). As with all cross-cultural therapy, it is not sufficient simply to append culturally relevant content to "regular" therapy. Culturally sensitive therapy requires development of a framework based on culture; culture is not an appendage but the body politic.

Valuing Disability Culture

It is not useful to acknowledge disability as a minority group with its own culture if one then devalues that culture. Disability culture has its own history, language, humor, heroes, and devils. You cannot presume to know a person with a disability without knowing that person's culture. Language is an important factor in the cohesion of a culture and in establishing insider–outsider identification. Therapists should be aware of the power of language and the nuances of language in a cultural context. It is not enough merely to be *told* what language to use; the process of discovering for oneself is a process of disability acculturation. We cannot escape the "fact that language and its use is not just a semantic issue; it is a political issue as well" (Oliver, 1996, p. 74).

Models of Disability

Therapists should understand the moral, medical, and minority models of disability. They should be cognizant of the treatment and psychological implications of each model, be aware of their own model, and know how to help clients understand the client's own models (see Chapter 2, in this volume).

Disability versus Impairment

Therapists should understand the distinction between impairment and disability and allow the client to be the expert on his or her disability. However, the therapist should take responsibility for learning about impairments (Harsh, 1993). Persons with disabilities carry an enormous burden to continually educate others; therapy should not duplicate this burden or it becomes another arena of oppression.

Values

Disability raises the "large questions" in life. These include the value and quality of life, morality, normality and deviance, justice and equity, interdependence and responsibility, and mortality. Therapists must be prepared to ask and answer difficult philosophical and practical questions. Examples include the following: (1) How do we understand the suffering of children with terminal diseases? (2) How do we reconcile the idea that we would never want to live "like that," when people "like that" want to live? (3) How do we balance long-term goals with taking enjoyment of each day because we can never know what will happen? (4) Should a mother refuse to allow her child to attend a program that is physically unaccessible to the mother? (5) What are the consequences of teaching clients to see themselves as members of an oppressed minority? (6) What are the clinical implications of teaching about social oppression to those with developmental and/or cognitive impairments? (7) Given the dearth of empirical guidance on clinical treatment of persons with disabilities, what guides do we use in designing a treatment plan? (8) What are the short and long-term effects on clients when therapists incorporate notions of self-advocacy and political activism as part of treatment? (9) What is the role of home care and institutional care in our society, and who has the right to decide? Must families "accept full and perpetual responsibility for the patient [sic] without support"? (Jackson & Haverkamp, 1991, p. 363).

Have you ever listened to reports of famine and killing in Rwanda and gone home and hugged your child? Facing disability in others can have that effect—we suddenly become hyperaware of our own faculties and those of our families. We temporarily have a heightened sense of enjoyment of the ordinary. How do we reconcile these feelings of thankfulness for what we retain (sight, hearing, health, etc.) without feeling pity for those who haven't? What, exactly, does "quality of life" mean? As we grapple with these questions we also hold beliefs about the therapy process. These beliefs shape our work with *all* clients. The question here is whether these beliefs are based on an assumption of nondisability as the "normal" state and whether we change these beliefs for clients with disabilities based on prejudices and stereotypes. We have a responsibility to make our values and assumptions and meta-cognitions about therapy known, at least to ourselves, and then to examine how we apply these to clients with and without disabilities.

Dialectics

Disability issues encompass many dialectics and enjoin us to formulate a coherent set of beliefs and values. In dialectical arguments, one end of the spectrum is always accorded a superior position over its opposite. (For a list of dialectics related to disability, see Table 13.1.) One of the tensions is between the notions of autonomy (with its attendant false sense of equity despite inequalities in power) and autocracy (benevolence). What is missing is a model for deciding *with*, not *for*, persons with disabilities. For example, the ADA requires an interactive process for selecting a reasonable accommodation. As Prilleltensky (1997) states, "Excesses or abuses of power . . . include assuming to know what is best for clients, minimizing clients' autonomy by excluding them from decision-making processes, stigmatizing individuals with deficit-oriented labels, defining problems exclusively in intrapsychic terms, and neglecting to consider social injustices" (p. 518).

Disability issues challenge us to grapple with these dialectics, not as abstracts but in everyday acts. For example, I am the faculty adviser to students with disabilities at a graduate professional school of psychology. Many students request that their meetings with me and their disability status be kept confidential. When I agree to do so I make their individual concerns and needs superordinate to those of the institution. In particular, I give up some power and opportunity for organizational multiculturalism—that is, I cannot take the public and political actions at the institutional level that would in fact most improve the lives of students with disabilities at our campus. We all make personal choices that carry political weight. We cannot shy away from the implications of our actions related to disability issues by relegating disability to a subordinate position.

The Sociopolitical

When working with a minority client, sociopolitical issues join the therapy. The relationship of laws and court rulings to the everyday lives of minorities is tangible. For minorities, issues of oppression, discrimination, stigma, poverty, immigration, stereotyping, and powerlessness are

TABLE 13.1. Dialectics Raised by Disability Issues

Impairment	Disability
Researcher	Researched
Individual	Society; collective
Objective	Subjective
Theory	Practice
Mind	Body
Child	Adult
Subjugation; victim	Activism; emancipation
Victimizer	Victim
Absence and dysfunction	Presence and function
Oppression	Empowerment
Personal tragedy	Social oppression
Instability or regression	Stability or progression
Outsider	Insider
Drain on society	Gainfully employed
Dependence versus independence	Interdependence
Pathos	Hero
Incompetence	Competence
Obligations	Rights
Secrecy and confidentiality	Publicity and unity
Expertise	Experience
Attitudes	Behaviors
Profession driven	Consumer driven
Control	Choice

not abstract concepts or only distally meaningful laws but quotidian events, protections, and civil rights. These sociopolitical elements have effects on our institutions of teaching, research, and clinical practice. Therapy with persons with disabilities must incorporate the sociopolitical into the therapeutic: "It serves the interests of neither professionals nor their clients-indeed, it perpetuates a myth-to ignore people's need for political and economic changes while offering them only clinical treatment" (Biklen, 1988, p. 137). It is difficult to work with populations of persons with disabilities without addressing sociopolitical questions. For example, Jackson and Haverkamp (1991) ask, to what extent should those involved in treatment advocate for social, economic, and political changes that will benefit persons with TBI and their families?

Therapists must be informed about the rights of persons with disabilities, and be prepared to help clients achieve their rights. For example, a client needs flexible leave over a 6-month period for intensive treatment for Hodgkin's disease, or a student with a learning disability requests an essay rather than a multiple-choice exam, or a supervisee with motor difficulties requests assistance with chart keeping. We may declare that we shouldn't give legal advice, but this maneuver won't absolve us of the responsibility for knowing basic laws and rights for persons with disabilities. (After all, we do advise clients about legal issues, such as actions that might be taken if a previous therapy involved a sexual relationship, or if a teenager may be seen in counseling without parental consent.) However, therapists must not induce clients to be forever tilting at windmills.

Countertransference

Therapists are human beings neither immune to nor above the negative socialization to disability. We must be open to honest self-examination of our own responses to clients with disabilities, including negative affect (e.g., anxiety or repulsion) and cognitions (e.g., "I would never live like that"). We must be able to accept clients' intense emotions, such as grief, terror, rage, physical and emotional pain. Persons with disabilities live in the shadow of uncertainty: "Will my impairment get worse?" "Will I have enough energy to do that task tonight?" "Will the building be accessible?" "Will there be handicapped parking?" Disability requires a high tolerance for this uncertainty, as well as for pain, powerlessness, discrimination, and oppression. It is easy for therapists to avoid these issues by downplaying their salience or impact or, conversely, to view the client as heroic for withstanding the onslaught of physical and emotional demands of disability. Disability forces us to recognize that the world is not just, that lightning can strike anyone, and thus we face our own vulnerabilities. Therefore, in addition to tolerating affect in our clients, we must tolerate in ourselves the strong emotional reactions generated by disability. We may experience aversion, repulsion, horror, terror, and sadness. Even those of us with disabilities are likely to hold prejudices and stereotypes against other types of disabilities. Our countertransference issues are likely to include a bias against deviance, defenses against the hopelessness of a disability with no "cure," and feelings of incompetence. We might bolster our professional esteem by convincing ourselves that we are good generalist therapists, and therefore can utilize our skills with most populations of clients. It takes the sturdy among us to face the countertransference and beliefs head on. There probably is no remedy for "able-ism" more powerful than immersing oneself in disability culture, viewing over time persons with disabilities in "normal" functional roles and social interactions. But this is possible only when we encounter the "other" on an equal basis, not as professional and client, helper and helpee.

Case Formulation

Therapists must strive to see the disability as one aspect, but not necessarily the defining aspect, of a human being who comprises many facets. Furthermore, disability should not be decontextualized—it is not a trait floating around on its own but, rather, occurs in the context of a person with other attributes; there is always the disability *and* _____ (gender, age, ethnicity, sexual orientation, etc.). We cannot understand the experience of disability for any one person outside of the context of the ands.

To ensure that disability is not playing an excessive role in case formulation, or an overly minuscule one, we should develop cultural competence in the skill of hypothesis generation at both etic and emic levels, with concomitant openness to disconfirming data. Presence of an impairment, no matter how severe, does not mean it is the presenting problem, or even a major part of the presenting problem. We also must guard against the possibility of the presence of impairment overshadowing other diagnoses (Reiss, Levitan, & Szyszko, 1982).

Competence

Therapists are ethically bound not to practice outside their areas of competence and bear a responsibility to increase knowledge, skills, and proficiencies such that they can formulate cases and develop appropriate intervention strategies for clients with disabilities. Saying that one doesn't treat clients with disabilities is rather like saying one doesn't treat depression—you never know when in the therapy the issue will arise, and the ability to provide treatment for this problem is fundamental to our work.

Therapists must be knowledgeable about how theory and techniques are culture bound, and the effects this has. Therapists must recognize how disability can shape the world view of clients and include understanding of issues of power, submission, subordination, alienation, anger, and wariness. If the therapist is able-bodied, he or she must be familiar with insider–outsider considerations. And it is vital that psychologists understand the effects of specific types of disabilities on standardized tests and assessments and not use tests normed on the able-bodied to derive overly pathologizing assessments of persons with disabilities.

Systems

Disability, like feminist theory, is about "the phenomenology of connection" (Brown, 1990, p. 227). Therapists should recognize that therapy is not just about the client with a disability but about broader systems, and he or she should know how to incorporate broader systems into the treatment. At the very least, therapy should be able to include the family. Jackson and Haverkamp (1991) raise a question about how clinicians should respond when disability sequelae (e.g., forgetfulness leading to leaving a stove on) violate the rights or safety of family members.

Therapists may have to incorporate even broader systems into the treatment, such as personal attendants, other types of caregivers, the medical service delivery system, orthotists, state departments of rehabilitation, and so on. In addition, the family will interact frequently and often in times of great stress with these service delivery systems. It is important to recognize that persons with disabilities and their families generally have a full and often negative history with these systems. It falls to the therapist to be able to integrate these systems, with their disparate cultures and goals, into a cohesive treatment approach.

There are even bigger systems, such as the American Psychological Association (APA) accreditation process for programs and internships, ethics codes, institutional and organizational systems, and funding sources. Not all psychologists see their work as incorporating these larger systems. But it is hard to work with families or students with disabilities without feeling the direct effects of such systems on the lives of persons with disabilities. For example, in our recent APA-accreditation site visit I raised the question of who holds the responsibility of providing reasonable accommodations to practica students and interns with disabilities. Because this question has been largely unaddressed, such students too easily fall through the cracks of service provision.

Disability and ?

We have a responsibility not to define away "minority status" by asserting that all people are different or dismissing the minority experience by stating that all people have "handicaps" of one kind or another and we must learn about each client individually. We must not trivialize the minority experiences of prejudice, stigma, discrimination, and devaluation. Nor should we do among ourselves what others do to us, by considering only one minority status at a time while excluding others. For example, the organized disability community is mostly Caucasian. At the disability conferences I've attended the blacks are from Africa, and African Americans and other ethnic minorities from the United States are notably scarce. Some attendees also complain that we duplicate in our organizational structure the hierarchy of acceptability of disabilities and exclusion of inconvenient disabilities.

Disability as Part of Diversity

The role of disability in diversity training should not be underplayed. We must bear the responsibility of ensuring that disability topics are richly incorporated into such training, and we must not wait for persons with disabilities to force the issue. There probably never will be a sufficient critical mass of faculty or students with disabilities to demand a place for disability issues in the curriculum. Most programs have one or no students with disabilities at any one time.

Many training programs and clinical training programs have made the choice to focus diversity training on race. The idea is that racism is so pervasive that we must start there before moving on to other minorities. But, precisely because racism is so pervasive, this issues will never be "finished." However, whenever people discuss opening up the minority arena to other groups (e.g., gays and lesbians, persons with disabilities, the elderly), there is a fear that this more broadly defined target group will be used to avoid or divert attention from the difficult issues of racism. This is a real concern. However, if the door that is opened a crack for race is not held open long enough to let disability squeeze through, disability will never become the subject of attention. As difficult as issues of race and racism are, the issues related to disability are also difficult. We must pay attention to disability issues, take the initiative, and do it now. We can mingle minorities in our training.

Teaching

Teaching is more than the imparting of knowledge:

> An implicit assumption in much educational research is that teaching centers around the transmission of information and the cultivation of certain cognitive skills. Yet we would argue that many transformations of central concern to teachers generally, and to teachers of psychology in particular, fall in the realm of belief and attitude change. That is, teaching is at a fundamental level a process of persuasion. (Friedrich & Douglass, 1998, p. 549)

The field of disability studies is about persuasion and is both an academic pursuit and a political act. It is owned by persons with disabilities. It asserts that the study of disability is mainstream: "Disability studies is no more an optional 'additive' to the liberal arts than is the study of gender or race." (Bérubé, 1998, p. x). Why do people on the privileged side of race, gender, and/or sexual orientation support laws and movements and studies that may never affect them directly, but view disability studies, which may one day pertain directly to them, as special? "The field of disability studies is even more marginal in the academic culture than disabled people are in the civic culture" (Linton, 1998, p. 3).

The modal number of courses on disability in APA-accredited clinical and counseling programs is zero (Olkin & Paquette, 1994). What is the meaning of this? "The curriculum is a manifest expression of the cultural values just as laws are manifest expressions of what a society deems to be right or wrong behavior" (Kliebard, cited in Linton, 1998, p. 1). Yet disability studies would seem to be a logical and intrinsic part of clinical psychology training. By omitting disability studies from training programs, our inaction is tantamount to a political stance that reinforces the marginalization of people with disabilities. If we hope to increase the representation of persons with disabilities in the profession, then as mentors and guides for a new generation of persons with disabilities we must show that we have set a place for them at the table.

Research

Regarding research, we have a responsibility to understand the different models and paradigms of research on disability (Olkin, 1997) and to be aware of how research is used and misused against those it studies. We should include persons with disabilities in all normative samples. Research is no longer needed that compares "disabled" and "normal" populations.

The "social relations of research production . . . are built upon a firm distinction between the researcher and the researched" (Oliver, 1992, p. 102). Traditionally, able-bodied persons have been the researchers and persons with disabilities have been the researched. This has allowed a disconnection between the authentic voices of persons with disabilities and the professional and academic empirical literature about such persons. We must bridge that gap by allowing persons with disabilities to be the researchers and the researched and by including voices of disability in research seemingly not about disability.

CLINICAL EXAMPLE AND A CHALLENGE
TO THERAPISTS

The ideas in this chapter may seem obvious and prosaic. But if they were easy to implement, people with disabilities would not experience such pervasive discrimination, and I would not hear such horror stories from clients with disabilities about what their previous therapists said to them. Before we declare that *we* are not like *that*, let me issue you a challenge to take responsibility for an assessment of your own values, beliefs, cognitions, perspectives, and behaviors as a therapist who might see clients with disabilities. Read the following clinical example, then respond to the questions that follow.

> Sally is a Latina married woman in her early 30s with two young children. She had polio as a child in Mexico. As a result, one leg is 2 inches shorter than the other, her back is severely curved in a hunched position, and her arms are smaller than expected and of limited utility. In recent years she has experienced an increase in pain, fatigue, and muscle weakness (the hallmarks of postpolio syndrome).
>
> Sally works in administration for a school district but feels that she is "hidden in the back room." Her face is of average prettiness, but her hair is cut in an unflattering short style because it is difficult for her to wash, brush, or style her hair. She mostly wears pantsuits to work to hide her leg length and girth differential and the brace on one leg, and she doesn't wear scarves or jewelry because they are too hard for her to put on. She has interviewed unsuccessfully for other positions and feels that her disability, particularly her deformed look, has prevented her from getting job offers. Her marriage is stable but unhappy; she has frequent thoughts of leaving but thinks she cannot leave the marriage because she depends on her husband for physical care and housekeeping tasks, could not support herself and her children on her salary alone, and is convinced that no other man would date her, so she would be alone for the rest of her life. She is worried about the effects of aging on her disability and her long-term survivability. She presents in therapy as someone who is angry and hopeless.

Questions

    1. Sally wants to apply to the clinical psychology program where you are on the faculty. What might be your reasons to admit her and not to admit her?

    2. How willing would you be to work with Sally as a client? In

what ways do you think you are competent to do so, and what are the areas in which you do not feel competent?

3. Make a list of what you believe are all of the presenting problems, then list them in order of priority in your opinion and in what you think would be Sally's opinion. How are the lists the same or different?

4. What role has discrimination, prejudice, and oppression played in Sally's current situation? What is the relative contribution of her ethnicity and disability status to these factors?

5. What is your case formulation, and what are the roles of disability, ethnicity, and gender in this formulation?

6. How receptive do you think Sally will be to therapy with you? What do you imagine to be the areas of alliance? of resistance? of countertransference?

7. Have any ideas in this book persuaded you to see this case differently than you might have before you read it? Why or why not?

CONCLUSIONS

Should persons who are members of a minority group, whether based on ethnicity, sexual orientation, gender, or disability status, be offered treatment that affirms their minority status as a positive and valued attribute? As it turns out, this is the easier question. The harder questions arise after we answer that first question "Yes, of course." It is in the implementation of minority-affirmative therapy that the complexities and conflicts are manifest, and where countertransference feelings, unspoken values, cherished beliefs, and therapeutic persuasions are most challenged.

On the final page of the novel *The Fixer* (Malamud, 1966, p. 271), Yakov, a hapless Jew in Czarist Russia, having undergone a systematic stripping of his liberty and dignity, thinks, "There's no such thing as an unpolitical man, especially a Jew. You can't be one without the other, that's clear enough. You can't sit still and see yourself destroyed." For minorities in the United States, there is no such thing as an unpolitical therapy.

FOURTEEN

Research on Disability: Shifting the Paradigm from Pathology to Policy

So many treatises end with a call for more research that the final section is almost invariably the semiobligatory list of three or four more urgently needed studies. This penultimate chapter focuses on research for a different reason: In place of a clarion call for more data I want to enter a plea for cessation of studies unless and until researchers approach the topic of disability from a different paradigm. Not only will more of the same fail to improve the state of our knowledge about disability or the lives of families with disabilities, but it will be counter-effective by perpetuating the prevailing models of disability. In fact, despite five decades of research on disability, "research findings, per se, seem not to have contributed appreciably to improving the living conditions of people with physical disabilities. Such a conclusion is not new" (Kerr & Bodman, 1994, p. 100).

If research on disability is to prove useful it should help our understanding in such a way that we can provide better services, prevent and ameliorate problems, and make better programmatic and policy decisions, all for the ultimate purpose of improving the lives of those we study. I would argue, as have Kupst (1994) and Harper (1991) about research in pediatric illness and disability, and Kerr and Bodman (1994) about disability research in general, that our research paradigms in the area of disability have not only failed to produce positive changes but have in fact perpetuated a "two-group mentality (normal—disabled)" (Harper, 1991, p. 541) that impedes progress.

The purpose of this chapter is to examine the paradigms that have guided research on disability over the past 50 years. The goal is to examine what questions have been asked, the purposes for which studies were conducted, and the paradigms that have guided the research. I propose five models of research, with a shift in paradigm occurring between the third and fourth models such that the first three models might be conceptualized as representing paradigm I and the latter two models as paradigm II. Paradigm I encompasses the moral and medical models of disability, and paradigm II reflects the minority model. The five models may be viewed as stages—that is, a series of models that seem to follow one another over time (though often getting stuck at model 3, unable to shift out of paradigm I). This pattern seems to characterize much of the research on any out-group (gays and lesbians, persons with disabilities). Sample studies are cited to illustrate the five models. Further, I propose three examples of how one topic can be examined from each of the five models, depending on how the questions are framed, the purpose of the examination, and the methods used. The factors that seem to delimit research on disability are outlined.

BEGINNING INQUIRY

Disability did not become a serious research topic until World War II, when the work force consisted of a greater number of persons with disabilities (and also women). Studies of employees with disabilities indicated that they were equal to or better than their able-bodied counterparts in terms of productivity, absenteeism, safety, lateness, and turnover (Yuker, 1994). Yet under- and unemployment of workers with disabilities again became a problem after the war. Employers continued to cite fears of accidents, absenteeism, reduced productivity, and higher insurance rates as factors in why they did not hire more persons with disabilities. Thus it seemed that *perception* of persons with disabilities was an important variable. Research on such perceptions began in earnest, beginning with the seminal dissertation of Mussen (1943) and the early work of Barker (1948).

Over the past 50 years the choice of research topics within disability has gone in waves, the impetus coming more from legislative activities and funding sources than from serious reflection on either the state of our knowledge or from solid theoretical or conceptual underpinnings, sacrificing importance to convenience. For example, during the 10 or so years (circa 1980) when a sex and disability clinic was funded at the University of California, San Francisco, a journal (*Sex and Disability*) was begun, and research on this topic flourished. When soft monies dried up and the clinic closed, the topic faded from professional inquiry. Indeed, almost all the literature on sex and disability still can be found in the one journal, most of it stemming from the era of this one clinic. Similarly, in the mid-1970s when the Education for All Handicapped Children Act (1975) was enacted, graduate students by the droves wrote dissertations on mainstreaming. But after about a dozen years the interest waned, and research on the topic decreased. Unfortunately, 12 years is inadequate time for a body of research to begin to gel, for dissenting voices to emerge, for critiques of early work to coalesce into improved questions and methods. A meaningful body of research can only develop over time. But time alone is insufficient unless there is also a breakthrough of new ideas, assumptions, questions, methods, or measures.

A typical research sequence is as follows. Initial studies undertake an investigation of a little researched population, say, persons with quiggle (see Chapter 3, in this volume). Quiggle is viewed as an undesirable state and assumed to cause suffering. Researchers therefore construct research questions and hypotheses around pathology, picking populations likely to manifest distress (e.g., inpatients with new diagnoses of quiggle) and measures designed to detect it. The basic questions of this early stage are, "How does quiggle affect persons with quiggle?" and, "What is the burden of quiggle on the family?" For example, early studies repeatedly found high levels of emotional distress in children with cystic fibrosis (CF; Silvers, 1996). After a series of similarly designed (and similarly flawed) studies, the findings are held to be immutable: Persons with quiggle show high rates of anxiety, depression, and distress, and their families show multiple signs of burden. Then someone decides to revisit the question, slightly altering questions, measures, and populations, and discovers that only some people with quiggle show distress while others do remarkably well. This leads to the question of why some people with quiggle do better than others, and the answer that people with quiggle with good mothers do better than those with bad mothers, and that the siblings of children with quiggle mirror marital distress when it is present and do well when it is absent. Now the focus becomes the burden of quiggle on the family, how the family copes, what supports the family utilizes, and the effects of quiggle on the marital relationship. For example, a revisitation of the question of children with CF (Gayton, Friedman, Tavormina, & Tucker, 1977) failed to support previous findings of high levels of distress. Instead, the authors found that most children with CF are not emotionally disturbed and the development of their siblings is not negatively affected. Similarly, it was not until a 1992 review (Bussing & Johnson) that it was concluded that men with hemophilia, as a group, do not differ from healthy controls on measures of psychological functioning.

It is usually at this point that the body of research refuses to grow. Much of the research on disability has stayed mired at this level. How does this cycle keep happening? For one thing, several methodological and conceptual problems riddle the earlier works. Many such studies are based on the assumption that disability creates difficulties in performing social and occupational roles, creating severe and chronic stress, which increases the risk of psychological distress. This assumption stems from the pervasive notion that disability causes suffering (see Chapter 3). Researchers then use a pathogenic filter which looks for and inevitably finds pathology. As Harper (1991) stated in a critique of literature on early-onset disability, the most endemic problem is the "dogma that a child's response to disease/disability is understood or 'framed' in a psychopathological model" (p. 535). Furthermore, data typically are collected from inpatient or outpatient rehabilitation settings and not from the community, and usually from small numbers of people. Often subjects are newly disabled, and the response to the acute stage of disability onset is confused with response over the long term. In keeping with the idea that when disability is present it overrides all other factors, age and gender of subjects are restricted (usually males, often in early adulthood), and ethnicity is almost never mentioned, from which one can infer that most subjects were Caucasian. Such data, coming from small numbers of homogeneous subjects, is not subject to rigorous analysis and instead is "analyzed" using the impressions of the researchers, who are outsiders to the experience of disability and who find what they set out to find. Prejudices, stereotypes, and myths about disability are infused into every stage of the research process until the inevitable outcome is to verify these misconceptions. Outcome measures are often undefined, subjective, or inappropriate for persons with disabilities, and interpretations of scores are made against norms that excluded persons with disabilities. Thus core questions readers should ask about any research related to disability include the following: What is the number of subjects? Was it a community or a clinical sample? What is the length of time since onset of the disability? What are the assumptions of the researchers? How is the data analyzed? What measures are used, do they measure only pathology, are they appropriate for the population, and are they able to be interpreted against appropriate norms? Whether we are constructors or consumers of research, we must not read with unconditional positive regard.

There is another possibility for how early research finds endemic pathology whereas later research fails to substantiate earlier findings. Suppose there are two distributions of "scores" on an infinite variety of measures of mental health (see Figure 14.1). One distribution represents the population of persons with disabilities and the other the population of

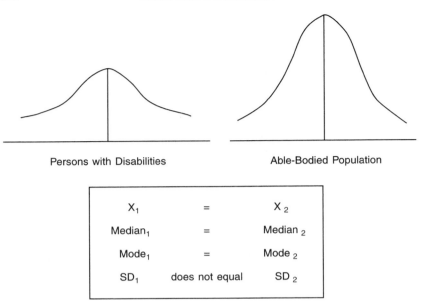

FIGURE 14.1. Hypothetical distribution of scores for the population of persons with disabilities and the able-bodied population.

able-bodied persons. Each distribution is a bell-shaped curve. However, the disabled distribution is flatter and wider than the other. Under these circumstances, the means, medians, and modes of the two distributions are equal but the standard deviation is not. Most important, for the disabled distribution a greater proportion of the population lies at the two extremes of the curve. Thus, a study that sampled from the lower end of the two population curves would find that more people with disabilities manifested symptoms of pathology. When early studies sample from clinical populations, this is indeed what they find. However, if the other end of the curve were sampled (e.g., people with high levels of achievement), this too would yield a higher proportion of persons with disabilities. For example, a recent study of siblings of ventilator-dependent children (Baldwin, 1997) found that these siblings were doing not just well but remarkably well. How can we understand both this result and earlier studies showing greater distress in such siblings? It can be explained by differences or flaws in methodology, by differences in populations sampled, or by conceptualizing the distribution of scores as just outlined.

One way to provide a panoramic view of research on persons with disabilities is to examine trends in dissertation topics over time (Table 14.1). These data give a flavor of the outside boundaries of the field. As can be seen, the least studied topics are technology, family studies, and social and cultural aspects of disability (the crux of the minority model). Technology studies were absent until 1986. This may at first seem obviously related to recent advances in technology including the advent of the personal computer, entrance into the information age, and home use of technology once purely hospital based (e.g., dialysis). But bear in mind that technologies such as wheelchairs, crutches, and prostheses have been around for a long time. Thus there may be a second explanation, which is that until these newer technologies became widely available no one simply thought to ask questions about the relationship of persons with disabilities and the technologies on which they relied. A second newer area of inquiry, "social and cultural aspects of disability," made its debut in 1984 and marks an important shift in disability research, signaling the critical passage from paradigm I to paradigm II.

FIVE MODELS OF RESEARCH

I propose five models of disability research as a way of organizing the literature in this area. The five models reflect how the questions are framed, the goals of the researchers, the perspective of the researchers on several key issues (e.g., pathologizing vs. exploration), the degree to which the voice of those with disabilities is honored or ignored, the methodology selected, and how the outcome is intended to and will be used. It is important to note that no issue is inherently linked to one

TABLE 14.1. Number and Percentage of Dissertations in 10 Categories, 1954–1993

Category	No. of studies	% of total
Predictive outcome studies	674	27%
Program and policy studies	407	16%
Intervention studies	396	16%
Attitudes and attitude change	343	14%
Professional issues	301	12%
Assessment instrumentation and development	175	7%
Family studies	110	4%
Social and cultural aspects of disability	30	1%
Technology studies	20	<1%
Miscellaneous	18	<1%

Note. Data combined and adapted from Leahy, Habeck, and Fabiano (1988, 1989); Leahy, Habeck, and VanTol (1992); Leahy, VanTol, Habeck, and Fabiano (1990); Lofaro (1983).

model or another; any issue can be examined from each of the five models. In the following discussion I describe the five models and provide examples. (Although I supply titles of papers, many of these titles are fictitious, and any copying of real titles is unintentional. However, the format of the titles, which are an amalgam of many studies, closely conforms to those in the literature.) To further illustrate the models, Table 14.2 presents three potential research issues and shows how they might be studied using each of the five models.

Models 1 through 3 can be grouped in paradigm I which can be characterized as follows: static, viewing difference as equaling deficit, pathology oriented, predominantly intrapsychic, guided mostly by psychodynamic theory, about but not by persons with disabilities, working toward amelioration or prevention of problems, sees those with disabilities as "high risk," and relies on methodology based on we–they, using either the able-bodied as norms or other outcast groups (e.g., convicts) as norms. The research questions, methods, and interpretations in paradigm I reflect the moral and medical models of disability. Paradigm II, which embodies models 4 and 5, reflects the minority model of disability. It shifts to a systemic perspective; views adaptation as a fluid process; inquires about health and resilience; considers disability as a culture; views the major problems of disability as prejudice, discrimination, and denial of civil rights; looks for information and solutions in public policy and legislation; and tends to be not only about but by persons with disabilities. These different assumptions inherent in the two paradigms are fundamental in guiding research. All too often "the way we see the problem . . . is the problem" (Harper, 1991, p. 534).

Model 1

This first stage focuses on the basic question, "Who are these people?" It explores how the reference group (i.e., people with disabilities) differs from the "norm" (here defined as able-bodied people). It asks, "What are the attributes of persons with disabilities?" Its basic inquiry is firmly entrenched in a two-group mentality, what Meyerson and Michael (1962) called "sheep and goats" research. It seeks differences and therefore not surprisingly finds them, then attributes these differences to the disability status. An assumption is that psychological theories (e.g., of development) are sufficient to describe all persons, and if they fail to apply to persons with disabilities it is because such persons are deviant. Standard assessments and instruments are used in a one-size-fits-all approach, despite the absence of persons with disabilities in groups used to establish norms on tests, unknown effects of disabilities on responses to specific test items, and misinterpretation of results. Although some

TABLE 14.2. Example of How Three Issues Could Be Studied from Each of Five Research Models

Research focus	Model 1	Model 2	Model 3	Model 4	Model 5
Under- and unemployment rates of persons with disabilities	Why some persons with disabilities are employed and others not: A comparison of those with internal and external locus of control	The marital impact of unemployment after SCI	Preparing persons with SCI for the workplace: a social skills model	Improving attitudes of employers toward hiring persons with SCI	Increasing employer compliance with Title I (employment) of the ADA
Students with disabilities in higher education	Predicting academic outcome and social adjustment for vocational rehabilitation clients	How students at two community colleges view their peers with disabilities	Provision of services to students with disabilities: a needs survey on two campuses	Problems in recruitment, admission and retention of persons with disabilities: removing obstacles to equal access	Increasing graduation rates of persons with disabilities from college by early intervention in the education pipeline: an analyses of where monies are best spent
Evaluation of a medical rehabilitation program	Predicting adjustment to SCI in young males: a regression analysis of five personality variables	From the rehabilitation hospital to the family: using the circumplex model to guide transfer of care to the family	Comparison of SCI patients with and without alcohol involvement in the accident: an analysis of the views of family and rehabilitation staff	Training medical residents in emergency room procedures for new SCI: importance of the first 12 hours	How managed care policy affects length of stay and rehospitalization rates of young males with SCI

research never leaves model 1, more often this line of inquiry is rescued by its own findings. After some amount of such research, it becomes clear that (1) persons with disabilities are more alike than unlike persons without disabilities, (2) there are more intra- than intergroup differences, and (3) some persons with disabilities are more well adjusted to their disabilities than are others.

Examples of model 1 research abound. Titles might include such articles as the following: "Self-Esteem of Children with Asthma, Diabetes, or No Disorder"; "Identity and Self-Concept of the Visually Impaired"; "Increased Galvanic Skin Response and Heart Rate in Interactions with Disabled Persons"; "Rorschach and TAT Responses of Normal, Homosexual, and Physically Disabled Undergraduates."

Model 2

This is essentially the model of mother bashing. In seeking to answer the question, "Why are some persons with disabilities more adjusted than other persons with disabilities?" it eventually reaches the obvious answer that persons with disabilities who receive good (or good enough) mothering do better on all measures than do persons with disabilities with more negative, distant, rejecting, or depressed mothers. This leads to research on the mother of the child with a disability, and a prominent question of model 2 is the terrible effects of a child with a disability on the family, a well-worked area. It begins with the assumption—and hence ends with the conclusion—that the person with a disability is a "burden" on the family.

Model 2 is quite prevalent. Recent titles might include such articles as the following: "Caregiver Burden: An Examination of Parental Stress in Caring for a Child with Cystic Fibrosis"; "The Effects of Mental Retardation on Normal Sibling(s)"; and "Infants' Responses to Normal and Distorted Faces: Effects of Mothers' Blindness on Mother–Infant Bonding."

Model 3

Having established how horrible it is for all those around the person with the disability, model 3 focuses on the family system and social environment, though still using a predominantly intrapsychic rather than systemic perspective. It asks about the social, financial, and emotional supports available and used by the family, evaluates coping skills, conducts surveys of persons with disabilities, and gives percentages of responses to each category (e.g., "72% of persons with disabilities depend on private autos for transport"; Fletcher, 1995). It provides data on rates of under- and unemployment, dropout from school, alcoholism and substance abuse, divorce rates of parents after birth of a child with a disability—and assumes that these outcomes stem from the disability. In creating a composite from the statistics generated, the picture that results is bleak. (One can readily see corollaries to research on other groups: number of black males in jail; rate of HIV transmission among gay Latino youth.) Although often conducted for benign or benevolent purposes, a basic assumption of this research is usually that the answers lie in changing "those people." Thus such research serves to further stigmatize the group and provides data that bolsters the view that the group is pathological, abnormal, and different from "us." Model 3 often asks about the attitudes of others toward this group. One frequent finding from model 3 research is that specific groups of people who interact frequently with persons with disabilities (e.g., rehabilitation counselors and special education teachers) have no special immunity to the pervasive negative views of disability, and their attitudes toward disability are as bad as (and in some cases worse than) the general public's. One result is articles designed to reassure us that "these people aren't so scary." An example might be a hearing counselor describing the work he or she did in providing therapy to a deaf client, using an interpreter; the author describes with some authority all that has been learned from this on-the-job training, yet he remains appallingly ignorant of Deaf culture.

Examples from literature of model 3 might include: "Dogmatism, Ethnocentrism, and Attitudes toward the Physically Handicapped"; "Acceptance or Rejection of Students with Disabilities by Special Education Teachers"; "Birth Order, Gender, Self-Concept, and Prejudice against the Physically Disabled"; "Superintendents' and Principals' Attitudes toward Special Education in the Least Restrictive Environment"; "Rates of Substance Abuse in SCI Patients at Five Hospitals"; and "A Poll of Persons with Disabilities Two Years after the ADA."

Major journals reflecting mostly paradigm I (models 1 through 3) include *Rehabilitation Psychology* and *Rehabilitation Counseling Bulletin*. Calls for shifts in paradigms are generally absent in journals devoted to treatment or rehabilitation of persons with disabilities, which usually are well entrenched in the assumptions of paradigm I. Yet in the research of model 3 lies the seeds of growth and change. Imagine, for example, research on rates of substance abuse among recently spinal-cord-injured men. This research might inquire about treatment efficacy at 100 substance abuse treatment centers in a large metropolitan area and in so doing be forced to note that none of these centers are physically accessible to persons with wheelchairs. This observation starts to raise questions about person–environment interaction in a new way, promoting bidirectional research. Further, it becomes repeatedly clear in multitudes of studies that the severity of the disability is not correlated with difficulties in adaptation. This again forces the recognition of contextual and systemic factors. But the leap to model 4 is, frankly, a paradigm shift, and as such requires first an attempt to make explicit the assumptions inherent in previous research and then an open examination of the rationale for those assumptions. Second, it calls for research to become programmatic and additive and to be guided by theory built on a solid conceptual basis.

Model 4

In keeping with the paradigm shift between models 3 and 4, the locus of attention now firmly shifts from persons with disabilities to the social, educational, legal, financial, occupational, and physical world around them. Instead of inquiring about the effects of persons with disabilities on others, the question is about the effects of others on persons with disabilities. Model 4 is interdisciplinary, focusing on bridges and interplay among systems. Analyses and interventions are aimed at the social environment, particularly attitudes (and too infrequently on behavior) of the able-bodied. Employment data might survey Fortune 500 company executives about their attitudes toward hiring employees with disabilities rather than studying how well the employee with the disability is doing on the job. Assessment measures are reexamined for inherent problems that skew results for respondents with disabilities, noting the lack of persons with disabilities in the normative groups and seeking to renorm data appropriate for specific disabilities (e.g., "The Moderating Effect of Spinal Cord Injury on MMPI-2 Profiles: A Clinically Derived T Score Correction Procedure," Rodevich & Wanlass, 1995); the goal is to depathologize the group by using more accurate measures.

Model 4 research is relatively scarce, and most of it is fairly recent. Examples might include the following: "Interventions with Superintendents and Principals to Improve Attitudes toward Special Education in the Least Restrictive Environment"; "An Examination and Renorming of Three Personality Measures Skewed by Disability"; "Deaf Children in Post-Mainstreaming Education: Failure of a System"; "How Cultural Beliefs and Values Affect Treatment of Persons with Disabilities"; and "A Survey of Application Procedures at APA-Accredited Clinical Programs from the Perspective of Applicants with Disabilities."

Model 5

Model 5 is the natural outgrowth of model 4. Having shifted the emphasis from persons with disabilities to the environment, systems controlling that environment are now the focus. These include laws, policies, and regulations and how these are implemented. Social change is the goal, so that persons with disabilities might achieve full access to and equity with the nondisabled world. Two recent journals (*Journal of Disability Policy Studies, Disability and Society*) reflect primarily models 4 and 5.

Examples of research might include the following: "An Evaluation of State Laws Affecting Persons with Disabilities: Recommendations for Legislation"; "Parental Rights of Persons with Disabilities: Why Isn't Parenting on the List of Activities of Daily Living?"; "Who Should Hire and Train Personal Attendants?"; "Using Universal Design to Increase Participation of the Elderly and Persons with Disabilities in Public Parks"; and "Financial Disincentives to Discontinue SSI: A Reevaluation of Policy."

FACTORS LIMITING RESEARCH ON DISABILITY

Kerr and Bodman (1994) argue that a key limitation of current research is the reliance on Aristotelian rather than Galilean modes of thought: "Aristotle was prone to view causes and effects from the perspective of the characteristics of the object itself. He did not place any import upon the characteristics of the environment of the objects. Conversely, Galileo studies the interaction between the characteristics of the object and the characteristics of the environment" (p. 101). These philosophies of science determine "conceptions of (a) lawful behavior; (b) causal variables; (c) useful research variables; (d) productive research questions; (e) appropriate data analyses; and (f) criteria for positive results. Today, this would be called a paradigm" (Kerr & Bodman, 1994, p. 101). In 1984, Asch wrote about factors that limit research on disability. It is disconcerting how many of the same factors remain. Following is a list of those factors that constrain current research on disability:

1. *Failure to include more disciplines.* Disability has been ghettoized into certain circumscribed areas, and virtually ignored in mainstream inquiries. Disability is "a narrow area of specialization outside the mainstream" (Kahn, 1984). There is a lack of cross-fertilization across disciplines. This results in loss of multiperspectives, preventing leaps in conceptualizations and rapid growth of knowledge.

2. *Underrepresentation of minorities.* The obvious disadvantage of this is the absence of minority perspectives and voices at every stage of inquiry. Further, investigation of dual minority status (one of which is disability) has been lacking. Research on minorities excludes disability, and research on disability excludes minorities; each of these stigmatized conditions is considered a defining characteristic and hence studied in isolation.

3. *Underrepresentation of people with disabilities.* It is phenomenal

how undeterred we are from pursuing "outsider" research by the able-bodied about disability. For no other out-group is the pervasive exclusion of voices from within so silent and stilled. Thus the loss to the field is significant, creates a rift between research and practice, and generates a schism between those studied and those doing the studying.

4. *An almost exclusive focus on the effects of persons with disabilities on others.* The perspective continually is from the vantage point of ABs looking from the outside at those with disabilities.

5. *Circumscribed funding.* Most funds are directed at large, well-known medical centers, usually university affiliated. This supports the input from large agencies, limits innovation, and almost guarantees the absence of all but a few token professionals with disabilities. Furthermore, most research and demonstration projects are solicited by governmental calls for proposals and less so from grass-roots or disability community groups.

6. *Exclusion of literature as a source for opinions and learning.* There is no recognized study of literature by persons with disabilities (analogous to black studies or women's studies, which often use literature in their endeavors). Thus a large and growing body of authentic voices is missing and hence does not influence research directions or policy.

7. *Significant problems in tests, measures, and norms.* Research is hampered by insufficient information about testing norms for persons with disabilities, knowledge about effects of specific disabilities on specific tests, and awareness of how interpretations might be altered by the fact of disability. Few tests are designed specifically with persons with disabilities in mind, and too many are pathology oriented.

8. *The focus of research has been too limited and narrow.* For example, there has been intense interest in the effects of disability on work productivity but not on parenting. This reflects the value in our society placed on the work ethic and productivity, and—despite lip service to family values notwithstanding—an undervaluing of parenting. There is a plethora of research on the effects of disability on social interactions: "No further research is needed to show that it is socially disadvantageous to be physically handicapped in initial social encounters . . . the disadvantage is powerful and pervasive" (Richardson, 1976, p. 32). Other topics are virtually ignored (e.g., Have APA-accrediting guidelines had any impact on accessibility of doctoral programs? What percentage of practica and internships have trainees with disabilities?)

9. *Failure to make the paradigm leap.* Research in paradigm I should cease, and resources should be redirected to paradigm II. This requires that people with disabilities be allowed a more prominent and influential role in research at every stage of the process, but most especially in determining the questions worth asking.

CONCLUSIONS

There is little need for further research in paradigm I, especially in models 1 and 2. Model 3 could yield useful survey data provided several assumptions are met: (1) disability should be categorized by function rather than diagnosis, (2) people with disabilities are the best judge of functional needs, (3) the voices of persons with disabilities should be given legitimacy and salience, (4) the goal should not be to examine ways that persons with disabilities are different from "us," and (5) the goal of the research is to examine and improve policies and practices. The presumption of a stage model of adjustment to disability has been discredited and should be replaced with a more fluid, developmental, and contextual model of "response." A greater focus on families is needed, but not from the perspective of the effect of disabilities on the family but rather from the vantage point of how services and policies can maximize family functioning and the effects of the family on the person with the disability. Both the word and the concept underlying the "burden" of people with disabilities on others should be dropped. We should be more explicit about social, political, financial, and educational policies that assume that people with disabilities are a burden and a drain on schools, counties and states, and medical and managed care systems. Collaborative and interdisciplinary models should be valued, promoted, and reinforced. Training of graduate students should incorporate attitudes, knowledge, and skills related to disability. Finally, we might do well to keep in mind the goal of making research on disability a moot point, because persons with disabilities are not "them" but "us."

FIFTEEN

For Teachers
and Supervisors

Students are unlikely to enter graduate training with any formal education about persons with disabilities. For example, a content analysis of introductory psychology textbooks from 1990 on (Hogben & Waterman, 1997) examined coverage of diversity, defined as "racism/prejudice, minority group members, sexual orientation, gender issues, age, AIDS, and multicultural/global issues" (p. 96). This list does not include disability because, as the authors state, they "intended to include issues pertaining to bisexuality and people with disabilities. Unfortunately, textbook coverage in these two areas was so sparse that we were unable to conduct any meaningful analysis" (p. 96). Another study (Bluestone et al., 1996) found that in one graduate psychology curriculum, physical disability received the lowest amount of coverage from a list of many diversity issues (ethnicity, gender, aging, sexual orientation, socioeconomic status, and religion). Indeed, "most professional programs do not include disability issues in their curricula" (Kemp & Mallinckrodt, 1996, p. 378). The modal number of courses on disability in APA-accredited programs is 0 (Olkin & Paquette, 1994).

This does not imply that students arrive at the topic as blank slates. Not only have they been subject to a host of negative and pathologizing messages about disability, but the very absence of persons with disabilities in psychology (in texts, normative groups, or as professors) is a powerful statement about the marginalization of those with disabilities. Thus instructors have to help students unlearn the old as they simultaneously learn the new.

Where is the place for disability in the graduate curriculum in mental health? Most programs are jammed with courses necessary to meet the requirements of accrediting bodies, licensing boards, and basic knowledge for entry-level competence. Shoehorning new content into an already overcrowded curriculum seems daunting, yet something must be done to remedy the situation, as "professional training programs do not adequately prepare students to serve this population [clients with disabilities]" (Kemp & Mallinckrodt, 1996, p. 378). Thus in this chapter I am making what I hope are realistic suggestions for the time frame most programs will have to devote to the topic. By choosing only one of the teaching suggestions, or by mixing and matching, you can create teaching modules ranging from 2 hours to a three-unit semester-long course. The 2-hour modules are designed with courses on "diversity training" in mind (i.e., to fit into existing one- to three-unit courses on diversity). As one study indicates (Bluestone et al., 1996), "multicultural training and training related to other areas of diversity can coexist . . . [c]ourses with the highest ratings for coverage of multicultural content also obtained high ratings across the remaining diversity dimensions . . . these findings . . . may potentially quell the fear . . . that focusing on a broader range of diversity issues will detract from multicultural competence within programs" (p. 398).

The in-class modules can be coupled with some of the suggestions for work outside the classroom (e.g., homework or fieldwork). Clearly these learning modules cannot substitute for supervised experience with clients with disabilities. They can't even substitute for interaction with peers with disabilities. As ever, classroom learning can only take students so far. However, it also shouldn't be given short shrift: "Multicultural training has historically focused on exposure to a diverse client caseload with much less emphasis on formal didactic courses, diverse faculty, supervisors, and multicultural supervision models" (Allison, Echemendia, Crawford, & Robinson (1996, p. 391). "Training," therefore, incorporates coursework, exposure to modeling and mentoring, appropriate and expert multicultural supervision, and clinical experience.

GOALS WITH STUDENTS AND SUPERVISEES

Those who teach future clinicians have an opportunity to profoundly influence the practice of their discipline. Even 2 hours of teaching on disability, if it is the right 2 hours, can open a window so firmly that it can never be closed. "It appears that even a small amount of training on issues of disability may be associated with significantly less bias in case conceptualization and treatment planning" (Kemp & Mallinckrodt, 1996, p. 383). Therefore the primary goal is to influence the cognitions students have about persons with disabilities and to help outsiders see from both the outsider and insider perspectives. That is, the goal is identical to that of this book, namely, to alter the way one thinks about disability. The goal is not attitude change. The perennial weak link between attitudes and behaviors that plagues social science suggests that a focus on attitudes is not the most fruitful target of our resources. Thus the focus is on how one frames disability (i.e., the model of disability), how one views the realm of possible solutions, and on enabling competent care of clients with disabilities in a cross-cultural context (disability–nondisabled). As Asch (1988) said, "psychology can help students shift from thinking of disabilities as 'flaws to be rehabilitated' to viewing the disabled [*sic*] as a minority group with civil rights" (p. 156). This shift can have profound implications for clinicians' treatment of clients with disabilities.

The goal also is not "tolerance." This word implies benign acceptance of the inevitable, as opposed to "appreciation" or "valuing." In an article on how diversity is taught by psychology educators (Murray, 1997), one instructor is quoted as saying that "if all we do is heighten people's awareness of their own prejudices, we've done something" (p. 52). I disagree. In fact, we may do more harm than good by allowing students to think they "get it" while still ignorant of how much they don't get.

In a discussion of the "culturally sensitive psychotherapist," Lopez et al. (1989) discuss the developmental stages of cultural awareness. They conclude that these are not in fact truly stages, that the relationship of ideas inherent in each stage is more fluid than a stage theory implies. However, their remarks on what constitutes a culturally sensitive therapist apply well to treatment of persons with disabilities. A culturally aware therapist should (1) have increased knowledge of the specific culture of the client; (2) be able to organize information more efficiently, with more linkages among concepts; (3) have a better balance of etic and emic views and be able to entertain both views simultaneously; (4) be able to generate more hypotheses, at both emic and etic levels, and know how to assess them; and (5) be more open to information disconfirming the hypotheses. These are valuable and culturally sensitive skills for those learning to work with clients with disabilities.

Another goal is to develop and mentor students and supervisees with disabilities such that more people with disabilities are able to enter the mental health field. Minority faculty are more likely than non-minority faculty to actively engage in minority issues in teaching and supervision. For example, in the review of textbooks in psychology cited previously (Hogben & Waterman, 1977), the authors found that female authors, more than male or mixed-gender authorships, "covered some diversity issues to a significantly greater extent" (p. 95). Another study, on graduate psychology curriculum (Bluestone et al., 1996), concluded that "the most profound implication of this study emanates from the dramatically superior coverage of diversity content by women and faculty of color" (p. 398). This makes a strong case for affirmative action in recruitment, retention, tenure, and promotion of minority faculty, who bring special competencies, interests and enthusiasms that enrich the field.

FOR SUPERVISORS OF STUDENTS
WITH DISABILITIES

The worst stories I've heard from students with disabilities relate to their experiences with clinical supervision. Supervisors, because they have ultimate responsibility for clients, may be using that charge as license to express prejudicial and discriminatory perspectives to the supervisees. Examples are legion. A blind student is told that clients will want to "take care of her." A student with a profound stutter is told that "talk therapy" is a poor choice for her, and no clients get assigned to her. A student with moderately severe physical disabilities is denied a placement at a college counseling center because it was felt that he wouldn't be able to relate to the social and sexual concerns of able-bodied college students. Often supervisees are asked to prove to the supervisor that they are able to "handle" the disability in a clinically appropriate manner before they can be assigned clients. This extra hoop does not exist for able-bodied students, who are expected to be novices at the practice of psychotherapy in their early years of supervision and are not asked to demonstrate skills before being given a chance to practice them with clients. My own experience is that the only people who were ever deeply bothered by my disability and saw it as a fundamental impediment to treatment were supervisors. I know only too well the no-win situation this presents for the supervisee. Protestations that the disability is not a problem for the clients inevitably lead the supervisor to pronounce that the supervisee is "denying" the disability. This is ironic, given that the supervisor is not letting the supervisee forget for one instant that he or she has a disability! Once this cycle of accusation and defense begins it can propel itself endlessly.

A review of client attitudes toward therapists with disabilities shows mixed results, but overall, clients do not mind if the therapist has a disability and in some circumstances prefer such a therapist over an able-bodied one. Clients' transference to therapists with disabilities often imputes to the therapist an intimate understanding of how it feels to be the outsider and underdog, to experience pain and struggle. None of the 1,000 or so clients I've seen have objected to my disability as a condition of treatment.

But perhaps they were unable to tell me, or felt they had to protect me? I like to think that I am a good enough clinician to tell if and when this was happening; after all, I am able to detect clues for other unconscious material. But you see how hard it is for me to try to convince you that *it is not a problem for clients*? Everything I say can be turned to make me sound as if I am in denial, closed to unconscious material of clients, oblivious of the impact of my disability on clients. As an experienced clinician, I am able to garner evidence to the contrary because I have clinical experience to draw on. Imagine how difficult it would be for me if I were a clinical tyro. This is the position in which many students with disabilities find themselves. My suggestion is simple: Give the supervisee with a disability the same right to try, and to be good, mediocre, or lousy, as you would any other supervisee. Rather than talk about disability as an abstract, listen to tapes of sessions and see if and when the disability seems to be a manifest part of the treatment. Disagreements then can be focused on specific incidents rather than on global concerns about the supervisee, and can be adjudicated by a consultant with expertise in disability. To do any less is to enact prejudice in such a way as to create a blockage in the path to joining the profession, one that will stop many budding professionals with disabilities in their tracks.

USING MULTIPLE METHODS

Goals common to teaching students to work with clients with disabilities are to reduce students' anxiety and increase their self-efficacy. Bandura (1977) hypothesized that self-efficacy beliefs could be acquired and modified through four routes: past performance, vicarious learning, social persuasion, and emotional or physiological arousal. Classroom methods that provide positive experiences with role-plays with "clients" with disabilities, demonstrate skills, impart new ways of conceptualizing people with disabilities, use persuasion to demystify and depathologize clients, and lower affective and physiological arousal in the presence of disability can all be expected to yield an increase in self-efficacy. Theoretically self-efficacy should be related to actual clinical performance, though at least one study found the opposite results (Rudolf, Manning & Sewell, 1983).

Lecture Topics

As every teacher knows, lecturing only gets you so far. But there are some topics within disability that lend themselves more readily than others to didactic presentation. The goal of lectures is to impart knowledge about persons with disabilities that students otherwise are unlikely to acquire. But it also is important for students to have contact with people with disabilities. Even if the instructor has a disability, students should not be allowed to assume that one person with a disability speaks for all. One way to achieve some minimal exposure is to have a panel of speakers with differing disabilities come to the class and present on similar topics, exposing students to varying perspectives and to allow them to see similarities and differences among persons with disabilities. Topics could include types of disability experiences, examples of discrimination and strategies for coping, impact of the family's views of disability, dating and sexuality, and communication about disability. Ideally the panel will comprise persons with varying disabilities, including blindness or low vision, deafness and sign language use, cognitive impairment, physical or mobility disability, learning disability, and a hidden physical or systemic disability. Speakers could include not only persons with disabilities but family members of persons with disabilities.

Textbooks and Other Readings

Texts should augment and complement, rather than supplant, lectures, class discussion, exercises, films, and other classroom activities. In addition, voices of people with disabilities should be included; instructors should guard against using only materials by able-bodied authors. Good texts include Charlton (1998), Davis (1997), Linton (1998), Nagler (1993), Quinn (1998), or Wright (1983). Particularly good books on specific disabilities include Ablon (1984), Finger (1990), Fries (1997), LeMaistre (1993), Mairs (1997), Mehta (1985), Preston (1994), Sacks (1989), and Zola (1982b).

It may be that students will spend only one class period on persons with disabilities. My tendency when time is so limited has been to have students read Olkin (1993) or Chapter 1 or 2 (in this volume) as homework and use the classroom time for more interactive activities (e.g., a panel, or the first exercise discussed under classroom activities.) I choose this article because it lays out many of the essential aspects of disability experience. However, I find that students are remarkably unpersuaded by this article, perhaps because it does not generate much affect, while actual contact with persons with disabilities arouses a great deal of affect. Thus it should be coupled with classroom activities that approach the topic in a more visceral way.

Experiential Learning

Another term for experiential learning is "sensitization," which Green (1996) defines as "helping students develop a comfortable awareness of 'not knowing everything,' and an enthusiasm for learning about and forming multiple identifications with a different cultural group" (pp. 390–391). Students do not always seem to embrace learning about different cultures with the enthusiasm and openness we might wish. Perhaps this is understandable from a developmental perspective: Students may resist learning about other cultures because this learning often comes at a point in their training when they are just beginning to consolidate a small but growing sense of competence which they are reluctant to give up so soon. One inducement to learning about disability is to reduce the anxiety that disability can engender and to increase students' sense of capabilities. Thus "sensitization" includes "desensitization"— the need for students to be able to look at persons with all types of disabilities without fear, visible shudders, marked discomfort, and obvious eye movement manipulations either to stare or to avoid staring. Because this is not likely to be the case at first, it is better if they can practice initially through movies, videotapes, and role-plays rather than with real clients with disabilities.

Experiential learning can take place through personal contact with persons with disabilities. As discussed in Chapter 3 (in this volume), personal contact is an essential means of reducing negative stereotypes about persons with disabilities and increasing positive attitudes. However, that contact must be as peers, cooperative and positive for beneficial effects to accrue. Limiting contacts to clients cannot be expected to improve attitudes. Thus instructors and supervisors have to instigate other types of contacts between students and persons with disabilities.

There are numerous experiential activities that incur a similar process: tremendous student anxiety and trepidation at first, followed by the actual doing of the task, resulting in great relief of anxiety. For example, I have had students make phone calls using a TTY (which we have available at our school), or call our TTY line using relay services (listed under State Relay Services in the phone book). They experience acute anxiety about using the TTY and are surprised at how much using it just a single time defuses the anxiety.

Other activities have a different effect: They increase frustration and provide a glimpse of some of the additional difficulties persons with disabilities encounter. For example, students can be asked to find out the exact procedures for applying as a client to the Department of Rehabilitation. Or, they can research specific information on access and services (e.g., How high should elevator buttons be? What is the correct slope of a ramp? Do temporary employees with disabilities have the same rights for accommodations as permanent employees? With what agency should a complaint about wrongful termination be lodged?). These exercises expose students to the "insider" world of issues, questions, services, laws, codes, and frustrations that are commonplace for persons with disabilities.

One type of experiential learning merits specific mention. This is the use of "simulation exercises" in which people simulate various disabilities for a period (cf. French, 1992). For example, someone might use a wheelchair for several hours, or people don masks over their eyes and rely on others to lead them, or place muffs over their ears to simulate loss of hearing. I most emphatically discourage the use of such exercises for a variety of reasons. First, they do not in fact simulate disability. For example, being blindfolded does not equal "blindness." Those who are blind have developed different brain pathways, are well practiced in alternate modes of navigation and communication, have developed multiple coping skills, and may have aligned their values in accordance with their status as a person with a disability. They are not inept, helpless, or dependent, as the blindfolded person is likely to be. Second, people who are blind will not regain their sight in an hour as will the person in the blindfold. Part of the experience of disability is the experience of "forever"—the disability and the person are joined for a lifetime. Simulating a disability for an hour, several hours, even all day in no way approaches the psychological impact of "forever." Third, these exercises focus on the physical aspects of a disability, that is, on the "impairment" or "handicap," not the "disability." This makes sense only to those who don't have disabilities—that is, ABs think of disability as losses of physical or sensory functions (e.g., deafness means not being able to hear; paraplegia means not being able to walk), but a major point in this book is that disability is a social construct. Fourth, the locus of the impairment in simulation exercises is most decidedly within the individual, whereas the minority model of disability emphasizes problems and solutions that reside in society. People with disabilities repeatedly assert that the interpersonal and social arenas are the main "handicaps" associated with disability. When you sit down in a wheelchair your world changes, not because you cannot walk but because from that moment on most people will treat you differently, and even small quotidian interactions are fraught with messages about your disability status. This pervasive and powerful experience cannot readily be simulated. Fifth, there is no evidence that simulation exercises "work," in the sense that they alter cognitions about or attitudes—much less behaviors—toward persons with disabilities. Two reviews of almost 60 studies on simulation exercises noted negligible effects (VanSickle, 1986) or even negative effects (in 29% of the 58 studies reviewed by Shaver, Curtis, Jesunathadas, & Strong, cited in Kiger, 1992). Such exercises can evoke hopelessness, discouragement, and pity—the very ideas these exercises hope to dispel (Asch, 1988). Although participants often use such words as "enlightening" and "meaningful" to describe their experiences, this view often is unaccompanied by changes on objective measures (Pfeiffer, 1989). Furthermore, Wright (1975) describes a study in which undergraduates who had undergone a simulation exercise had ratings on a semantic differential scale indicating that their feelings while in the wheelchair during simulation were "weak, bad, and anxious"—the very stereotypes one would hope to overcome. Sixth, a serious problem is that students who've undergone disability simulation may think they now "get it" and arrest their further exploration of disability. Seventh, several ethical issues are raised in using these exercises (see Kiger, 1992), requiring thought about our responsibilities to those who participate, those in the community with whom they interact, and the institution in which the exercise takes place. Eighth, but certainly not least important, I find it rude for people to "imitate" me as a way of understanding my minority status. It implies that only through direct experience can one come to understand "minority status," as if the word of people with disabilities isn't good enough. For no other minority status do we direct students to use imitation as a means of enlightenment.

Classroom Activities

I find that one of the most useful initial activities is for me to give a brief lecture on the three models of disability and then have students generate a list on the blackboard of ways in which disability is like other minority groups. Doing the exercise together as a class has much greater impact than reading lists of similarities and differences, because in generating items students actually think about the concepts, and they are much more likely to understand at a deeper level what it means to call people with disabilities a "minority group."

Having student debates is useful, assigning positions on the debate randomly. Students should be asked to prepare for the debate rather than simply using their own thoughts on the subject. Topics that lend themselves to this kind of activity are ones that generate a certain amount of affect. These tend to include physician-assisted suicide, genetic testing, whether laws can alter attitudes, and public transportation (e.g., should all buses, or only some, be required to be accessible, the use of paratransit as an alternative to public transportation, and whether people with disabilities should get reduced fares on rapid transit systems).

Small-group activities often encourage more intimate sharing of ideas, are less threatening to some students, and encourage quieter students to participate more. Good topics for this venue include body image (where it comes from, norms, how body image affects self-esteem), analysis of case studies, sharing of personal experience with disability, and discussion of vignettes. Students in small groups can design a brochure for an organization (the school, internship site, community agency, etc.)

to help recruit persons with disabilities either as clients, students, or therapists. In doing so they must consider how to make the information available in alternate formats for persons with varying disabilities.

Role-plays are an essential aspect of training therapists to work with clients with disabilities. However, when students with disabilities are in the class, they are unfairly burdened with continually playing the client, and if there are no students with disabilities, the analog therapy situation too remotely mirrors the real one. It is hard for students without disabilities to role-play clients with disabilities realistically. Yet students need to first observe and then practice assessment and intervention strategies and techniques with clients with disabilities. They especially need to practice asking about the disability, questioning whether the disability plays a role in presenting problems, and discussing specific aspects of how disability might affect treatment. A way out of this dilemma is to hire students with disabilities (not necessarily in your program or agency) willing to role-play or to hire persons with disabilities (in Los Angeles or New York, just open your front door and yell, "Actor needed!").

Reading of fiction or short personal essays related to disability is a good way to enter the subject less cerebrally and more viscerally. Students can read the work before class, but reading the piece out loud in class is often quite affecting. Discussion can start with students' personal reactions but should not stop there. The point is not to discover what students feel but to examine how these feelings affect case formulation and treatment.

Structured student presentations, individually or in groups, is a useful tool for getting students immersed in the literature. Topics should be specific, and instructors need to give prior approval to topics to avoid students choosing areas in which there is either too little or too much literature. For example, the topic "attitudes toward disability" is enormous. More manageable subtopics would be "attitudes of doctors toward patients with disabilities," "classroom strategies to alter attitudes toward disability," and "comparison of instruments used to measure attitudes toward disability." Other topics might include effective strategies for school-to-work transition; changes made in the most recent reauthorization of the Individuals with Disabilities Education Act and their implications for the profession; positive effects on siblings of a child with a disability; adapted baby-care equipment for mothers with visual impairments; use of measures of depression with Deaf clients; and disability pride. What is key is that students adopt a minority model perspective in their reviews.

I usually allow students to write any question they have always wanted to ask a person with a disability on an index card and turn it in (anonymously). I try to answer the question, I may have the class try to generate answers, I may have them do library research to find the answer, or fieldwork to collect answers from different people. We also talk about why the question is so hard to ask, and how as clinicians they can use this process to understand both their own and clients' process in therapy—how they might avoid asking clients about topics that are anxiety provoking, and how clients might avoid bringing up material that is embarrassing.

Videos, Films, and Other Media

The way in which the media depict persons with disabilities is an important topic in itself. Like other minority groups, the disability community has complained that its image in the media is mostly notable for its absence but then is distorted and inaccurate in the little attention that is paid to it. A good exercise is to have students collect all discussion, pictures, images, stories, and so on, about people with disabilities, for a 1-month period. This exercise yields current examples, which is important in showing that not as much has changed as students may think. For example, students can be given the *Guidelines for Reporting and Writing about People with Disabilities* (Research and Training Center on Independent Living, 1990), and then they use these guidelines to assess current magazine and newspaper features. Another activity is to have students contrast the images of people with disabilities in the media with information learned from a panel of guest speakers with disabilities.

Students can view a half-hour segment of the most recent Jerry Lewis Telethon for muscular dystrophy (on TV in the fall each year) and write a brief reaction paper. They can then read several articles by members of the disability community about why we hate these telethons. Student can then view the same half hour of the telethon and again write about their reactions. (Don't worry about which half hour the student chooses; they're all about the same. But for your own sake, avoid the really bad comedians.)

Second, good use of media makes available many more images of persons with disabilities than can usually be obtained in the classroom. A number of videos are available, but many of them perpetuate negative stereotypes of disability. And there are too few videos of clinical interviews with persons with disabilities or counseling strategies and techniques with clients with disabilities. But videos are a good way to expose students to disability culture. For example, some instructional videos that teach sign language also talk about the Deaf culture and the role of signing in the culture. *Vital Signs: Crip Culture Talks Back* is an excellent introduction to disability culture. *Mending Spirits: Native Americans with Disabilities* shows disability in the context of Native American culture. *Little People* is one of the better videos I've seen; it shows the culture of little people of America and doesn't shy away from the more complex issues of disability. Good popular films include *Coming Home, Rain Man, Mask, My Left Foot,* and *Children of a Lesser God.*

Field Experiences

Interviews are a good choice of field experience. The interview could be with a person with a disability, and questions could include how the disability has affected, if at all, the areas of education, work, transportation, housing, relationships, sexuality, parenting, self-esteem, political views, and friendships. Students can try to ascertain the model of disability inherent in the information given to them in the interview. Learning is increased if more than one person is interviewed using the same semistructured interview, either by the same interviewer or by different interviewers from the class who then compare data. It is also enlightening to interview family members separately about the effects of the disability on the family. A longer-term project would be to assign a student to one family for the course of a semester. In this way the student can examine greater complexity of disability issues, and the context of the disability (i.e., gender, ethnicity, and SES) becomes more salient.

Informational interviews with service providers can help students learn about the professional roles of persons who provide treatment to people with disabilities. Students can combine their interview data to create a more composite picture of a profession: What is the prevailing stance toward clients with disabilities in that profession? What services does that profession provide? How are clients thought of (as consumers, patients, clients, etc.)? How many people with disabilities does the professional see in a week? What are the frustrations of the service providers? How does the culture of that profession complement or clash with disability culture?

Because I do not use simulation exercises with students, I rely on other methods of conveying some of the problems of physical access. One goal of these exercises on access is to refocus students from the perspective of the person with the disability as the problem to ways in which the physical world fails to accommodate persons with disabilities. For example, I have students measure my scooter and its turning radius (a wheelchair would do as well) and then have them take a tape measure everywhere they go for 1 week, to measure each bathroom, doorway, table height, aisle, parking space, and so on, with which they come into contact during the week and keep records of accessibility. They are also to note curb cuts, ramps, steps, and handicapped parking. Another exercise to raise awareness about access issues is as follows: Imagine that a friend who uses an electric wheelchair is arriving at the local airport at 8 P.M. Then, make arrangements to get the friend to your house or to a hotel via public transportation. What were the alternatives? What if it were snowing? Was the hotel shuttle accessible? Did the hotel have accessible rooms?

Another assignment related to access issues is for students to evaluate the accessibility at a particular site (e.g., their practicum site), keeping in mind an array of types of disabilities. To do this assignment the students have to figure out how to obtain state guidelines for building access, find or make a checklist, and then perform the assessment. Or, they can get a list of Alcoholics Anonymous meetings for 1 week and ascertain how many meetings are held in places with wheelchair access. Or, they can call a dozen substance abuse programs and ask whether sign language interpretation is available.

Other Homework Assignments

Other assignments that have proven useful include having students keep a journal of ideas, thoughts, feelings, and reactions to issues presented in class and to stimuli related to disability outside class or write reaction papers to specific topics or readings. They can do a case study of one person with a disability, trying to understand how the disability is part of a complex composite picture of a person and his or her family. Or, they might write a paper on how laws have directly affected their own lives and compare and contrast this with the impact of laws on the lives of people with disabilities.

EVALUATING RESEARCH

As students and supervisees enlarge their understanding of disability issues they will be reading research by and about persons with disabilities. They should not be passive consumers of this research. Much of the research perpetuates stereotypes about persons with disabilities and contributes to a rationale for continued discrimination and segregation.

A first step would be for instructors and students to read Chapter 14 and then evaluate current research on disability. I suggest they select three articles from three of the main disability journals[1] and for each article answer a series of questions:

---

[1]*Disability and Society; Journal of Disability Policy Studies; Journal of Applied Rehabilitation Counseling; Journal of Rehabilitation; Journal of Rehabilitation Administration; Rehabilitation Counseling Bulletin; Rehabilitation Education; Rehabilitation Psychology.*

1. What is the purpose of the study?
2. What are the specific questions of the study?
3. What assumptions underlie the research?
4. What measures were used, are these measures appropriate for use with people with disabilities, and do the normative samples include persons with disabilities?
5. What are the main findings, and how do these fit with what we know from other (nonresearch) sources?
6. What are the policy and legal implications of the findings?
7. What are the likely uses of the research results?
8. How might the results of the study be misused, or used in a way that would be harmful for persons with disabilities?

Four other assignments are useful. In each case the goal of the assignment is to get students immersed in the literature while utilizing their critical faculties to understand and evaluate the assumptions, methods, findings, and implications of the research. The first assignment can be to identify a body of current and important studies in the field (i.e., not those about disability). Then students can evaluate the role (if any) of persons with disabilities as participants in these studies. Were the methods and measures of the study accessible to participants with different types of disabilities? From this exercise, students are likely to become aware that persons with disabilities are rarely included in studies that are not directly about disability issues.

The second assignment would be to investigate the normative groups used for common measurement instruments. These could include the Minnesota Multiphasic Personality Inventory—II (MMPI), the Child Behavior Checklist, the Rorschach, Derogatis Sexual Functioning Inventory, the Beck Depression Inventory, the Dyadic Adjustment Scale, and so on. For each measure the composition of the normative group should be discussed, and an item analysis can be conducted looking for items that might be skewed by the presence of disability. An example from the MMPI is, "Do you experience tingling in your fingers or toes?"—an item which has different meanings if you do or do not have MS or a SCI.

The third assignment is to examine studies of persons with disabilities and look at two factors: (1) To what extent are other minority statuses included (e.g., ethnicity, sexual orientation, and gender)? (2) What comparison groups are used, and in what ways are these appropriate (or not)?

The fourth assignment is to ask students (perhaps working in groups) to take one topic within the broad area of "disability studies" and investigate our present state of knowledge in that topic. Topic areas should be well defined and circumscribed and viewed from a minority model perspective. Examples of topics might include sexuality and women with adult-onset disabilities, effects of simulation exercises on attitudes toward disability, ways to reduce the frequency with which able-bodied drivers park illegally in handicapped parking spots, and rates of depression in early- versus late-onset disability. Once students can articulate the state of the research in a given area, they should develop a list of the important questions to ask. Finally, students can be asked to design studies in that defined area from each of the five research models discussed in Chapter 14 (in this volume).

SUPERVISED EXPERIENCE WITH CLIENTS WITH DISABILITIES

Three elements are essential to training supervisees to work with clients with disabilities: (1) doing the actual work with clients with disabilities, (2) ensuring that those clients are diverse in all the ways that clients without disabilities are (e.g., ethnicity, gender, sexual orientation, and age), and (3) supervision by someone expert in working with clients with disabilities, and who has personal experience with disability. I am especially leery of able-bodied therapists supervising able-bodied trainees to conduct therapy with clients with disabilities. Although it is not necessary to be one to treat one, it is necessary to have had direct training and supervised experience with families with disabilities to be competent to supervise trainees in this area. In my experience the most damaging group (in terms of misinformation, false expertise, and conveyance of damaging stereotypes) are those teachers and supervisors who have just a little experience with disability and therefore feel that they qualify as someone with expertise. In one study (Allison et al., 1996), from a list of 13 cultural groups based on ethnicity, sexual orientation, or disability, practicing psychologists rated their own levels of competence with clients with motor or sensory impairments in the bottom half of the list. Also disturbing was that "a small but troubling number of respondents reported seeing clients despite reporting low levels of competence with that client group" (p. 386). Without training in working with clients with disabilities, therapists are less likely to recognize appropriate themes in treatment. Kemp and Mallinckrodt (1996) have said that "the ability of therapists to recognize potential themes that may be related to disability is an ethical issue" (p. 382). In their study, even small amounts of training in this area improved practitioners' abilities.

In listing skills that therapists must develop to work with clients with disabilities, both the *impairment* and the *disability* must be considered. The following set of skills comes from commingling my own list with two other lists from rehabilitation education (Hosie, Patterson, & Hollingsworth, 1989; Livneh & Thomas, 1997):

1. Understanding of the impact of the political, social, and physical environment on persons with disabilities.
2. Recognition of stigma, prejudice, discrimination, and the role and status of persons with disabilities in our society.
3. Familiarity with the disability rights movement, major laws related to disability, and disability culture.
4. Awareness of the types of disabling conditions, how they differ, and how they affect the psychosocial experience of the person with the disability.
5. Knowledge of the medical, developmental, psychological, familial, sociocultural, ethnic, cultural, political, and spiritual contexts of disabilities and the effects on the person and family with a disability. This includes knowledge of the synergistic effects of dual or triple minority status.
6. Interdisciplinary collaboration and understanding of the roles and culture of other professions involved in services to families with disabilities.
7. Expertise in assessment, diagnosis, case formulation, psychosocial intervention, applications, and evaluation.
8. Specific knowledge of ILM, supported employment, and strategies for transition from school to work.
9. Knowledge of technological advances, assistive devices and technology, and the person-technology interface.
10. Ethical knowledge and practices related to families with disabilities and working within one's area of competence.

MODELING AND MENTORING

Multilayers of modeling are necessary. First, as Green (1996) points out, the organizational structure in which the teaching or supervision is conducted must model sensitivity to issues related to disability, hire and value employees with disabilities, look to appropriate expert consultants for guidance, and uphold the letter and spirit of the ADA and other applicable laws. Second, the supervisee with a disability needs role models of therapists, teachers, and supervisors with disabilities. Third, able-bodied supervisees need positive models of active, working, nonpathological adults with disabilities in order to be able to conceptualize the disability as only one aspect of a client. Fourth, able-bodied teachers and supervisors should model acceptance of the limits of their own expertise in working with diverse clients and demonstrate a process for increasing awareness, knowledge, and skills. Fifth, attention to multicultural issues in general must accompany a focus on disability. "Although the counseling profession has paid considerable attention to infusing multicultural issues in their professional code, the rehabilitation counseling profession has not kept pace" (McGinn, Flowers, & Rubin, 1994, p. 261). Thus ethnicity and disability are rarely discussed together.

One of the ways we continuously provide the wrong modeling comes from the omission of disability in lists of "multicultural" issues. For example, Allison et al. (1996) conducted a study of professionals' training and experience with multicultural populations, including persons with disabilities. Nonetheless, they call for "aggressive recruitment and training of *ethnic minority psychologists*" (p. 386, emphasis added). Where is the clarion call for aggressive recruitment and training of psychologists with disabilities?

DISABILITY IN THE GHETTO

A perennial problem in psychology training has been that multicultural content is rarely fully integrated into curricula (Allison et al., 1996). Diversity training is often in a separate course, and issues related to disability are not usually included. When they are, they are segregated from other topics, even other diversity topics. But "disabilities should *not* be presented as a separate section on 'abnormal' or 'exceptional' people, or only addressed in those sections, which serves only to perpetuate myths and stereotypes" (Asch, 1988; p. 157). Obviously it is best if learning about disability is woven throughout a program and not segregated into one lecture ("Now class, we're going to learn all about people with disabilities in the next 2 hours."). Nor can you simply append culturally relevant content on to the "regular" format because cultural sensitivity requires that the development of the "regular" format is based on culture; the structure must be shaped by culture, not just plastered on afterwards. Nonetheless, I am aware of the difficulty of trying to get up to speed in a new area while maintaining currency in the topics in which one teaches, supervises, researches, and provides therapy. The intent of this chapter is to impart some practical tools for getting started. The time allotted can be as short as 2 hours or expanded well beyond that. My hope is that the ideas presented here will aid you in making good use of the time, however limited.

References

Abberley, P. (1991). Disabled people: Three theories of disability. *Occasional Papers in Sociology*, no. 10, Department of Economics and Social Science, Bristol Polytechnic.

Ablon, J. (1984). *Little people in America: The social dimensions of dwarfism*. New York: Praeger.

Abroms, K., & Kodera, T. (1978). Expectancies underlying the acceptability of handicaps: The pervasiveness of the medical model. *Southern Journal of Educational Research, 12*, 7–21.

Albrect, G., Walker, B., & Levy, J. (1982). Social distance from the stigmatized: A test of two theories. *Social Science and Medicine, 16*, 1319–1327.

Allen, H., Peterson, J., & Keating, G. (1982). Attitudes of counselors toward alcoholics. *Rehabilitation Counseling Bulletin, 26*, 162–164.

Allen, K., Linn, R. T., Gutierrez, H., & Willer, B. S. (1994). Family burden following traumatic brain injury. *Rehabilitation Psychology, 39*, 29–48.

Allessi, D. F., & Anthony, W. A. (1969). The uniformity of children's attitudes toward physical disabilities. *Exceptional Children, 35*, 543–545.

Allison, K., Echemendia, R., Crawford, I., & Robinson, W. L. (1996). Predicting cultural competence: Implications for practice and training. *Professional Psychology: Research and Practice, 27*, 386–393.

Alston, P., & Daniel, H. (1972). Perceived relative impact of disabilities on vocational, educational, and social functioning. *Journal of Applied Rehabilitation Counseling, 3*, 53–59.

Altman, B. (1981). Studies of attitudes toward the handicapped: The need for a new direction. *Social Problems, 28*, 321–337.

Americans with Disabilities Act of 1990, Public Law 101-336, 42 U.S.C. 12111, 12112.

American Psychiatric Association. (1987). *Diagnostic and statistical manual of mental disorders* (3rd ed., rev.). Washington, DC: Author.

American Psychiatric Association. (1994). *Diagnostic and statistical manual of mental disorders* (4th ed.). Washington, DC: Author.

An act to add Section 13660 to, and to repeal Section 13412 of, the Business and Professions Code, relating to disability, California AB 1277, October 10, 1997.

Annon, J. (1974). *The behavioral treatment of sexual problems: Vol. 1. Brief therapy: Vol. II. Intensive therapy*. New York: Harper & Row.

Antaki, C., & Rapley, M. (1996). Questions and answers to psychological assessment schedules: Hidden troubles in "quality of life" interviews. *Journal of Intellectual Disability Research, 40*, 421–437.

Antonovsky, A. (1979). *Health, stress, and coping.* San Francisco: Jossey-Bass.

Antonovsky, A. (1987). *Unraveling the mystery of health: How people manage stress and stay well.* San Francisco: Jossey-Bass.

Architectural Barriers Act, Public Law 90-480, August 12, 1968, 82 Stat. 718 (Title 42, Sec. 4151 et seq.).

Asbury, C., Walker, S., Belgrave, F., Maholmes, V., & Green, L. (1994). Psychosocial, cultural, and accessibility factors associated with participation of African-Americans in rehabilitation. *Rehabilitation Psychology, 39*, 113–121.

Asbury, C. A., Walker, S., Maholmes, V., Rackley, R., & White, S. (1992). *Disability prevalence & demographic association among race/ethnic minority pops in the United States: Implications for the 21st century.* Washington, DC: Howard University Research and Training Center for Access to Rehabilitation and Economic Opportunity.

Asch, A. (1984). The experience of disability: A challenge for psychology. *American Psychologist, 39*, 529–536.

Asch, A. (1988). Disability: Its place in the psychology curriculum. In P. Bronstein & K. Quina (Eds.), *Teaching a psychology of people: Resources for gender and sociocultural awareness.* Washington, DC: American Psychological Association.

Asch, S. E. (1946). Forming impressions of personality. *Journal of Abnormal and Social Psychology, 41*, 258–290.

Badeau, D. (1995). Illness, disability and sex in aging. *Sexuality and Disability, 13*, 219–237.

Baker, B. (1983). Communication disabilities: An overview. *Rehabilitation/World, 7*, 3–7.

Baker, B., Stump, R., Nyberg, E., & Conti, R. (1991). Augmentative communication and vocational rehabilitation. *Vocational Rehabilitation, 1*, 72–83.

Baker, B. L., Landen, S. J., & Kashima, K. J. (1991). Effects of parent training on families of children with mental retardation: Increased burden or generalized benefit? *American Journal of Mental Retardation, 96*, 127–136.

Baldwin, G. (1997). *Experiences of siblings of in-home technology-dependent children.* Unpublished doctoral dissertation, California School of Professional Psychology, Alameda.

Bandura, A. (1977). Self-efficacy: Toward a unifying theory of behavioral change. *Psychological Review, 84*, 191–215.

Barker, R. G. (1948). The social psychology of physical disability. *Journal of Social Issues, 4*, 28–38.

Barnes, C. (1994). Institutional discrimination, disabled people and professional care. *Journal of Interprofessional Care, 8*, 203–212.

Barret, M. (1990). Resources on sexuality and physical disability. In M. Nagler (Ed.), *Perspectives on disability* (1st ed.). Palo Alto, CA: Health Markets Research.

Batavia, A., & Hammer, G. (1990). Toward the development of consumer-based criteria for the evaluation of assistive devices. *Journal of Rehabilitation Research and Development, 27*, 425–436.

Batten, S., Follette, V., & Hayes, S. (1997). Experiential avoidance as a model for understanding psychological correlates of HIV and AIDS: Review, theory, and treatment implications. *Behavior Therapist, 20*, 99–100, 102–103.

Beatty, W. W. (1996). Multiple sclerosis. In R. Adams, O. Parsons, J. Culbertson, & S. J. Nixon (Eds.), *Neuropsychology for clinical practice.* Washington, DC: American Psychological Association.

Beck, R., Janikowski, T., & Stebnicki, M. (1996). Doctoral dissertation research in rehabilitation: 1992–1993. *Rehabilitation Counseling Bulletin, 39*, 165–188.

Beck, R., Janikowski, T., & Stebnicki, M. (1994). Doctoral dissertation research in rehabilitation: 1990–1991. *Rehabilitation Counseling Bulletin, 38,* 2–26.

Beckham, J. C., Burker, E. J., Rice, J. R., & Talton, S. L. (1995). Patient predictors of caregiver burden, optimism, and pessimism in rheumatoid arthritis. *Behavioral Medicine, 20,* 171–178.

Beckham, K., & Giordano, J. A. (1986). Illness and impairment in elderly couples: Implications for marital therapy. *Family Relations, 35,* 257–264.

Begley, S. (1996, July 1). To stand and raise a glass: New research in treatment of paralysis. *Newsweek, 128*(l), 52–54.

Belcastro, F. P. (1987). Hearing impaired. In V. Van Hasselt & M. Hersen (Eds.), *Psychological evaluation of the developmentally and physically disabled.* New York: Plenum Press.

Belgrave, F. Z. (1998). *Psychosocial aspects of chronic illness and disability among African Americans.* Westport, CT: Auburn House.

Belinkoff, C. (1960). Community attitudes toward mentally retarded. *American Journal of Mental Deficiency, 65,* 221–226.

Benedict, M. I., Wulff, L. M., & White, R. B. (1992). Current parental stress in maltreating and nonmaltreating families of children with multiple disabilities. *Child Abuse and Neglect, 16,* 155–163.

Benshoff, J., Janikowski, T., Taricone, P., & Brenner, (1990). Alcohol and drug abuse: A content analysis of the rehabilitation literature. *Journal of Applied Rehabilitation Counseling, 21,* 9–12.

Beresford, B. A. (1993). Easing the strain: Assessing the impact of a Family Fund grant on mothers caring for a severely disabled child. *Child Care and Health Development, 19,* 369–378.

Bérubé, M. (1998). Foreword: Pressing the claim. In S. Linton, *Claiming disability: Knowledge and identity.* New York: New York University Press.

Biklen, D. (1988). The myth of clinical judgment. *Journal of Social Issues, 44,* 127–140.

Blotzer, M. A., & Ruth, R. (1995). *Sometimes you just want to feel like a human being: Case studies of empowering psychotherapy with people with disabilities.* Baltimore: Brookes.

Bluestone, H. H., Stokes, A., & Kuba, S. A. (1996). Toward an integrated program design: Evaluating the status of diversity training in a graduate school curriculum. *Professional Psychology: Research and Practice, 27,* 394–400.

Bogdan, R., & Taylor, S. (1989). Relationships with severely disabled people: The social construction of humanness. *Social Problems, 36,* 135–148.

Bolton, B., & Brookings, J. (1998). Development of a measure of intrapersonal empowerment. *Rehabilitation Psychology, 43*(2), 131–142.

Boyle, P. S. (1993). Training in sexuality and disability: Preparing social workers to provide services to individuals with disabilities. *Journal of Social Work and Human Sexuality, 8,* 45–62.

Bracken, M., & Shepard, M. (1980). Coping and adaptation following acute spinal cord injury: A theoretical analysis. *Paraplegia, 18,* 74–85.

Braden, J. P., & Pacquin, M. (1985). A comparison of WISC-R and WAIS-R Performance Scales in deaf adolescents. *Journal of Psychoeducational Assessment, 3,* 285–290.

Brantlinger, E. (1992). Professionals' attitudes toward the sterilization of persons with disabilities. *JASH, 17,* 4–18.

Brauer, B. A. (1992). The signer effect on MMPI performance of deaf respondents. *Journal of Personality Assessment, 58,* 380–388.

Brauer, B. A. (1993). Adequacy of a translation of the MMPI into American Sign Language for use with deaf individuals: Linguistic equivalency issues. *Rehabilitation Psychology, 38,* 247–260.

Breske, S. (1996). The forgotten ADL. *Advance/Rehabilitation, 5,* 43–48.

Briccetti, K. (1994). Emotional indicators of deaf children on the Draw-a-Person test. *American Annals of the Deaf, 39,* 500–505.

Brooks, N. (1990). Users' perceptions of assistive devices. In *Rehabilitation engineering.* Boca Raton, FL: CRC Press.

Brown, L. (1990). What female therapists have in common. In D. Cantor (Ed.), *Women as therapists.* New York: Springer.

Bruyere, S. M., & O'Keefe, J. (Eds.) (1994). *Implications of the Americans with Disabilites Act for psychology.* New York: Spring Publication Company.

Buchanan. A., & Wilkins, R. (1991). Sexual abuse of the mentally handicapped: Difficulties in establishing prevalence. *Psychiatric Bulletin, 15,* 601–605.

Buck, F. (1980). *The influence of parental disability on children: An exploratory investigation of the adult children of spinal cord injured fathers.* Unpublished doctoral dissertation, University of Arizona.

Buck, F., & Hohmann, G. (1981). Personality, behavior, values, and family relations of children of fathers with spinal cord injury. *Archives of Physical Medicine and Rehabilitation, 62,* 432–438.

Buck, F., & Hohmann, G. (1982). Child adjustment as related to severity of paternal disability. *Archives of Physical Medicine and Rehabilitation, 63,* 249–253.

Buck, F. M., & Hohmann, G. (1983). Parental disability and children's adjustment. *Annual Review of Rehabilitation, 3,* 203–241.

Bussing, R., & Johnson, S. B. (1992). Psychosocial issues in hemophilia before and after the HIV crisis: A review of current research. *General Hospital Psychiatry, 14,* 387–403.

Byrd, E., Byrd, P., & Emener, W. (1977). Student, counselor, and employer perceptions of employability of the severely disabled. *Rehabilitation Literature, 38,* 102–108.

Callahan, J. (1989). *Don't worry. He won't get far on foot.* New York: Vintage Books.

Campodoni, J., & McGlynn, S. (1995). Assessing awareness of deficits: Recent research and applications. In L. Cushman & M. Scherer (Eds.), *Psychological assessment in medical rehabilitation.* Hyattsville, MD: American Psychological Association.

Carpiniello, B., Piras, A., Pariante, C. M., Carta, M. G., & Rudas, N. (1995). Psychiatric morbidity and family burden among parents of disabled children. *Psychiatric Services, 46,* 940–942.

Center for the Future of Children. (1996), *6,* 2.

Chan, F., Lam, C., Wong, D., Leung, P., & Fang, X. F. (1988). Counseling Chinese-Americans with disabilities. *Journal of Applied Rehabilitation Counseling, 19,* 21–25.

Charlton, J. I. (1998). *Nothing about us without us: Disability oppression and empowerment.* Berkeley: University of California Press.

Cherry, L., & Tusler, A. (1991). *National policy and leadership development symposium: Stanford, 1991.* Unpublished manuscript, Institute on Alcohol, Drugs, and Disability.

Cohen, J. (1963). Employer attitudes toward hiring mentally retarded individuals. *American Journal of Mental Deficiency, 67,* 705–713.

Cohen, L. J. (1998). *Mothers' perceptions of the influence of their physical disabilities on the developmental tasks of children.* Unpublished doctoral dissertation, California School of Professional Psychology, Alameda.

Cohen, S. B. (1986). Parents' attributions of exceptionality: Social distancing effects in the mainstreamed classroom. *Remedial and Special Education, 7,* 48–53.

Cohen, T. (1996). *Variables predicting out-of-home placement of adults with mental retardation: A comparison among Latino, African-American, and Caucasian parents.* Unpublished doctoral dissertation, California School of Professional Psychology, Alameda.

Collins, K. D. (1997). I teach. *New Mobility*, May, p. 12.

Condeluci, A. (1989). Empowering people with cerebral palsy. *Journal of Rehabilitation, 55*, 15–16.

Conley-Jung, C. (1996). *The early parenting experiences of mothers with visual impairments and blindness*. Unpublished doctoral dissertation, California School of Professional Psychology, Alameda.

Cornelius, XX (1995). Continuity of care for minorities with disabilities. Paper presented at the annual meeting of the Western SSA (XX). XX

Crandell, J. M., & Streeter, L. (1977, Spring). The social adjustment of blind students in different educational settings. *9*, 1–7.

Crewe, N. (1993). Spousal relationships and disability. In F. P. Haseltine, S. Cole, & D. Gray (Eds.), *Reproductive issues for persons with physical disabilities*. Baltimore: Brookes.

Crewe, N., Athelstan, G. T., & Krumberger, J. (1979). Spinal cord injury: A comparison of preinjury and postinjury marriages. *Archives of Physical Medicine and Rehabilitation, 60*, 252–256.

Crewe, N., Krause, J. (1988). Marital relationships and spinal cord injury. *Archives of Physical Medicine and Rehabilitation, 69*, 435–438.

Crewe, N., & Krause, J. (1990). An eleven-year follow-up of adjustment to spinal cord injury. *Rehabilitation Psychology, 35*, 205–210.

Crewe, N., & Krause, J. (1992). Marital status and adjustment to spinal cord injury. *Journal of the American Paraplegia Society, 15*, 14–18.

Danek, M. (1992). The status of women with disabilities revisited. *Journal of Applied Rehabilitation Counseling, 23*, 7–13.

Davidson, P. W., & Dolins, M. (1993). Assessment of the young child with visual impairment and multiple disabilities. In J. Culbertson & D. Willis (Eds.), *Testing young children: A reference guide for developmental, psychoeducational, and psychosocial assessments*. Austin, TX: Pro-Ed.

Davis, L. J. (Ed.). (1997). *The disability studies reader*. New York: Routledge.

Dean, J., Fox, A., & Jensen, W. (1985). Drug and alcohol use by disabled and nondisabled persons: A comparative study. *International Journal of the Addictions, 20*, 629–641.

Dell Orto, A., & Marinelli, R. (1995). *Encyclopedia of disability and rehabilitation*. New York: Simon & Schuster.

DeLoach, C. P. (1989). Gender, career choice and occupation outcomes among college alumni with disabilities. *Journal of Applied Rehabilitation Counseling, 20*, 8–12.

DeLoach, C. P. (1992). Career outcomes for college graduates with severe physical and sensory disabilities. *Journal of Rehabilitation, 58*, 57–63.

DeLoach, C. P. (1994). Attitudes toward disability: Impact on sexual development and forging of intimate relationships. *Journal of Applied Rehabilitation Counseling, 25*, 18–25.

Dembo, T., Leviton, G. L., & Wright, B. A. (1975). Adjustment to misfortune: A problem of social-psychological rehabilitation. *Rehabilitation Psychology, 22*, 1–100.

De Miranda, J., & Cherry, L. (1989). California responds: Changing treatment systems through advocacy for the disabled. *Alcohol Health and Research World, 13*, 154–157.

DeVivo, M., & Fine, P. (1982). Employment status of spinal cord injured patients three years after injury. *Archives of Physical Medicine and Rehabilitation, 63*, 200–203.

DeVivo, M., Rutt, R., Stover, S., & Fine, P. (1987). Employment after spinal cord injury. *Archives of Physical Medicine and Rehabilitation, 68*, 494–498.

DiNitto, D., & Krishef, C. (1984). Drinking patterns of mentally retarded persons. *Alcohol Health and Research World, 7,* 40–42.

Dion, K., Berscheid, E., & Walster, E. (1972). What is beautiful is good. *Journal of Personality and Social Psychology, 24,* 285–290.

Dosen, A., & Menolascino, F. J. (Eds.). (1990). *Depression in mentally retarded children and adults.* Leiden: Logon.

Dunn, M. (1977). Social discomfort in the patient with spinal cord injury. *Archives of Physical Medicine and Rehabilitation, 58,* 257–260.

Dunne, T., & Power, A. (1990). Sexual abuse and mental handicap: Preliminary findings of a community based study. *Mental Handicap Research, 3,* 111–125.

Dworkin, A., & Dworkin, R. (Eds.). (1976). *The minority report.* New York: Praeger.

Dykens, E. (1995). The Draw-a-Person task in persons with mental retardation: What does it measure? *Research in Developmental Disabilities, 17,* 1–13.

Edgerton, R. (1986). Alcohol and drug use by mentally retarded adults. *American Journal of Mental Deficiency, 90,* 602–609.

Edmonson, B. (1988). Disability and sexual adjustment. In V. Van Hasselt, P. Strain, & M. Hersen (Eds.), *Handbook of developmental and physical disabilities.* New York: Pergamon Press.

Education of All Handicapped Children Act of 1975, Public Law 94-142.

Education of the Handicapped Acts Amendments, Public Law 99-457, 1986, 20 U.S.C. (Sec. 1400 et seq.).

Elliott, T. R., & Umlauf, R. L. (1991). Measurement of personality and psychopathology following acquired physical disability. In L. A. Cushman & M. Scherer (Eds.), *Psychological assessment in medical rehabilitation.* Hyattsville, MD: American Psychological Association.

Enders, A. (1991). Rehabilitation and technology: Self-help approaches to technology: An independent living (IL) model for rehabilitation. *International Journal of Technology and Aging, 4,* 141–152.

English, R. W. (1971). Correlates of stigma towards physically disabled persons. *Rehabilitation Research and Practice Review, 2*(1), 1–17.

Euthanasia world directory. (1996). Online. http://www.FinalExit.org/kervorkian.html. Internet. http://www.efn.org/-ergo/kevorkian.html.

Everaerd, W. (1983). A case of apotemnophilia: A handicap as sexual preference. *American Journal of Psychotherapy, 37,* 285–293.

Fay, L. (1993). An account of the search of a woman who is verbally impaired for augmentative devices to end her silence. *Women and Therapy, 14,* 105–115.

Feigin, R. (1994). Spousal adjustment to a post-marital disability in one partner. *Family Systems Medicine, 12,* 235–247.

Fewell, R. R. (1991). Trends in the assessment of infants and toddlers with disabilities. *Exceptional Children, 58,* 166–173.

Fine, M., & Asch, A. (Eds.). (1988). *Women with disabilities: Essays in psychology, culture, and politics.* Philadelphia: Temple University Press.

Fine, M., & Asch, A. (1993). Disability beyond stigma: Social interaction, discrimination, and activism. In M. Nagler (Ed.), *Perspectives on disability.* Palo Alto, CA: Health Markets Research.

Finkelhor, D. (1984). *Child sexual abuse: New theory and research.* New York: Free Press.

Finger, A. (1990). *Past due: A story of disability, pregnancy and birth.* Seattle: Seal Press.

Fletcher, D. (1995). A five-year study of effects of fines, gender, race, and age on illegal parking in spaces reserved for people with disabilities. *Rehabilitation Psychology, 30,* 203–210.

Florian, V. (1982). Cross-cultural differences in attitudes towards disabled persons: A study of Jewish and Arab youth in Israel. *International Journal of Intercultural Relations, 6*, 291–299.

Florian, V., & Katz, S. (1991). The other victims of traumatic brain injury: Consequences for family members. *Neuropsychology, 5*, 267–279.

Florian, V., Weisel, A., Kravetz, S., & Shurka-Zernitsky, E. (1989). Attitudes in the kibbutz and city toward persons with disabilities: A multifactorial comparison. *Rehabilitation Counseling Bulletin, 32*, 210–218.

Ford, J. A., & Moore, D. (1992). Identifying substance abuse in persons with disabilities. *SARDI [Substance Abuse Resource and Disability Issues] Training Manual for Professionals, 4*, 8–9. (Adapted version reprinted in Helwig, A., & Holicky, R. (1994). Substance abuse in persons with disabilities: Treatment considerations. *Journal of Counseling and Development, 72*, 227–233.)

Frank, R. G., Elliott, T. R., Corcoran, J. R., & Wonderlich, S. A. (1987). Depression after SCI: Is it necessary? *Clinical Psychology Review, 7*, 611–630.

Fredrick, J., & Fletcher, D. (1985). Facilitating children's adjustment to orthotic and prosthetic appliances. *Teaching Exceptional Children, 17*, 228–230.

Freedman, D. A., Feinstein, C., & Berger, K. (1988). The blind child and adolescent. In C. J. Kestenbaum & D. T. Williams (Eds.), *Handbook of clinical assessment of children and adolescents. Vol. II.* New York: New York University Press.

Freeman, A. C., Ferreyra, N., & Calabrese, C. (1997). *Fostering recovery for women with disabilities: Eliminating barriers to substance abuse programs.* Oakland, CA: Berkeley Planning Associates.

French, S. (1992). Simulation exercises in disability awareness training: A critique. *Disability, Handicap, and Society, 7*, 257–266.

Frieden, A. L. (1990). Substance abuse and disability: The role of the independent living center. *Journal of Applied Rehabilitation Counseling, 21*, 33–36.

Friedrich, J., & Douglass, D. (1998). Ethics and the persuasive enterprise of teaching psychology. *American Psychologist, 53*, 549–462.

Fries, K. (1997). *Body, remember.* New York: Dutton.

Gaeth, J., & Lounsbury, E. (1966). Hearing aids and children in elementary school. *Journal of Speech and Hearing Disorders, 31*, 283–289.

Gainer, K. (1992, September/October). I was born colored and crippled. Now I am black and disabled. *Mouth: The Voice of Disability Rights*, p. 31.

Gallagher, H. (1985). *FDR's splendid deception.* New York: Dodd Mead.

Gass, C. (1991). MMPI-2 interpretation and closed head injury: A correction factor. *Psychological Assessment, 3*, 27–31.

Gayton, W., Friedman, S., Tavormina, J., & Tucker, F. (1977). Children with cystic fibrosis: Psychological test findings of patients, siblings, and parents. *Pediatrics, 59*, 888–894.

Gill, C. (1994). A bicultural framework for understanding disability. *The Family Psychologist, 10*, 13–16.

Gill, C. (1997). Psychological solutions. *One Step Ahead: The Resource for Active, Healthy, Independent Living, 4*, 12.

Glaser, G. (1964). The problem of psychosis in psychomotor temporal lobe epileptics. *Epilepsia, 5*, 271–278.

Glass, E. J. (1980/1981). Problem drinking among the blind and visually impaired. *Alcohol Health and Research World, 5*, 20–25.

Gleeson, B. J. (1997). Disability studies: A historical materialist view. *Disability and Society, 12*, 179–202.

Goffman, E. (1963). *Stigma: Notes on the management of spoiled identity.* Englewood Cliffs, NJ: Prentice-Hall.

Goodyear, R. K. (1983). Patterns of counselors' attitudes toward disability groups. *Rehabilitation Counseling Bulletin, 26*, 36–46.

Gordon, R. P., Stump, K., & Glaser, B. A. (1996). Assessment of individuals with hearing impairments: Equity in testing procedures and accommodations. *Measurement and Evaluation in Counseling and Development, 29,* 111–118.

Gordon, S. G. (1971). Missing in special education: Sex. *Journal of Special Education, 5,* 351–354.

Grady, A., Kovach, L., Lange, M., & Shannon, L. (1991). Promoting choice in selection of assistive technology devices. In *Proceedings of the Sixth Annual Conference on technology and persons with disabilities.* Los Angeles: California State University, Northridge.

Gray, J., M., Shepherd, M., McKinlay, W. W., & Robertson, I. (1994). Negative symptoms in the traumatically brain-injured during the first year post-discharge, and their effect on rehabilitation status, work status and family burden. *Clinical Rehabilitation, 8,* 188–197.

Green, R-J. (1996). Why ask, why tell? Teaching and learning about lesbians and gays in family therapy. *Family Process, 35,* 389–400.

Greene, B. F., Norman, R., Searle, M., Daniels, M., & Lubeck, R. (1995). Child abuse and neglect by parents with disabilities: A tale of two families. *Journal of Applied Behavior Analysis, 28,* 417–434.

Greer, B. (1986). Substance abuse among persons with disabilities: A problem of too much accessibility. *Journal of Rehabilitation, 52,* 34–38.

Greer, B., Roberts, R., & Jenkins, W. (1990). Substance abuse among clients with other primary disabilities: Curricular implications for rehabilitation education. *Rehabilitation Education, 4,* 33–44.

Greer, B., & Walls, R. (1997). Emotional factors involved in substance abuse in a sample of rehabilitation clients. *Journal of Rehabilitation, 63,* 5–8.

Gunther, M. (1969). Emotional aspects. In R. Reuge (Ed.), *Spinal cord injuries.* Springfield, IL: Charles C Thomas.

Gutierrez, L., & Ortega, R. (1991). Developing methods to empower Latinos: The importance of groups. *Social Work with Groups, 14,* 23–43.

Gwin, L. (1995, January/February). Big apple, bigger worm: How state spending for persons with disabilities gets gobbled up by programs and providers. *Mouth: The Voice of Disability Rights,* pp. 7–9.

Hahn, H. (1991). Alternative views of empowerment: Social services and civil rights. *Journal of Rehabilitation, 57,* 17–19.

Hahn, H. (1993). The politics of physical differences: Disability and discrimination. In M. Nagler (Ed.), *Perspectives on disability.* Palo Alto, CA: Health Markets Research.

Hahn, H. (1993). Can disability be beautiful? In M. Nagler (Ed.), *Perspectives on disability.* Palo Alto, CA: Health Markets Research.

Hallissy, E. (1993, August 3). Elizabeth Martinez—Radio career cut by gunman's bullet. *San Francisco Chronicle,* p. 20.

Halstead, L. (Ed.). (1998). *Managing post-polio: A guide to living well with post-polio syndrome.* Washington, DC: National Rehabilitation Hospital Press.

Hansen, J., & Coppersmith, E. I. (Eds.). (1984). *Families with handicapped members.* Rockville, MD: Aspen.

Hanson, S., Buckeleew, S. P., Hewett, J., & O'Neal, G. (1993). The relationship between coping and adjustment after spinal cord injury; A 5-year follow-up study. *Rehabilitation Psychology, 38*(1), 41–52.

Harper, D. (1991). Paradigms for investigating rehabilitation and adaptation to childhood disability and chronic illness. *Journal of Pediatric Psychology, 16,* 533–542.

Harris, L., & Associates. (1986). *Disabled Americans' self-perceptions: Bringing disabled Americans into the mainstream.* A survey conducted for the International Center for the Disabled. New York.

Harsh, M. (1993). Women who are visually impaired or blind as psychotherapy clients: A personal and professional perspective. *Women and Therapy, 14,* 55–64.

Heinemann, A. W. (1991). Substance abuse and spinal cord injury. *Paraplegia News, 45*(7), 16–17.

Heinrich, R., & Tate, D. (1996). Latent variable structure of the Brief Symptom Inventory in a sample of persons with spinal cord injuries. *Rehabilitation Psychology, 41,* 131–148.

Heller, T., & Factor, A. (1993). Aging family caregivers: Support resources and changes in burden and placement desire. *American Journal of Mental Retardation, 98,* 417–426.

Heller, B. W., & Harris, R. I. (1987). Special considerations in the psychological assessment of hearing impaired persons. In B. W. Heller, L. M. Flohr, & L. S. Zegans (Eds.), *Psychosocial interventions with sensorially disabled persons.* Orlando, FL: Grune & Stratton.

Helwig, A. A., & Holicky, R. (1994). Substance abuse in persons with disabilities: Treatment considerations. *Journal of Counseling and Development, 72,* 227–233.

Hepner, R., Kirshbaum, H., & Landes, D. (1980/1981). Counseling substance abusers with additional disabilities: The Center for Independent Living. *Alcohol Health and Research World, 5,* 11–15.

Herrick, S., Elliott, T., & Crow, F. (1994). Social support and the prediction of health complications among persons with spinal cord injuries. *Rehabilitation Psychology, 39,* 231–250.

Hersen, M., & Van Hasselt, V. B. (Eds.). (1990). *Psychological aspects of developmental and physical disabilities: A casebook.* Newbury Park, CA: Sage.

Hevey, D. (1992). *The creatures time forgot: Photography and disability imagery.* New York: Routledge.

Hillyer, B. (1993). *Feminism and disability.* Norman: Oklahoma University Press.

Hockenberry, J. (1995). *Moving violations.* New York: Hyperion.

Hogben, M., & Waterman, C. K. (1997). Are all of your students represented in their textbooks? A content analysis of coverage of diversity issues in introductory psychology textbooks. *Teaching of Psychology, 24,* 95–100.

Hohenshil, T. H. (Ed.). (1979). Counseling persons with disabilities and their families [Special issue]. *Journal of Counseling and Development, 58*(4).

Horne, M., & Ricciardo, J. (1988). Hierarchy of response to handicaps. *Psychological Reports, 62,* 83–86.

Hosie, T. W., Patterson, J. B., & Hollingsworth, D. K. (1989). School and rehabilitation counselor preparation: Meeting the needs of individuals with disabilities. *Journal of Counseling and Development, 68,* 171–176.

House Judiciary Constitution Subcommittee. (1996). Physician assisted suicide and euthanasia in the Netherlands. *One Step Ahead, 3,* 9–10.

Huang, A. M. (1981). The drinking patterns of the educable mentally retarded and the non-retarded student. *Journal of Alcohol and Drug Education, 26,* 41–50.

Hubbard, R. (1997). Abortion and disability. In L. J. Davis (Ed.), *The disability studies reader.* New York: Routledge.

Huebner, R. A., & Thomas, K. R. (1995). The relationship between attachment, psychopathology, and childhood disability. *Rehabilitation Psychology, 40,* 111–124.

Hurley, A. D. (1993). Conducting psychological assessments. In F. L. Rowley-Kelly & D. H. Reigel (Eds.), *Teaching the student with spina bifida.* Baltimore: Brookes.

Inanami, M., Ogura, T., Rodgers, C., & Nishi, N. (1994). Parental stress from caring for children with disabilities. *Japanese Journal of Special Education, 32,* 11–21.

Individuals With Disabilites Education Act, Public Law 101-476, 1990, 104 Stat. 1103 (Title 20, Sec. 1400 et seq.)

Jackson, A., & Haverkamp, B. (1991). Family response to traumatic brain injury. *Counseling Psychology Quarterly, 4,* 355–366.

James, M., DeVivo, M., & Richards, J. (1993). Postinjury employment outcomes among African-American and White persons with spinal cord injury. *Rehabilitation Psychology, 38,* 151–164.

Jancar, J., & Gunaratne, I. J. (1994). Dysthymia and mental handicap. *British Journal of Psychiatry, 164,* 691–693.

Jaques, M., Linkowski, D. C., & Seika, F. (1970). Cultural attitudes towards disability: Denmark, Greece, and the United States. *International Journal of Social Psychiatry, 16,* 54–62.

Johnson, F. A., & Greenberg, R. P. (1978). Quality of drawing as a factor in the interpretation of figure drawings. *Journal of Personality Assessment, 42,* 489–495.

Jones, R. L. (1974). The hierarchical structure of attitudes toward the exceptional. *Exceptional Children, 40,* 430–435.

Jordan, J. E., & Friesen, E. D. (1967). Attitudes of rehabilitation personnel toward physically disabled persons in Colombia, Peru, and the U.S. *Journal of Social Psychology, 74,* 151–161.

Jurkovic, G. J. (1997). *Lost childhoods: The plight of the parentified child.* Philadelphia: Brunner/Mazel.

Kagan, J., Henker, B., Hen-Tov, A., Levine, J., & Lewis, M. (1966). Infants' differential reactions to familiar and distorted faces. *Child Development, 37,* 519–532.

Kahn, A. S. (1984). Perspectives on persons with disabilities. *American Psychologist, 39,* 516–517.

Kahn, S. (1986). *Fact sheet for Third Generation Hardiness Test.* Arlington-Heights, IL: Hardiness Institute.

Kallianes, V., & Rubenfeld, P. (1997). Disabled women and reproductive rights. *Disability and Society, 12,* 203–221.

Kamenetz, H. (1969). A brief history of the wheelchair. *Journal of the History of Medicine and Allied Sciences, 24,* 205–210.

Kaplan, L., Grynbaum, B., Rush, H., Anastasia, T., & Gassler, S. (1966). Reappraisal of braces and other mechanical aids in patients with spinal cord dysfunction: Results of follow-up study. *Archives of Physical Medicine and Rehabilitation, 47,* 393–405.

Karchmer, M., & Kirwin, L. (1977). *Use of hearing aids by hearing impaired students in the U.S.* Washington, DC: Gallaudet College Press.

Keany, K. M-H., & Glueckauf, R. (1993). Disability and value change: An overview and reanalysis of acceptance of loss theory. *Rehabilitation Psychology, 38,* 199–210.

Keiser, S. (1998). Test accommodations: An administrator's view. In M. Gordon & S. Keiser (Eds.), *Accommodations in higher education under the Americans with Disabilities Act.* New York: Guilford Press.

Kelly, S. D. M., & Lambert, S. S. (1992). Family support in rehabilitation: A review of research, 1980–1990. *Rehabilitation Counseling Bulletin, 36,* 98–119.

Kelly, T. B., & Kropf, N. P. (1995). Stigmatized and perpetual parents: Older parents caring for adult children with life-long disabilities. *Journal of Gerontological Social Work, 24,* 3–16.

Kemp, N. T., & Mallinckrodt, B. (1996). Impact of professional training on case conceptualization of clients with a disability. *Professional Psychology: Research and Practice, 27,* 378–385.

Kendall, P., Edinger, J., & Eberly, C. (1978). Taylor's MMPI correction factor for spinal cord injury: Empirical endorsement. *Journal of Consulting and Clinical Psychology, 46,* 370–371.

Kent, D. (1987). Disabled women: Portraits in fiction and drama. In A. Gartner & T. Joe (Eds.), *Images of the disabled, disabling images.* New York: Praeger.

Kerr, N., & Bodman, D. A. (1994). Disability research methods: An argument for the use of Galileian modes of thought in disability research. *Journal of Social Behavior and Personality, 9*, 99–122.

Kewman, D., Warschausky, S., Engel, L., & Warzak, W. (1997). Sexual development of children and adolescents. In M. L. Spipski & C. J. Alexander (Eds.), *Sexual function in people with disability and chronic illness: A health practitioner's guide.* Gaithersburg, MD: Aspen.

Kiger, G. (1992). Disability simulations: Logical, methodological, and ethical issues. *Disability, Handicap and Society, 7*, 71–78.

Kirshbaum, M. (1988). Parents with physical disabilities and their babies. *Zero to Three, 8*, 8–15.

Kirshbaum, M. (1994). Family context and disability culture reframing: Through the looking glass. *Family Psychologist, 10*, 8–12.

Kirshbaum, M., & Preston, P. (1998). *Keeping our families together: A report of the national task force on parents with disabilities and their families* (National Institute of Disability and Rehabilitation Research grant # H133B30076). Berkeley, CA: Research and Training Center, Through the Looking Glass.

Kirshbaum, M., & Rinne, G. (1985). The disabled parent. In M. Aurenshine & M. Enriguez (Eds.), *Maternity nursing: Dimensions of change.* Belmont, CA: Wadsworth.

Knight, S. (1989). Sexual concerns of the physically disabled. In B. Heller & L. Flohr (Eds.), *Psychosocial interventions with physically disabled persons.* New Brunswick: Rutgers University Press.

Kobasa, S. (1979). Stressful life events, personality, and health: An inquiry into hardiness. *Journal of Personality and Social Psychology, 37*, 1–11.

Kobasa, S., Maddi, S., & Courington, S. (1981). Personality and constitution as mediators in the stress-illness relationship. *Journal of Health and Social Behavior, 22*, 368–378.

Kobasa, S., Maddi, S., & Kahn, S. (1982). Hardiness and health: A prospective study. *Journal of Personality and Social Psychology, 42*, 168–177.

Kobasa, S., Maddi, S., Puccetti, M., & Zola, M. C. (1985). Effectiveness of hardiness, exercise and social support as resources against illness. *Journal of Psychosomatic Research, 29*, 525–533.

Kobasa, S., & Puccetti, M. (1983). Personality and social resources in stress resistance. *Journal of Personality and Social Psychology, 45*, 839–850.

Kobe, F. H., & Hammer, D. (1994). Parenting stress and depression in children with mental retardation and developmental disabilities. *Research in Developmental Disabilities, 15*, 209–221.

Kolk, C. J. V. (1987). Psychosocial assessment of visually impaired persons. In B. W. Heller, L. M. Flohr, & L. S. Zegans (Eds.), *Psychosocial interventions with sensorially disabled persons.* Orlando, FL: Grune & Stratton.

Koren, P. E., DeChillo, N., & Friesen, B. J. (1992). Measuring empowerment in families whose children have emotional disabilities: A Brief questionnaire. *Rehabilitation Psychology, 37*(4), 305–321

Kotchick, B., Forehand, R., Armistead, L., Klein, K., & Wierson, M. (1996). Coping with illness: Interrelationships across family members and predictors of psychological adjustment. *Journal of Family Psychology, 10*, 358–370.

Kravetz, S., Drory, Y., & Florian, V. (1993). Handiness and sense of coherence and their relation to negative affect. *European Journal of Personality, 7*, 233–244.

Krents, E., Schulman, V., & Brenner, S. (1987). Child abuse and the disabled child: Perspectives for parents. *Volta Review, 89*, 78–95.

Kreuter, M., Sullivan, M., & Siosteen, A. (1994a). Sexual adjustment after spinal cord injury (SCI) focusing on partner experiences. *Paraplegia, 32*, 225–235.

Kreuter, M., Sullivan, M., & Siosteen, A. (1994b). Sexual adjustment after spinal cord injury-comparison of partner experiences in pre- and postinjury relationships. *Paraplegia, 32,* 759–770.

Kreuter, M., Sullivan, M., & Siosteen, A. (1996). Sexual adjustment and quality of relationships in spinal paraplegia: A controlled study. *Archives of Physical Medicine and Rehabilitation, 77,* 541–548.

Kupst, M. J. (1994). Coping with pediatric cancer: Theoretical and research perspectives. In D. J. Bearison & R. K. Mulhern, *Pediatric psychooncology: Psychological perspectives on children with cancer.* New York: Oxford University Press.

Lane, A. (1997, May 12). Reds in bed. *New Yorker Magazine,* p. 104.

LaPlante, M. (1993). State estimates of disability in America (# 1993 0-339-986). *Disability Statistics Abstract No. 3.* Washington, DC: National Institute on Disability and Rehabilitation Research.

LaPlante, M. (1996). Health conditions and impairments causing disability. *Disability Statistics Abstract No. 16.* Washington, DC: National Institute on Disability and Rehabilitation Research.

LaPlante, M., Miller, S., & Miller, K. (1992). People with work disability in the U.S. *Disability Statistics Abstract No. 4.* Washington, DC: National Institute on Disability and Rehabilitation Research.

La Rue, A., & Watson, J. (1998). Psychological assessment of older adults. *Professional Psychology: Research and Practice, 29,* 5–14.

Leahy, M. J., Habeck, R., & Fabiano, R. (1988). Doctoral dissertation research in rehabilitation: 1982–1983. *Rehabilitation Counseling Bulletin, 32,* 161–187.

Leahy, M. J., Habeck, R., & Fabiano, R. (1989). Doctoral dissertation research in rehabilitation: 1984–1985. *Rehabilitation Counseling Bulletin, 32,* 346–382.

Leahy, M. J., Habeck, R., & VanTol, B. (1992). Doctoral dissertation research in rehabilitation: 1988–1989. *Rehabilitation Counseling Bulletin, 35,* 253–288.

Leahy, M. J., VanTol, B., Habeck, R., & Fabiano, R. (1990). Doctoral dissertation research in rehabilitation: 1986–1987. *Rehabilitation Counseling Bulletin, 33,* 315–356.

LeClere, F., & Kowalewski, B. (1994). Disability in the family: The effects on children's well-being. *Journal of Marriage and the Family, 56,* 457–468.

Lefebvre, K. A. (1990). Sexual assessment planning. *Journal of Head Trauma Rehabilitation, 5,* 25–30.

LeMaistre, J. (1993). *Beyond rage: Mastering unavoidable health changes* (2nd ed.). Oak Park, IL: Alpine Guild.

Leung, P. (1991). Older workers with disabilities: A minority perspective. In L. Perlman & C. Hansen (Eds.), *Aging, disability and the nation's productivity.* Reston, VA: National Rehabilitation Association.

Levine, E. S. (1974). Psychological tests and practices with the deaf: A survey of the state of the art. *Volta Review, 76,* 298–319.

Lichtenberg, P. (1997). The DOUR project: A program of depression research in geriatric rehabilitation minority inpatients. *Rehabilitation Psychology, 42,* 103–114.

Lindemann, J. E. (1981). *Psychological and behavioral aspects of physical disability: A manual for health practitioners.* New York: Plenum Press.

Linton, S. (1998). *Claiming disability: Knowledge and identity.* New York: New York University Press.

Lintula, P. & Miezitis, S. (1977). A classroom observation-based consultation approach to early identification. *Ontario Psychologist, 9,* 29–38.

Livneh, H. (1982). On the origins of negative attitudes towards persons with disabilities. *Rehabilitation Literature, 43,* 338–347.

Livneh, H. (1997). Psychosocial aspects of disability. *Rehabilitation Education, 11,* 173–183.

Livneh, H., & Thomas, K. R. (1997). Psychosocial aspects of disability. *Rehabilitation Education, 11*(3), 173–183.

Llewellyn, G. (1995). Relationships and social support: Views of parents with mental retardation/intellectual disabilities. *Mental Retardation, 33*, 349–363.

Lofaro, G. A. (1983). Doctoral research in rehabilitation. *Rehabilitation Counseling Bulletin, 26*, 221–304.

Lollar, D. J. (1994). Therapeutic intervention with families in which a child has a disability. *Family Psychologist, 10*, 23–25.

Longmore, P. (1987). Elizabeth Bouvia, assisted suicide and social prejudice. *Issues in Law and Medicine, 3*, 141–168.

Lopez, S. R., Grover, K. P., Holland, D., Johnson, M. J., Kain, C. D., Kanel, K., Mellins, C. A., & Rhyne, M. C. (1989). Development of culturally sensitive psychotherapists. *Professional Psychology: Research and Practice, 20*(6), 1–8.

Mairs, N. (1997). *Waist high in the world: A life among the nondisabled.* New York: Beacon Press.

Majerovitz, S., & Revenson, R. (1994). Sexuality and rheumatic disease: The significance of gender. *Arthritis Care and Research, 7*, 29–34.

Malamud, B. (1966). *The fixer.* New York: Farrar, Straus & Giroux.

Marin Institute for the Prevention of Alcohol and Other Drug Problems. (1993, Winter). *Sell a case, save a kid?* Marin, CA: Author.

McCarthy, M., & Thompson, D. (1993). *Sex and the three Rs: Rights, responsibilities and risks.* Brighton, England: Pavilion.

McDaniel, S., Hepworth, J., & Doherty, W. (1992). *Medical family therapy: A biopsychosocial approach to families with health problems.* New York: Basic Books.

McDermott, S., Valentine, D., Anderson, D., Gallup, D., & Thompson, S. (1997). Parents of adults with mental retardation living in-home and out-of-home: Caregiving burdens and gratifications. *American Journal of Orthopsychiatry, 67*, 323–329.

McGhee, H. (1995). An evaluation of modified written and American Sign Language versions of the Beck Depression Inventory with the prelingually deaf. *Dissertation Abstracts International, 56*(11-B), 6456.

McGinn, R., Flowers, C., & Rubin, S. (1994). In quest of an explicit multicultural emphasis in ethical standards for rehabilitation counselors. *Rehabilitation Education, 7*, 261–268.

McGrath, P., Goodman, J., Cunningham, J., MacDonald, B., Nichols, T., & Unruh, A. (1985). Assistive devices: Utilization by children. *Archives of Physical Medicine and Rehabilitation, 66*, 430–432.

McGuire, G. B., & Greenwood, J. (1990). Effects of an intervention aimed at memory on perceived burden and self-esteem after traumatic head injury. *Clinical Rehabilitation, 4*, 319–323.

McNeff, E. A. (1997). Issues for the partner of the person with a disability. In M. Sipski & C. J. Alexander (Eds.), *Sexual function in persons with disabilities and chronic illness.* Gaithersburg, MD: Aspen.

McNeil, J. M. (1993). *Americans with disabilities: 1991–92* (Current Population Reports P70-33). Washington, DC: U.S. Bureau of the Census.

McShane, S. L., & Karp, J. (1993). Employment following spinal cord injury: A covariance structure analysis. *Rehabilitation Psychology, 38*(1), 27–40

Meadow-Orlans, K. (1995). Parenting with a sensory or physical disability. In M. Bornstein (Ed.), *Handbook of parenting: Vol. 4. Applied and practical parenting.* Mahwah, NJ: Erlbaum.

Mehta, V. (1985). *Sound shadows of the new world.* New York: Norton.

Meyerink, L., Reitan, R., & Selz, M. (1988). The validity of the MMPI with multiple sclerosis patients. *Journal of Clinical Psychology, 44*, 764–768.

Meyerson, L., & Michael, J. L. (1962). A behavioral approach to counseling and guidance. *Harvard Educational Review, 32,* 382–402.

Milam, L. (1993). *Crip Zen: A manual for survival.* San Diego: Mho & Mho Works.

Miller, M., Armstrong, S., & Hagan, M. (1981). Effects of teaching on elementary students' attitudes toward handicaps. *Education and Training of the Mentally Retarded, 16,* 110–113.

Miller, S., & Morgan, M. (1980). Marriage matters: For people with disabilities too. *Sexuality and Disability, 3,* 203–211.

Miller, T. W., Houston, L., & Goodman, R. W. (1994). Clinical issues in psychosocial rehabilitation for spouses with physical disabilities. *Journal of Developmental and Physical Disabilities, 6,* 43–53.

Mittenberg, W., Theroux-Fichera, S., Zielinski, R. E., & Heilbronner, R. L. (1995). Identification of malingered head injury on the Wechsler Adult Intelligence Scale—Revised. *Professional Psychology: Research and Practice, 26,* 491–498.

Milligan, M. S., & Neufeldt, A. H. (1998). Postinjury marriage to men with spinal cord injuries: Women's perspectives on making a commitment. *Sexuality And Disability, 16,* 117–132.

Moore, D., Greer, B. G., & Li, L. (1994). Alcohol and other substance use/abuse among people with disabilities. *Journal of Social Behavior and Personality, 9,* 369–382.

Moore, D., & Polsgrove, L. (1991). Disabilities, developmental handicaps, and substance abuse: A review. *International Journal of the Addictions, 26*(2), 65–90.

Morgan, A., & Vernon, M. (1994). A guide to the diagnosis of learning disabilities in deaf and hard-of-hearing children and adults. *American Annals of the Deaf, 139,* 358–370.

Morgan, S. R. (1987). *Abuse and neglect of handicapped children.* Boston: Little, Brown.

Mueller, S., & Girace, M. (1988). Use and misuse of the MMPI, a reconsideration. *Psychological Reports, 63,* 483–491.

Murray, B. (1997, April). How is diversity taught by psychology educators? *American Psychological Association Monitor, 28*(4), 52.

Mussen, P. H. (1943). *Cripple stereotypes and attitudes toward cripples.* Unpublished doctoral dissertation, Stanford University.

Mussen, P. H., & Barker, R. (1944). Attitudes toward cripples. *Journal of Abnormal and Social Psychology, 39,* 351–355.

Nagler, M. (Ed.). (1993). *Perspectives on disability* (2nd ed.). Palo Alto, CA: Health Markets Research.

Nakdimen, K. A. (1984). The physiognomic basis of sexual stereotyping. *American Journal of Psychiatry, 141,* 499–503.

National Clearinghouse for Alcohol and Drug Information. (1987). *NCADI update: Alcohol and other drugs and the physically/mentally impaired.* Rockville, MD: Author.

National Institute on Disability and Rehabilitation Research. (1990). *Rehab Brief: Bringing research into effective focus.* Washington, DC: Office of Special Education and Rehabilitation Services.

National Institute of Handicapped Research. (1985). *Summary of data on handicapped children and youth.* Washington, DC: U.S. Government Printing Office.

Nestor, M. A. (1993). Psychometric testing and reasonable accommodation for persons with disabilities. *Rehabilitation Psychology, 38,* 75–84.

Nosek, M. (1995). Sexual abuse of women with physical disabilities. *Physical Medicine and Rehabilitation: State of the Art Reviews, 9,* 487–502.

Nosek, M., Fuhrer, C., & Potter, C. (1995). Life satisfaction of people with physical disabilities: Relationship to personal assistance, disability status, and handicap. *Rehabilitation Psychology, 40,* 191–202.

Nosek, M., & Howland, C. (1997). Sexual abuse and people with disabilities. In M. Sipski & C. J. Alexander (Eds.), *Sexual function in people with disability and chronic illness.* Gaithersburg, MD: Aspen.

Nosek, M., Young, M. E., Rintala, D., Howland, C., Foley, C. C., & Bennett, J. L. (1995). Barriers to reproductive health maintenance among women with physical disabilities. *Journal of Women's Health, 4,* 505–518.

Oliver, M. (1992). Changing the social relations of research production. *Disability, Handicap and Society, 7,* 101–114.

Oliver, M. (1996). *Understanding disability: From theory to practice.* New York: St. Martin's Press.

Olkin, R. (1981). *Attitudes toward visible physical disabilities.* Unpublished doctoral dissertation, Santa Barbara, CA.

Olkin, R. (1993). Crips, gimps and epileptics explain it all to you. *Readings, 8,* 13–17.

Olkin, R. (1995). Matthew: Therapy with a teenager with a disability. In M. A. Blotzer & R. Ruth (Eds.), *Sometimes you just want to feel like a human being: Empowering therapy with persons with disabilities.* Baltimore: Brookes.

Olkin, R. (1997, Spring). Five models of research on disability: Shifting the paradigm from pathology to policy. *Newsletter of the American Family Therapy Academy, 67,* 27–32.

Olkin, R. (1998). "Psychosocial dimensions of polio and post-polio syndrome" and "Polio/PPS and specific life tasks." In L. Halstead (Ed.), *Managing post-polio: A guide to living well with post-polio syndrome.* Washington, DC: National Rehabilitation Hospital Press.

Olkin, R., & Howson, L. (1994). Attitudes toward and images of physical disability. *Journal of Social Behavior and Personality, 9,* 81–96.

Olkin, R., & Paquette, T. J. (1994, August). *Disability: A model for evaluating graduate clinical psychology programs.* Paper presented at the annual conference of the American Psychological Association, Los Angeles, CA.

Olsen, R. (1996). Young carers: Challenging the facts and politics of research into children and caring. *Disability and Society, 11,* 41–54.

Orona, C. J. (1989). Moral aspects of giving care. *Generations (AIDS and An Aging Society), 13,* 60–62.

O'Toole, C., & Bregante, J. (1993). Disabled lesbians: Multicultural realities. In M. Nagler (Ed.), *Perspectives on disability.* Palo Alto, CA: Health Markets Research.

O'Toole, C., & Martinez, K. (1991). Disabled women of color. *New Directions for Women, 20,* .

Palfrey, J., Walker, D., Haynie, M., Singer, J., Porter, S., Bushey, B., & Cooperman, P. (1991). Technology's children: Report of a statewide census of children dependent on medical supports. *Pediatrics, 87,* 611–618.

Panda, K., & Bartel, N. (1972). Teacher perception of exceptional children. *Journal of Special Education, 6,* 261–266.

Parker, G. (1993). Disability, caring and marriage: The experience of younger couples when a partner is disabled after marriage. *British Journal of Social Work, 23,* 565–580.

Pavkov, T. W., Lewis, D. A., & Lyons, J. S. (1989). Psychiatric diagnoses and racial bias: An empirical investigation. *Professional Psychology: Research and Practice, 20*(6), 364–368.

Pelka, F. (1997). *The ABC-CLIO companion to the disability rights movement.* Santa Barbara: ABC-CLIO.

Peterson, Y. (1979, January). The impact of physical disability on marital adjustment: A literature review. *Family Coordinator, 28,* 47–51.

Pfeiffer, D. (1989). Disability simulation using a wheelchair exercise. *Journal of Post-Secondary Education and Disability, 7,* 53–60.

Phelps, L., & Ensor, A. (1986). Concurrent validity of the WISC-R using deaf norms and the Hiskey–Nebraska. *Psychology in the Schools, 23,* 138–141.

Phillips, B., & Zhao, H. (1993). Predictors of assistive technology abandonment. *Assistive Technology, 5,* 36–45.

Pollard, R. Q. (1994). Public mental health service and diagnostic trends regarding individuals who are deaf or hard of hearing. *Rehabilitation Psychology, 39,* 147–160.

Preston, P. (1994). *Mother father deaf: Living between sound and silence.* Cambridge, MA: Harvard University Press.

Prilleltensky, I. (1997). Values, assumptions, and practices: Assessing the moral implications of psychological discourse and action. *American Psychologist, 52,* 517–535.

Quinn, P. (1998). *Understanding disability: A lifespan approach.* Thousand Oaks, CA: Sage.

Quittner, A., Opipari, L., Regoli, M. J., Jacobsen, J., & Eigen, H. (1992). The impact of caregiving and role strain on family life: Comparisons between mothers of children with cystic fibrosis and matched controls. *Rehabilitation Psychology, 37,* 275–290.

Ragosta, M. (1980). *Handicapped students and the SAT: Final report* (#RDR 80-81, No. 1). Princeton, NJ: Educational Testing Service.

Rape, R. N., Bush, J. P., & Slavin, L. A. (1992). Toward a conceptualization of the family's adaptation to a member's head injury: A critique of developmental stage models. *Rehabilitation Psychology, 37,* 3–22.

Ravid, R. (1992). Disclosure of mental illness to employers: Legal recourses and ramifications. *The Journal of Psychiatry and Law, 20,* 85–102.

Ravid, R., & Menon, S. (1993). Guidelines for disclosure of patient information under the Americans with Disabilities Act. *Hospital and Community Psychiatry, 44,* 280–281.

Ray, M. H. (1946). *The effect of crippled appearance on personality judgment.* Unpublished master's thesis, Stanford University.

Rehabilitation Act of 1973, Public Law 93–112.

Reiss, S., Levitan, G., & Szyszko, J. (1982). Emotional disturbance and mental retardation: Diagnostic overshadowing. *American Journal of Mental Deficiency, 86,* 567–574.

Research and Training Center on Independent Living for Underserved Populations. (1996). *Guidelines for reporting and writing about persons with disabilities* (5th ed.). (Available from the Research and Training Center on Independent Living, 4089 Dole Building, University of Kansas, Lawrence KS 66045)

Resources for Rehabilitation. (1997a). *A man's guide to coping with disability.* Lexington, MA: Author.

Resources for Rehabilitation. (1997b). *A woman's guide to coping with disability.* Lexington, MA: Author.

Rhine, S. A. (1993). Genetic counseling and evaluation of recurrence for people with physical disabilities. In F. P. Haseltine, S. S. Cole, & D. B. Gray (Eds.), *Reproductive issues for persons with physical disabilities.* Baltimore: Brookes.

Richardson, S. A. (1976). Attitudes and behaviors toward the physically handicapped. *Birth Defects: Original Articles Series, 12,* 15–34.

Rintala, D., Young, M. E., Hart, K., Clearman, R., & Fuhrer, M. (1992). Social support and the well-being of persons with spinal cord injury living in the community. *Rehabilitation Psychology, 37,* 155–164.

Robinson, R. G. (1993). Diagnosis of depression in neurologic disease. In S. Starkstein & R. G. Robinson (Eds.), *Depression in neurologic disease.* Baltimore: Johns Hopkins University Press.

Rodevich, M., & Wanlass, R. (1995). The moderating effect of spinal cord injury on MMPI-2 profiles: A clinically derived *T* score correction procedure. *Rehabilitation Psychology, 40,* 181–190.

Rodgers, J., & Calder, P. (1990). Marital adjustment: A valuable resource for the emotional health of individuals with multiple sclerosis. *Rehabilitation Counseling Bulletin, 34*(1), 24–32.

Rogers, J., & Matsumura, M. (1991). *Mother to be: A guide to pregnancy and birth for women with disabilities.* New York: Demos Publications.

Rohe, D. E., & DePompolo, R. (1985). Substance abuse policies in rehabilitation medicine departments. *Archives of Physical Medicine and Rehabilitation, 66,* 701–703.

Rokeach, M. (1973). *The nature of values.* New York: Free Press.

Rolland, J. (1994). *Families, illness and disability.* New York: Basic Books.

Romeo, A. J., Wanlass, R., & Arenas, S. (1993). A profile of psychosexual functioning in males following spinal cord injury. *Sexuality and Disability, 11,* 269–276.

Rosen, A. (1967). Limitations of personality inventories for assessment of deaf children and adults as illustrated by research with the Minnesota Multiphasic Personality Inventory. *Journal of Rehabilitation of the Deaf, 1,* 47–52.

Rousso, H. (1982). Special considerations in counseling clients with CP. *Sexuality and Disability, 5*(2), 78–88.

Rudolf, S. R., Manning, W., & Sewell, W. (1983). The use of self-efficacy scaling in training student clinicians: Implications for working with stutterers. *Journal of Fluency Disorders, 8,* 55–75.

Saad, S. C. (1997). Disability and the lesbian, gay man, or bisexual individual. In M. L. Sipski & C. J. Alexander (Eds.), *Sexual function in people with disability and chronic illness: A health professional's guide.* Gaithersburg, MD: Aspen.

Sacks, O. (1989). *Seeing voices: A journey into the world of the deaf.* New York: Harper Perennial.

Saddler, A., Hillman, S., & Darling, R. B. (1993). The influence of disabling condition visibility on family functioning. *Journal of Pediatric Psychology, 18,* 425–439.

Sanders, G. L. (1984). Relationships of the handicapped: Issues of sexuality and marriage. *Family Therapy Collections, 11,* 63–74.

Scheinberg, L. C. (Ed.). (1983). *Multiple sclerosis: A guide for patients and their families.* New York: Raven Press.

Scherer, M. (1988). Assistive device utilization and quality-of-life in adults with spinal cord injuries or cerebral palsy. *Journal of Applied Rehabilitation Counseling, 19,* 21–30.

Scherer, M. (1993). *Living in the state of stuck: How technology impacts the lives of people with disabilities* (2nd ed.). Cambridge, MA: Brookline Books.

Scherer, M. (1995). Technology and disability. In A. E. Dell Orto & R. P. Marinelli (Eds.), *Encyclopedia of disability and rehabilitation.* New York: Simon & Schuster.

Scherer, M. (1996). *Living in the state of stuck: How technology impacts the lives of people with disabilities* (2nd ed.). Cambridge, MA: Brookline Books.

Schneider, C., & Anderson, W. (1980). Attitudes toward the stigmatized: Some insights from recent research. *Rehabilitation Counseling Bulletin, 23,* 299–313.

Sequeira, E. M., Madhu, R. P., Subbakrishna, D. K., & Prabhu, G. G. (1990). Perceived burden and coping styles of the mothers of mentally handicapped children. *National Institute of Mental Health and Neurological Sciences, 8*(1), 63–67.

Shadish, W., Hickman, D., & Arrick, M. C. (1981). Psychological problems of spinal cord injury patients: Emotional distress as a function of time and locus of control. *Journal of Consulting and Clinical Psychology, 49*(2), 297.

Shakespeare, T. (Ed.). (1998). *The disability reader: Social science perspectives.* New York: Cassell.

Shears, L., & Jensema, C. (1969). Social acceptability of anomalous persons. *Exceptional Children, 36,* 91–96.

Shepperdson, B. (1988). The control of sexuality in young people with Down's syndrome. *Child: Care, Health & Development, 21,* 333–349.

Shiloh, S. (1996). Genetic counseling: A developing area of interest for psychologists. *Professional Psychology: Research and Practice, 27,* 475–486.

Silvers, B. (1996). *Sexuality, early-onset physical disability, and sense of coherence.* Unpublished doctoral dissertation, California School of Professional Psychology, Alameda.

Singer, G. H. S., & Powers, L. E. (Eds.). (1993). *Families, disability and empowerment: Active coping skills and strategies for family interventions.* Baltimore: Brookes.

Singhi, P. D., Goyal, L., Pershad, D., Singhi, S., & Walia, B. N. (1990). Psychosocial problems in families of disabled children. *British Journal of Medical Psychology, 63,* 173–182.

Sipski, M., & Alexander, C. J. (Eds.). (1997). *Sexual function in people with disability and chronic illness.* Gaithersburg, MD: Aspen.

Sisco, K. (1991). Employment of the older workers with a disability: An overview. In L. Perlman & C. Hansen (Eds.), *Aging, disability and the nation's productivity.* Reston, VA: National Rehabilitation Association.

Sisson, L. A., & Van Hasselt, V. B. (1987). Visual impairment. In V. B. Van Hasselt & M. Hersen (Eds.), *Psychological evaluation of the developmentally and physically disabled.* New York: Plenum Press.

Sobsey, D. (1994a). Sexual abuse of individuals with intellectual disability. In A. Craft (Ed.), *Practice issues in sexuality and learning disabilities.* London: Routledge.

Sobsey, D. (1994b). *Violence and abuse in the lives of people with disabilities: The end of silent acceptance?* Baltimore: Brookes.

Sobsey, D., & Doe, T. (1991). Patterns of sexual abuse and assault. *Sexuality and Disability, 9,* 243–260.

Sobsey, D., Gray, S., Wells, D., Pyper, D., & Reimer-Heck, B. (1991). *Disability, sexuality, and abuse: An annotated bibliography.* Baltimore: Brookes.

Sobsey, D., Wells, D., Lucardie, R., & Mansell, S. (Eds). (1995). *Violence and disability: An annotated bibliography.* Baltimore: Brookes.

Solnit, A. (1989). Preparing for uncertainty: Family reactions to a seriously impaired child. In B. Heller, L. Flohr, & L. Zegans (Eds.), *Psychosocial intervention with physically disabled persons.* New Brunswick, NJ: Rutgers University Press.

Sparadeo, F., & Gill, D. (1989). Effects of prior alcohol use on head injury recovery. *Journal of Head Trauma Rehabilitation, 4,* 75–82.

Stainback, W., & Stainback, S. (1982). Nonhandicapped students' perceptions of severely handicapped students. *Education and Training of the Mentally Retarded, 17,* 177–182.

Standards for educational and psychological testing. (1985). Washington, DC: American Educational Research Association, American Psychological Association, National Council on Measurement in Education.

Stein, P. N., Gordon, W. A., Hibbard, M., & Sliwinski, M. (1992). An examination of depression in the spouses of stroke patients. *Rehabilitation Psychology, 37,* 121–130.

Strohmer, D. C., Leierer, S. J., Cochran, N. A., & Arokiasamy, C. V. (1996). The importance of counselor disability status. *Rehabilitation Counseling Bulletin, 40,* 96–115.

Sunshine, L., & Wright, J. W. (1988). *The hundred best treatment centers for alcohol and drug abuse.* New York: Avon Press.

Szymanski, E. M. (1988). Supported employment and time-limited transitional employment training: Options for rehabilitation counselors. *Journal of Applied Rehabilitation Counseling, 19,* 11–15.

Tangri, P., & Verma, P. (1992). A study of social burden felt by mothers of handicapped children. *Journal of Personality and Clinical Studies, 8,* 117–120.

Tate, D., Forchheimer, M., Maynard, F., Davidoff, G., & Djikers, M. (1993). Comparing two measures of depression in spinal cord injury. *Rehabilitation Psychology, 38*(1), 53–62.

Taylor, G. P. (1970). Moderator-variable effect on personality-test-item endorsements of physically disabled patients. *Journal of Consulting and Clinical Psychology, 35,* 183–188.

Technology-Related Assistance of Individuals with Disabilities Act of 1988. Public Law 100-407 (reauthorized in 1994).

Tharinger, D., Horton, C. B., & Millea, S. (1994). Sexual abuse and exploitation of children and adults with mental retardation and other handicaps. In M. Nagler (Ed.), *Perspectives on disability* (2nd ed.). Palo Alto, CA: Health Markets Research.

Thompson-Hoffman, S., & Storck, I. F. (Eds.). (1991). *Disability in the United States: A portrait from national data.* New York: Springer.

Thurman, S. K. (Ed.) (1985). *Children of handicapped parents: Research and clinical perspectives.* New York: Academic Press.

Toms Barker, L. T., & Maralani, V. (1997). *Challenges and strategies of disabled parents: Findings from a national survey of parents with disabilities.* Oakland, CA: Berkeley Planning Associates.

Traustadottir, R. (1990). *Women with disabilities: Issues, resources, connections.* New York: Syracuse University Center on Human Policy.

Trieschmann, R. (1980). *Spinal cord injuries: Psychological, social and vocational adjustment.* New York: Pergamon Press.

Tringo, J. L. (1970). The hierarchy of preference toward disability groups. *Journal of Special Education, 4,* 295–306.

Tripp, A. (1988). Comparison of attitudes of regular and adapted physical educators toward disabled individuals. *Perceptual and Motor Skills, 66,* 425–426.

Tseng, W., & Streltzer, J. (Eds.). (1997). *Culture and psychopathology: A guide to clinical assessment.* New York: Brunner/Mazel.

Turnbull, H. R., & Turnbull, A. P. (1985). *Parents speak out: Then and now* (2nd ed.). Columbus, OH: Merrill.

Turner, R. J., & McLean, P. D. (1989). Physical disability and distress. *Rehabilitation Psychology, 34,* 225–242.

U.S. Congress, Office of Technology Assessment. (1987). *Technological dependent children: Hospital v. homecare: A technical memorandum* (OTA-TM-38). Washington, DC: U.S. Government Printing Office.

Uswatte, G., & Elliott, T. R. (1997). Ethnic and minority issues in rehabilitation psychology. *Rehabilitation Psychology, 42,* 61–71.

VanSickle, R. (1986). A quantitative review of research on instructional simulation gaming: A twenty-year perspective. *Theory and Research in Social Education, 14,* 245–264.

Vargo, F. A. (1983). Adaptation to disability by the wives of spinal cord males—A phenomenological approach. *Journal of Applied Rehabilitation Counseling, 15,* 28–32.

Vash, C. (1981). *Psychology of disability.* New York: Springer.

Vash, C. (1983). Psychological aspects of rehabilitation engineering. In *Technology for independent living II.* Washington, DC: American Association for the Advancement of Science.

Vash, C. (1991). More thoughts on empowerment. *Journal of Rehabilitation, 57,* 13–16.

Walster, E. (1966). Assignment of responsibility for an accident. *Journal of Personality and Social Psychology, 3,* 73–79.

Waltz, M. (1986). Marital context and post-infarction quality of life: Is it social support or something more? *Social Science Medicine, 22,* 791–805.

Watson, E. W., Boros, A., & Zrimec, G. (1979/1980). Mobilization of services for deaf alcoholics. *Alcohol Health and Research World, 4,* 33–38.

Waxman Fiduccia, B., & Saxton, M. (1997). Disability feminism: A manifesto. *New Mobility, 8,* 60–61.

Weinberg, N. (1978). Preschool children's perceptions of orthopedic disability. *Rehabilitation Counseling Bulletin, 21,* 183–189.

Weissman, M. M., & Myers, J. K. (1978). Affective disorders in a US urban community: The use of Research Diagnostic Criteria in an epidemiological survey. *Archives of General Psychiatry, 35,* 1304–1311.

Wenger, B. L., Kaye, H. S., & LaPlante, M. P. (1996, March). Disabilities among children. *Disability Statistics Abstract No. 15.* Washington, DC: National Institute on Disability and Rehabilitation Research.

Wertlieb, E. C. (1985). Minority group status of the disabled. *Human Relations, 38,* 1047–1063.

Westbrook, M. T., Legge, V., & Pennay, M. (1993). Attitudes towards disabilities in a multicultural society. *Social Science Medicine, 36,* 615–623.

Wickham-Searl, P. (1992). Mothers with a mission. In P. M. Ferguson, D. L. Ferguson, & S. J. Taylor (Eds.), *Interpreting disability.* New York: Teachers College Press.

Willingham, W., Ragosta, M., Bennett, R., Braun, H., Rock, D., & Powers, D. (1988). *Testing handicapped people.* Boston: Allyn & Bacon.

Wilson, S. L. (1987). Cognitive assessment in clinical rehabilitation. *Clinical Rehabilitation, 1,* 257–263.

Wilson, S. L. (1990). Psychological assessment and severe physical disability. In R. West, M. Christie, & J. Weinman (Eds.), *Microcomputers, psychology and medicine.* New York: Wiley.

Wireless: A catalog for fans and friends of public radio. (1998). Gaelic blessing plaque. St. Paul, MN: Minnesota Public Radio.

Woodbury, B., & Redd, C. (1987). Psychosocial issues and approaches. In J. Garber & N. Seligman (Eds.), *Spinal cord injury concepts and management approaches.* Baltimore: Williams & Wilkins.

Woollett, S. L., & Edelmann, R. J. (1988). Marital satisfaction in individuals with multiple sclerosis and their partners; its interactive effect with life satisfaction, social networks and disability. *Sexual and Marital Therapy, 3,* 191–196.

World Health Organization. (1980). *International classification of impairments, disabilities and handicaps: A manual of classification relating to the consequences of disease.* Geneva: World Health Organization.

World Health Organization. (1993). *International classification of impairments, disabilities and handicaps: A manual of classification relating to the consequences of disease.* Geneva: World Health Organization.

Wright, B. A. (1963). *Physical disability: A psychological approach.* New York: Harper & Row.

Wright, B. A. (1975). Sensitizing outsiders to the position of the insider. *Rehabilitation Psychology, 22,* 129–135.

Wright, B. A. (1983). *Physical disability: A psychosocial approach* (2nd ed.). New York: Harper & Row.

Yoshida, K. (1994). Intimate and marital relationships: An insider perspective. *Sexuality and Disability, 12,* 179–189.

Young, E., Marcus, F., Drought, T., Mendiola, M., Ciesielski-Carlucci, C., Alpers, A., Eaton, M., Koenig, B., Loewy, E., Raffin, T., & Ross, C. (1997). Report of the Northern California Conference for Guidelines in aid-in-dying: Definitions, differences, convergences, conclusions. *Western Journal of Medicine, 166,* 381–388.

Yu, J. (Producer and Director). (1996). *Breathing lessons: The life and work of Mark O'Brien* [Film and videotape]. (Available from Fanlight Productions)

Yuker, H. E. (Ed.). (1988). *Attitudes toward persons with disabilities.* New York: Springer.

Yuker, H. E. (1994). Variables that influence attitudes toward persons with disabilities: Conclusions from the data. *Psychosocial Perspectives on Disability, A Special Issue of the Journal of Social Behavior and Personality, 9,* 3–22.

Zea, M., Belgrave, F., Townsend, T., Jarama, S., & Banks, S. (1996). The influence of social support and active coping on depression among African Americans and Latinos with disabilities. *Rehabilitation Psychology, 41,* 225–242.

Zieziula, F. R. (Ed.). (1988). *Assessment of hearing impaired people.* Washington, DC: Gallaudet College Press.

Zimmerman, M. A. (1990). Taking aim on empowerment research: On the distinction between psychological and individual conceptions. *American Journal of Community Psychology, 18,* 169–177.

Ziolko, M. E. (1993). Counseling parents of children with disabilities: A review of the literature and implications for practice. In M. Nagler (Ed.), *Perspectives on disability.* Palo Alto, CA: Health Markets Research.

Zirpoli, T. J. (1986). Child abuse and children with handicaps. *Remedial and Special Education, 7,* 39–48.

Zola, I. (1982a). Involving the consumer in the rehabilitation process: Easier said than done. In *Technology for independent living.* Washington, DC: American Association for the Advancement of Science.

Zola, I. (1982b). *Missing pieces: A chronicle of living with a disability.* Philadelphia: Temple University Press.

Index